The Year in Neurology 2

ANNALS OF THE NEW YORK ACADEMY OF SCIENCES

Volume 1184

The Year in Neurology 2

Edited by

Richard T. Johnson

The Johns Hopkins University School of Medicine, and
Bloomberg School of Public Health
Baltimore, Maryland

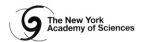

The New York
Academy of Sciences

Published by Blackwell Publishing on behalf of the New York Academy of Sciences
Boston, Massachusetts
2010

The Annals of the New York Academy of Sciences, (ISSN: 0077-8923 [print]; ISSN: 1749-6632 [online]) is published 32 times a year on behalf of the New York Academy of Sciences by Wiley Subscription Services, Inc., a Wiley Company, 111 River Street, Hoboken, NJ 07030-5774.

Mailing: The *Annals* is mailed standard rate.

Postmaster: Send all address changes to *Annals of the New York Academy of Sciences,* Journal Customer Services, John Wiley & Sons Inc., 350 Main Street, Malden, MA 02148-5020.

Disclaimer: The publisher, the New York Academy of Sciences and editors cannot be held responsible for errors or any consequences arising from the use of information contained in this publication; the views and opinions expressed do not necessarily reflect those of the publisher, the New York Academy of Sciences and editors.

Journal Customer Services: For ordering information, claims, and any inquiry concerning your subscription, please go to interscience.wiley.com/support or contact your nearest office:
  Americas: Email: cs-journals@wiley.com; Tel: +1 781 388 8598 or 1 800 835 6770 (Toll free in the USA & Canada).
  Europe, Middle East and Asia: Email: cs-journals@wiley.com; Tel: +44 (0) 1865 778315.
  Asia Pacific: Email: cs-journals@wiley.com; Tel: +65 6511 8000.
  Japan: For Japanese speaking support, Email cs-japan@wiley.com; Tel: +65 6511 8010 or Tel (toll-free): 005 316 50 480.
  Visit our Online Customer Self-Help available in 6 languages at www.interscience.wiley.com/support.

Information for Subscribers: The *Annals* is published in 32 volumes per year. Subscription prices for 2010 are:

Print & Online: US$4984 (US), US$5429 (Rest of World), €3518 (Europe), £2770 (UK). Prices are exclusive of tax. Australian GST, Canadian GST and European VAT will be applied at the appropriate rates. For more information on current tax rates, please go to www3.interscience.wiley.com/aboutus/journal_ordering_and_payment.html#Tax. The price includes online access to the current and all online back files to January 1, 1997, where available. For other pricing options, including access information and terms and conditions, please visit www.interscience.wiley.com/journal-info.

Delivery Terms and Legal Title: Prices include delivery of print publications to the recipient's address. Delivery terms are Delivered Duty Unpaid (DDU); the recipient is responsible for paying any import duty or taxes. Legal title passes to the customer on despatch by our distributors.

Production Editor: nyas@wiley.com.

Commercial Reprints: Lydia Supple-Pollard (email: lsupple@wiley.com).

Membership information: Members may order copies of *Annals* volumes directly from the Academy by visiting www.nyas.org/annals, emailing membership@nyas.org, faxing +1 212 298 3650, or calling 1 800 843 6927 (toll free in the USA), or +1 212 298 8640. For more information on becoming a member of the New York Academy of Sciences, please visit www.nyas.org/membership. Claims and inquiries on member orders should be directed to the Academy at email: membership@nyas.org or Tel: 1 800 843 6927 (toll free in the USA) or +1 212 298 8640.

Printed in the USA.

The *Annals* is available online at Wiley InterScience. Visit www.interscience.wiley.com to search the articles and register for table of contents e-mail alerts.

Access to the *Annals* is available free online within institutions in the developing world through the AGORA initiative with the FAO, the HINARI initiative with the WHO and the OARE initiative with UNEP. For information, visit www.aginternetwork.org, www.healthinternetwork.org, www.oarescience.org.

The *Annals* accepts articles for Open Access publication. Please see http://www.wiley.com/bw/journal.asp?ref=0077-8923&site=1 and select "Author Guidelines" for further information about Online Open.

ISSN: 0077-8923 (print); 1749-6632 (online)

ISBN-10: 1-57331-780-2; ISBN-13: 978-1-57331-780-1

ANNALS OF THE NEW YORK ACADEMY OF SCIENCES
Volume 1184

The Year in Neurology 2

Editor

Richard T. Johnson

Preface
By Richard T. Johnson . . . . *vii*

Sleep disorders in children
By Timothy F. Hoban *1*

REM sleep behavior disorder: Updated review of the core features, the REM sleep behavior
disorder-neurodegenerative disease association, evolving concepts, controversies, and
future directions
By Bradley F. Boeve *15*

Lewy body pathology in fetal grafts
By Yaping Chu and Jeffrey H. Kordower *55*

Congenital heart disease and brain development
By Patrick S. McQuillen and Steven P. Miller *68*

The tuberous sclerosis complex
By Ksenia A. Orlova and Peter B. Crino *87*

Neurological complications of immune reconstitution in HIV-infected populations
By Tory Johnson and Avindra Nath *106*

Vertebrobasilar dilatative arteriopathy (dolichoectasia)
By Min Lou and Louis R. Caplan *121*

Dermatomyositis and polymyositis: Clinical presentation, autoantibodies, and
pathogenesis
By Andrew L. Mammen *134*

Advances in the treatment of neurodegenerative disorders employing nanotechnology
By Girish Modi, Viness Pillay, and Yahya E. Choonara *154*

Neurologic Wilson's disease
By Matthew T. Lorincz *173*

The progression of pathology in Parkinson's disease
  By Glenda Margaret Halliday and Heather McCann *188*

Familial pain syndromes from mutations of the Na$_v$1.7 sodium channel
  By Tanya Z. Fischer and Stephen G. Waxman *196*

Epilepsy in the elderly
  By Ilo E. Leppik and Angela K. Birnbaum *208*

Flightless Flies: *Drosophila* models of neuromuscular disease
  By Thomas E. Lloyd and J. Paul Taylor *E1*
  (available online)

Ann. N.Y. Acad. Sci. ISSN 0077-8923

Preface

This is the second volume in *The Year in Neurology* series. The first volume was well received, so the focus has stayed the same—to present reviews covering interesting or novel approaches to understanding neurological diseases. As in the first volume, some topics and authors were suggested by the Editorial Advisory Board and others were chosen by me from the panoply of new and intriguing topics in clinical neuroscience. These topics range from an update of vertebrobasilar dolichoectasia, which intrigued me as a resident 50 years ago, to neurological nanotechnology, a topic of the future.

I wish to thank Ellen Dicks at the Johns Hopkins University Bloomberg School of Public Health for editorial assistance, and Douglas Braaten, PhD, director and executive editor of the *Annals of the New York Academy of Sciences*.

RICHARD T. JOHNSON
The Johns Hopkins University School of Medicine
and Bloomberg School of Public Health
Baltimore, Maryland, USA

Ann. N.Y. Acad. Sci. ISSN 0077-8923

Sleep disorders in children

Timothy F. Hoban

The Michael S. Aldrich Sleep Disorders Center, Departments of Pediatrics and Neurology, University of Michigan, Ann Arbor, Michigan, USA

Address for correspondence: Timothy F. Hoban, MD, L3227 Women's Hospital, 1500 East Medical Center Drive, SPC 5203, Ann Arbor, Michigan 48109-5203. Voice: 734-936-4179; fax: 734-763-7551. thoban@umich.edu

Although sleep disorders such as insomnia and obstructive sleep apnea are common in both children and adults, the clinical features and treatments for these conditions differ considerably between these two populations. Whereas an adult with obstructive sleep apnea typically presents with a history of obesity, snoring, and prominent daytime somnolence, a child with the condition is more likely to present with normal body weight, tonsillar hypertrophy, and inattentiveness during school classes. The adult with suspected sleep apnea almost always undergoes a baseline polysomnogram and proceeds to treatment only if this test confirms the diagnosis, while many children with suspected sleep apnea are treated empirically with adenotonsillectomy without ever receiving a sleep study to verify the diagnosis. This article reviews sleep disorders in children, with a particular focus on age-related changes in sleep, conditions that primarily affect children, and disorders for which clinical manifestations and treatment differ substantially from the adult population.

Keywords: pediatric sleep disorders; insomnia; circadian rhythm disorders; night waking; parasomnias; obstructive sleep apnea; restless legs syndrome; periodic limb movement disorder; rhythmic movement disorder

Evolution of normal sleep during infancy and early childhood

Healthy term infants spend in excess of 15 h asleep each day in the form of brief 2–4 h sleep periods. Periods of sleep and wakefulness are initially distributed equally across daytime and nighttime hours with little day-to-day consistency. Longer periods of wakefulness develop by 6 weeks of age, and by the age of 3 months, these periods are predictably distributed during the daytime or early evening hours.[1] As circadian regulatory mechanisms become stronger and entrained by recurring environmental and social cues, sleep lengthens and consolidates during nighttime hours in a process known as *settling*. Although 70% of infants settle by 3 months of age, 10% do not achieve sustained nighttime sleep during the first year of life.[2]

The toddler and preschool years are characterized by additional declines in daily sleep duration from an average of 13.9 h at 1 year of age to 11.4 h at age 5.[3] Daytime napping begins to subside during the second year of life, with most children giving up regular naps around age 3.

The quantitative changes of sleep during early childhood are accompaniment by significant qualitative changes in sleep architecture, which are demonstrable on electroencephalography (EEG) and polysomnography (PSG). Rapid eye movement (REM) sleep constitutes 50% of total sleep time during early infancy, declining by age 5 to 20%, the proportion exhibited by older children and adults.[4] Ultradian sleep cycles of REM and non-REM sleep states are substantially shorter for infants (50–60 min) than for adults (90–100 min).

Night waking and insomnia in younger children

It is important to recognize that some degree of nighttime waking is normal in young children, particularly during early infancy, when circadian mechanisms are still immature and nighttime feedings a necessity for most infants until about 6 months of age.[5] Among a cohort of children aged 11 to 27 months with no reported sleep problems, actigraphic monitoring of nighttime sleep revealed an average of two awakenings per night.[6] Night waking is considered problematic when it is excessively prolonged or frequent for age, or when it is excessively disruptive to other members of the household. Overall, about 20% of children below age 2 years exhibit night waking considered concerning by parents.[7]

A variety of predisposing influences may be associated with problematic night waking, some of which relate to expected developmental changes during early childhood. Nighttime feeding represents a biological need for younger infants until 6 months of age, which may persist as a learned behavior beyond that time. Near 1 year of age, separation anxiety may disrupt previously well-established sleep schedules and result in significant distress during episodes of night waking. Cosleeping with a parent is also associated with increased risk for arousal and awakening during nighttime sleep.[8]

Insomnia in younger children usually takes the form of bedtime resistance, in which a child may cry, repeatedly attempt to leave the room, or engage in other behaviors intended to forestall sleep onset. These behaviors often result in considerable distress and frustration for both child and parent. Although bedtime struggles are at least occasionally observed in most younger children, frequent or sustained bedtime resistance is exhibited by 20% of children between 1 and 3 years of age, and by 10% of 4-year-olds.[9]

Several factors exhibit strong influences upon settling problems at bedtime. Children whose temperamental characteristics are not conducive to self-settling are at increased risk for bedtime struggles. Children who lack structured bedtime routines or have irregular sleep habits represent another high-risk population. Other extrinsic influences that may impede settling at bedtime include anxiety, acute illness, medication side effects, and coexisting medical conditions such as attention deficit hyperactivity disorder, cerebral palsy, autism, and other developmental disabilities.[10]

Many young children exhibiting habitual bedtime struggles or night waking for at least 3 months duration meet diagnostic criteria for behavioral insomnia of childhood (Table 1).[11] The essential feature of this condition is that the difficulty falling asleep or staying asleep is related to an identified behavioral etiology—either inappropriate sleep onset associations or inadequate limit setting. In the sleep-onset association type, a young child habitually settles to sleep under circumstances such as being rocked, watching television, or having a parent present. Affected children become so reliant upon these habitual sleep associations that they are unable to fall asleep in their absence. Absence of the desired circumstances then results in emotional distress, which can disrupt sleep onset both at bedtime and following the physiological awakenings that punctuate normal childhood sleep.

The limit-setting type of behavioral insomnia of childhood occurs when parental or caregiver response to bedtime resistance or night waking is

---

Table 1. Diagnostic criteria for behavioral insomnia of childhood

1. Symptoms must meet criteria for insomnia based on parent or caregiver report
2. The child's symptoms are consistent with either the sleep-onset association or limit-setting types of insomnia defined below:
   a. Sleep-onset association type includes each of the following:
      i. Falling asleep is a protracted process requiring special conditions.
      ii. Sleep-onset associations are highly demanding or problematic.
      iii. In the absence of the typical associated conditions, sleep onset is substantially delayed or disrupted.
      iv. Nighttime awakenings require intervention by the parent or caregiver for the child to return to sleep.
   b. Limit-setting type includes each of the following:
      i. The child has difficulty initiating or maintaining sleep.
      ii. The child stalls or refuses to go to bed at an appropriate time or refuses to return to bed following nighttime waking.
      iii. The parent or caregiver demonstrates inappropriate or insufficient limit setting relative to the child's bedtime or sleep behavior.
3. The sleep disturbance is not better explained by another sleep, medical, neurological, or behavioral disorder.

Adapted from the *International Classification of Sleep Disorders*, second edition.[11]

either suboptimal or inconsistent. Whereas firm, consistent limit setting by parents in response to bedtime struggles ultimately reduces the duration and severity of the episodes, inappropriate or inconsistent caregiver response to the child's behavior tends to perpetuate or worsen the problem.

Treatment of sleeplessness during early childhood

Treatment for milder forms of sleeplessness in infants and young children begins with establishing good "sleep hygiene." Use of a structured, age-appropriate bedtime routine helps younger children settle into a quiet but relaxed state conducive to sleep onset. Routines for younger children may include bathing, changing, tooth brushing, reading stories, and being "tucked in." Potentially stimulating activities such as watching television and vigorous play should be avoided during the lead-in to bedtime.

Establishing a regular sleep schedule and an appropriate sleep environment are additional important elements of sleep hygiene for younger children. Maintaining regular bedtime and waking times 7 days per week may strengthen and entrain circadian mechanisms to promote rapid sleep onset near the desired bedtime. Eliminating daytime sleep except for age-appropriate naps may also augment sleepiness at bedtime. The optimal sleep environment for most young children is one that is quiet and kept at a stable, comfortable temperature. Although dark sleep environments are most conducive to sleep, use of dim night lights is appropriate for young children who are fearful of the dark.

Treatments for behavioral insomnia of and other persistent forms of sleeplessness during early childhood consist primarily of structured behavioral interventions.[12] Interventions considered to be well established for use in younger children include:

Extinction (systematic ignoring). This technique involves placing the child in bed and then ignoring any agitation or inappropriate behaviors that the child exhibits until morning with the exception of legitimate concerns regarding safety or illness.

Graduated extinction. This technique, described by Douglas and Richman[13] and popularized by Ferber,[14] specifies schedules by which parents ignore tantrums or inappropriate behavior for gradually increasing intervals before briefly checking on and reassuring the child.

Positive routines/faded bedtime with response cost. This technique couples a quiet but enjoyable bedtime routine with fading of bedtime toward the child's time of habitual sleep onset. Response cost involves taking the child briefly out of bed if not falling asleep, an application of stimulus control.

Parent education and anticipatory guidance. This technique, usually coupled with other specific behavioral interventions, educates parents and caregivers about early childhood sleep and the treatable influences that may promote or disrupt it.

A systematic review[15] and practice parameters[16] regarding behavioral treatments of sleep problems in infants and young children reported that several varieties of extinction-based therapies, positive routines with bedtime fading, and parent education were all individually effective therapies but found that there was insufficient evidence to recommend one therapy over another.

Drug treatment of sleeplessness in infants and young children has received remarkably little scientific study despite reportedly frequent use of such agents in this age group.[17] Controlled trials of trimeprazine tartrate, a sedating antihistamine, for treatment of night waking in young children have yielded conflicting results.[18,19] Although melatonin, diphenhydramine, and chloral hydrate are been used for treatment of sleep problems in younger children, reports of efficacy are largely anecdotal apart from a single placebo-controlled trial of diphenhydramine in infants which did not identify significant short-term benefits for treatment of night waking.[20,21]

Evolution of normal sleep during later childhood and adolescence

The sleep of school-age and adolescent children evolves at a more modest pace than that of younger children. Average daily sleep duration declines from 11 h at 6 years of age to 10 h at age 9, 9 h at age 13, and 8 h at age 16.[3] Maturation of sleep architecture is characterized by gradual reductions in the proportion of deep non-REM sleep and compensatory increases in the proportion of light non-REM sleep stages.

Normal sleep in preadolescent children is accompanied by high degrees of baseline alertness during daytime as measured by the multiple sleep latency test (MSLT). Mean sleep latency for healthy children on the MSLT averages 19 ± 1.6 min, considerably higher than the 10–13 min range considered normal for adults.[22] Given this high level of baseline alertness, prominent sleepiness in a preadolescent child is seldom encountered except in the context of a severe underlying sleep disorder or significant sleep deprivation.

During adolescence, daytime sleepiness as measured by the MSLT increases, which may reflect the effects of average sleep duration being insufficient relative to overall sleep needs. [23] In addition, many healthy adolescents demonstrate tendencies toward delayed circadian phase, trending toward progressively later bedtimes and—particularly on nonschool days—waking times.

Insomnia in older children and adolescents

Insomnia, daytime sleepiness, and other subjectively reported sleep problems remain common for school-aged children and adolescents, affecting 10–30% of elementary schoolchildren and a similar proportion of adolescents.[24–26] Social, environmental, and developmental influences have significant impact on sleep for this age group. For example, older children and adolescents gain increasing autonomy regarding their bedtime and sleep schedule compared with younger children, often resulting in irregular sleep habits and chronically insufficient sleep. The widespread availability of televisions, music players, and computers in the bedrooms of school-age children and the frequent use of these devices during nighttime hours is associated with increased risk for a variety of sleep disturbances.[27,28] Use of mobile telephones after bedtime is prevalent among secondary schoolchildren and associated with increased risk for daytime sleepiness.[29]

Another strong influence on the sleep patterns of older school-age children is the well-recognized tendency toward delayed circadian sleep phase that develops near adolescence.[26] Circadian rhythm disorder, delayed sleep phase type, formerly called *delayed sleep phase syndrome*, may be diagnosed when this tendency results in chronic or recurrent inability of the child to fall asleep and wake up at conventional and socially acceptable times.[11] When this condition results in chronically insufficient sleep, it is often accompanied by daytime napping, which may make it more difficult for the child to fall asleep at the desired

bedtime. Habitually later bedtime and waking time on nonschool nights—common in adolescents—tend to perpetuate or worsen the tendency toward delayed sleep phase.[30] Delayed sleep phase can be mimicked or exacerbated when medication or caffeine use result in insomnia with chronic sleep deprivation or when homework or other late-evening activities habitually delay sleep onset.

Psychophysiological insomnia in older children is characterized by chronic preoccupation with and excessive anxiety regarding sleep, which results in heightened arousal that delays sleep onset.[11] Affected children often report anxiety or identifiable rumination in conjunction with insomnia when trying to fall asleep at bedtime but are sometimes able to fall asleep easily during sedentary activities or when away from home.

Treatment of insomnia in older children and adolescents

Treatment of insomnia during later childhood is seldom effective unless all pertinent contributory influences are identified and addressed in the treatment plan. For adolescents in particular, it is common to identify multiple concurrent influences such as irregular sleep schedule, excessive caffeine use, insufficient time allotted for sleep, and tendency toward delayed sleep phase.

Establishing or optimizing appropriate "sleep hygiene" is a necessary foundation for other aspects of treatment. Optimal bedtime and waking time should be identified based on the child's age, school schedule, and individual sleep needs. Because regularity of sleep schedule helps maintain circadian entrainment, delayed bedtimes and "sleeping in" on nonschool days should be avoided whenever possible. Potentially stimulating activities such as vigorous exercise, video gaming, and consumption of caffeinated beverages should be discouraged during the evening hours. Eliminating use of electronic devices such as televisions, music players, and portable telephones in the bedroom near bedtime helps promote optimal sleep onset associations and a dark, quiet environment more conducive to sleep initiation and maintenance.

Insomnia related primarily to delayed circadian sleep phase can be treated in several ways. Mildly delayed sleep phase often responds to consistent enforcement of the desired sleep schedule by maintaining target bedtime and waking times 7 days weekly while eliminating any daytime napping. An alternative and comparably effective strategy consists of gradually advancing the child's bedtime and waking time earlier by 10–15 min each day until the target schedule is achieved.

More severe or resistant forms of delayed sleep phase often respond to chronotherapy, a process by which bedtime and waking time are delayed by 2–3 h nightly until the desired sleep schedule is attained.[31] Although this treatment is safe, highly effective, and does not require use of medication, the effects of treatment are typically maintained only if the target sleep schedule is maintained rigorously 7 days weekly following completion of the treatment protocol. Light therapy, a treatment designed to influence circadian rhythmicity via structured daily exposure to high-intensity light, has also been reported to be effective in treating delayed sleep phase in children and adolescents.[32,33]

Drug treatment for insomnia in older children and adolescents has received extremely limited scientific study despite reports that 10–12% of adolescents use medication for treatment of sleep problems.[17,34,35] Melatonin has been reported to be effective for treatment of insomnia in school-aged children and adolescents in both uncontrolled[36,37] and placebo-controlled[38] studies. Although reports of melatonin treatment for insomnia in children have assessed doses ranging from 0.3 to 20 mg,[39] the side effects, long-term safety, and optimal dosing of this agent for pediatric use have not been well established.

Numerous other medications are used off label for the treatment of insomnia in older children in spite of a paucity of scientific data assessing overall safety and efficacy. These include antihistamines, benzodiazepines, tricyclic agents, alpha-adrenergic agonists, antipsychotics, herbal preparations, and newer short-acting hypnotics.[17] Pharmacology and dosing for these agents relative to pediatric sleep disorders were recently reviewed by Pelayo and Dubik.[21]

Non-rapid eyemovement arousal parasomnias: night terrors and sleepwalking

Night terrors, sleepwalking, and confusional arousals in children are thought to represent forms of incomplete arousal from deep non-REM sleep. These aberrant arousals are associated with a spectrum of behaviors that may range from quiet somnambulism to extreme agitation. Episodes occur most commonly during the early hours of night-time sleep, when deep non-REM sleep stages are predominantly distributed, particularly in younger children. Children are difficult to awaken during the event, and if awakened, demonstrate little or no recall for the episode.

Exacerbations of non-REM arousal parasomnias are often triggered by sleep deprivation or intercurrent illness. Reports of human leukocyte antigen associations and familial clustering for patients with arousal parasomnias suggest that these disorders are subject to strong genetic influences.[40,41] Limited evidence suggests that obstructive sleep apnea or restless legs syndrome may represent a treatable precipitant of these parasomnias for some children.[42]

Night terrors and confusional arousals affect up to 17% of children[43] but are most commonly observed in toddlers and preschoolers. The semiology of events ranges from moaning or quiet crying with the child remaining in bed to extreme agitation accompanied by attempts to flee the room. Episodes may last as long as 1 hr, but most typically remit within minutes. Affected children usually have little or no subsequent recollection of events.

Although 40% of children exhibit at least one episode of sleepwalking, frequent sleepwalking affects only 2–3%, with peak prevalence near 10 years of age.[43,44] Episodes consist of quiet ambulation lasting several minutes, which may include semipurposeful activities such wandering to the parent's room or urinating in inappropriate locations. Sleepwalking children seldom sustain serious injury in their familiar home environment, but risk for injury increases when children leave the house during an episode or are sleeping in an unfamiliar environment.

Treatment of the non-REM arousal parasomnias in children should commence with the identification and treatment of precipitants such as sleep deprivation or obstructive sleep apnea. It is important to safeguard the child's sleep environment and limit the child's access to potentially hazardous areas inside and outside the house through judicious use of locks or alarms. Use of scheduled awakenings is often effective for children whose sleepwalking or night terrors occur at predictable times of the night.[45,46] Drug treatment using clonazepam may effective for children having particularly frequent or severe forms of sleepwalking and night terrors.[47,48]

Other childhood parasomnias: nightmares and enuresis

Nightmares arise from REM sleep and are thought to result from awakening during a frightening dream. Agitation following awakening is sometimes considerable, but the fact that the child awakens fully, responds to consolation by the parent, and has recollection of dream content helps distinguish nightmares from night terrors. Nightmares usually arise during the latter half of the child's nighttime sleep period, when REM periods are usually longest and most prevalent. Nightmares during childhood are common, affecting over half of early school-aged children on an occasional basis but only 3% of children more than once weekly.[49]

Occasional nightmares in otherwise healthy children represent a self-limited problem that seldom requires further assessment or treatment. Persistent nightmares which are unexpectedly frequent, prolonged, or violent in content, however, may signal a need for further investigation of potential medical and psychological causes.

Sleep enuresis in children is characterized by recurrent involuntary voiding during sleep at a level that is inappropriate for age, defined by the International Classification of Sleep Disorders as more than twice weekly for children older than 5 years of age.[11] Sleep enuresis is defined as primary if the child has never remained consistently dry during sleep and secondary if the child had previously been consistently dry for at least 6 months. Nocturnal enuresis becomes less common with advancing age, affecting 15% of 3- to 10-year-olds, but only 2% of 13-year-olds.[43] Boys are affected three times as frequently as girls. Postulated causes of primary enuresis include immaturity of arousal mechanisms, reduced functional bladder capacity, and genetic predisposition.

Treatment of primary sleep enuresis in children varies depending on age and severity. Most younger children with primary enuresis outgrow the condition by adolescence without treatment. Children with frequent or persistent forms of primary enuresis often respond to behaviorally based therapies and conditioning programs that incorporate fluid restriction, planned awakenings, bladder training exercises, behavioral incentives, and enuresis alarms either independently or in combination.[50,51] Drug treatment using desmopressin[52] and imipramine[53] is also effective for many children with sleep enuresis, but reports of hyponatremia[54] and other potentially serious mediation-related side effects[53] suggest that these agents are best used within the context of a comprehensive and closely supervised treatment program.

Children with secondary sleep enuresis or refractory primary enuresis sometimes require evaluation for underlying urological or sleep disorders. Sleep enuresis is frequently associated with symptoms of obstructive sleep apnea in children.[55,56] In one series of 144 children with PSG-confirmed obstructive sleep apnea, 42 (29%) demonstrated sleep enuresis prior to treatment.[57] Among the 27 children with enuresis treated with adenotonsillectomy, 11 (41%) experienced resolution of bedwetting within 1 month following surgery.

Sleep-related movement disorders: restless legs syndrome and rhythmic movement disorder

Restless legs syndrome (RLS) and periodic limb movement disorder (PLMD) are distinct but related conditions only recently recognized in the pediatric age group. Symptoms of RLS in children include dysesthesias or urges to move the legs, which are usually most prominent at night and relieved by movement.[11] Children with growing pains often meet diagnostic criteria for RLS as well.[58] Childhood PLMD is characterized by excessive periodic limb movements occurring over five times per hour of sleep during PSG, accompanied by clinical complaints of disturbed sleep.[11] Although RLS and PLMD are often comorbid conditions in both children and adults, the association is not obligate and either condition may present independently.

Leg restlessness and growing pains affect up to 17% and 8% of children, respectively,[59] but only 2% of children meet diagnostic criteria for clinically definite RLS.[60] Multiple studies have reported association between childhood RLS/PLMD and symptoms of attention deficit hyperactivity disorder (ADHD);[61–63] however, the strength and clinical significance of this association remains incompletely defined. Several reports suggest that genetic

Table 2. Diagnostic criteria for pediatric obstructive sleep apnea

1. Parent or caregiver report of snoring or other obstructive symptoms during sleep
2. Parent or caregiver report of at least one associated symptom:
    a. Paradoxical chest wall motion during inspiration
    b. Movement arousals
    c. Excessive perspiration
    d. Unusual sleeping positions, for example, neck hyperextension
    e. Daytime symptoms: hyperactivity, aggressive behavior, or sleepiness
    f. Impaired growth
    g. Headache upon waking
    h. Secondary enuresis
3. PSG documents at least one scoreable respiratory event per hour of sleep (events lasting at least two respiratory cycles in duration)
4. PSG demonstrates either a or b:
    a. At least one of the following findings:
        i. Frequent arousals associated with increased respiratory effort
        ii. Desaturation with apneic events
        iii. Hypercapnia in sleep
        iv. Excessively negative esophageal pressure fluctuations
    b. Periods of abnormal gas exchange during sleep (hypoxemia, hypercapnea, or both) with snoring, paradoxical chest wall motion, and at least one of the following:
        i. Frequent arousals during sleep
        ii. Excessively negative esophageal pressures swings
5. The disorder is not better explained by other sleep disorders, medical or neurological conditions, or by medication or substance use

Adapted from the *International Classification of Sleep Disorders*, second edition.[11]

influences[64] and iron deficiency states[65] may play a causative role in childhood RLS. Treatment options for childhood RLS/PLMD consist of iron supplementation for children with low ferritin levels or other evidence of iron deficiency,[66,67] or judicious use of dopaminergic agonists.[68,69]

Sleep-related rhythmic movement disorder (RMD) is characterized by recurrent and well-stereotyped rhythmic behaviors associated with sleep.[11,70] Common behaviors include head banging (jactatio capitis nocturna), head or body rolling, and body rocking. Movements typically involve the large muscle groups of the head, trunk, or limbs at a frequency of 0.5 to 2 Hz, often accompanied by synchronous humming or moaning vocalizations. Episodes of rhythmic movement typically last for several minutes but may recur throughout the night. RMD is unique among the parasomnias insofar as episodes may commence during wakefulness but persist during and following transition into sustained sleep.

Sleep-related rhythmic behaviors are observed in a majority of infants, but these behaviors subside before 5 years of age in most children.[71] By early adolescence, only 3% of children manifest prominent rhythmic behaviors associated with sleep.[43] For most affected children, RMD is a self-limited condition that does not require treatment. For children exhibiting particularly prolonged or violent forms of RMD, treatment options include benzodiazepines, behavioral therapies, or use of padding and protective helmets.[72]

Sleep-disordered breathing in children

The first modern description of obstructive sleep apnea (OSA) in children was provided by Guilleminault and colleagues in 1976.[73] This and subsequent reports have characterized childhood OSA as a condition characterized by upper airway obstruction that disturbs sleep quality, sometimes associated with recurrent oxyhemoglobin desaturation or (less commonly) hypercapnia.

Table 3. Clinical features of obstructive sleep apnea in children compared to adults

	Children	Adults
Physical characteristics		
Gender	Younger children: sexes equally affected	Primarily males, postmenopausal females
	Adolescents: males > females	
Peak age	2–8 years	Middle age and older
Body weight	Usually normal, occasionally overweight	Most often obese
Upper airway	Adenotonsillar enlargement frequent	Adenotonsillar enlargement occasional
	Redundant soft tissue occasional	Redundant soft tissue frequent
Symptoms during sleep		
Snoring	Frequent, continuous or intermittent	Frequent, often interrupted by pauses
Witnessed apnea	Occasional	Frequent
PSG characteristics		
Obstruction	Prolonged partial obstruction > intermittent	Cyclical intermittent obstruction
Sleep architecture	Normal > fragmented	Frequent arousals with sleep fragmentation
Secondary symptoms		
Daytime sleepiness	Most often absent or intermittent	Frequent, usually prominent
Neurobehavioral	Inattention, hyperkinesis, disturbed behavior	Cognitive slowing, increased accident risk
Cardiovascular	Hypertension, cor pulmonale	Hypertension, heart disease, stroke

Criteria for the diagnosis of childhood OSA, summarized in Table 2, were established by the *International Classification of Sleep Disorders*, second edition.[11] This classification, however, did not specify criteria for other varieties of sleep-disordered breathing sometimes observed in children. Children with neuromuscular disorders, underlying lung disease, or severe varieties of partial airway obstruction sometimes exhibit sleep-related hypoventilation, characterized by persistent hypercapnia during sleep.[74] Upper airway resistance syndrome (UARS), a condition in which prolonged partial airway obstruction during sleep disturbs sleep quality in the absence of apnea or desaturation, has also been described in children.[75]

It is estimated that about 2% of children suffer from OSA.[76] The condition may develop at any time during childhood but is most frequent between 2 and 8 years of age, the age range when adenotonsillar size is largest relative to size of the airway. OSA is equally frequent in boys and girls until adolescence, when the condition becomes more common in males. Other genetic, neurological, and craniofacial conditions are associated with increased risk for the development of childhood OSA, particularly Down syndrome, in which half of children may be affected.[77,78]

The clinical features of OSA in children are distinct from those of adults, as summarized in Table 3. Snoring is usually present in affected children, but frequency and severity are highly variable. Other common symptoms during nighttime sleep include mouth breathing, restlessness, diaphoresis, and unusual sleeping positions. Symptoms upon waking may include sore throat, dry mouth, headache, and transient grogginess. Daytime somnolence is seldom prominent in younger children with OSA unless obstruction is particularly severe.

A number of studies suggest that disturbances of attention, behavior, and academic performance are commonly associated with childhood OSA and may improve following treatment. Sleep-disordered breathing was identified in 18% of 297 first-grade children with poor academic achievement in one study.[79] Upon reassessment 1 year later, the 24 affected children who had been treated with adenotonsillectomy demonstrated significant academic improvement ($P < 0.001$) compared with untreated and unaffected children. In a more recent study of 78 children undergoing adenotonsillectomy for suspected sleep-disordered breathing, 22 (28%) met *DSM-IV* criteria for the diagnosis of ADHD preoperatively, but only half of these children still met criteria for the diagnosis of ADHD 1 year following surgery.[80]

The long-term effects and clinical sequelae of childhood OSA remain incompletely understood. Multiple reports suggest associations between childhood OSA and hypertension.[81,82] Reversible cor pulmonale has also been reported in severely affected children.[83,84]

The physical examination of children with OSA is often normal, but findings such as tonsillar hypertrophy, narrow upper palate, and low-lying soft palate are frequently identified. Mouth breathing with elongated facial appearance is sometimes apparent in children with underlying adenoidal hypertrophy. Other occasionally encountered physical features associated with increased risk for sleep-related airway obstruction include maxillary or mandibular hypoplasia, macroglossia, or nasal septal deviation. Although body weight is normal for most children with OSA, obesity nevertheless represents a clearly identifiable risk factor, particularly in adolescents.[85,86]

The diagnosis of childhood OSA (Table 2) is established on the basis of both clinical and polysomnographic criteria.[87] Lab-based PSG is now widely but not universally available for children, but the number of sleep laboratories having substantial experience in pediatric studies remains limited. Specific norms for the interpretation of PSG in children have been established,[74,88] which are distinct from adult norms and reflect the fact that adult criteria often fail to identify children with serious obstruction.[89] PSG can be customized through addition of end-tidal carbon dioxide or esophageal pressure monitoring if sleep-related hypoventilation or upper airway resistance syndrome are clinically suspected. A variety of techniques are available for making PSG more "child friendly."[90]

Adenotonsillectomy (AT) is the most common treatment of childhood OSA. This procedure has been used for decades to alleviate upper airway obstruction in children with suspected or documented OSA.[91] Although previously issued practice guidelines[92] and meta-analysis of published research[93] had estimated that the procedure was effective in curing childhood OSA in over 75% of cases, these estimates were limited by substantial variability in the criteria used to define childhood OSA and measure outcome. Several large, recent studies using contemporary criteria and PSG techniques to study the efficacy of AT in treating childhood OSA reported that complete normalization of the PSG may occur in only 25%[94] to 50%[95] of treated children. These and other data suggest that healthcare practitioners should remain vigilant for residual or recurrent[96,97] OSA in children treated with AT.

Nasal CPAP (continuous positive airway pressure) is an alternative first-line treatment for OSA in children of all ages.[98] Advantages of CPAP include the facts that the treatment is nonsurgical, generally safe, and effective for treatment of sleep-disordered breathing related to factors independent from adentonsillar hypertrophy. Limitations of this treatment include the fact that some children—especially those who are young or have concurrent developmental disabilities—may not acclimate easily to use of the device, although specific desensitization techniques are often helpful in these patients.[99]

Alternative and investigational medical treatments for childhood OSA include use of supplemental oxygen and positional therapy. Use of nasal steroid preparations may be effective in some cases;[100,101] however, the long-term efficacy and safety of this treatment in children have not been established. Surgical treatments sometimes used for treatment of children with complicated OSA include uvulopaltopharyngoplasty (UPPP), distraction osteogenesis, and mandibular or maxillary advancement procedures. Tracheostomy is used only as a last resort in children whose OSA is both severe and refractory to more conventional therapies.

Childhood hypersomnias

Excessive daytime sleepiness in children is most often secondary to other sleep problems such as insufficient sleep or more severe forms of obstructive sleep apnea. Nevertheless, primary hypersomnias such as narcolepsy and Kleine-Levin syndrome are occasionally observed in children.

As is the case for adults, narcolepsy in children is characterized by excessive daytime somnolence, which may be accompanied by cataplexy, sleep paralysis, and hallucinations at sleep onset or offset. Onset of symptoms most commonly occurs during the second decade,[102] usually in the form of isolated sleepiness, which can develop in either an abrupt or insidiously progressive fashion. Cataplexy, sleep paralysis, and other associated symptoms of narcolepsy, when present, may develop months to years after the child becomes somnolent. Evolution of severe somnolence or cataplexy at an especially young age or in an atypical fashion is sometimes observed in children with other medical conditions such as Niemann-Pick disease type C[103] or Prader-Willi syndrome.[104]

The diagnosis of narcolepsy in children is based on the presence of typical clinical features, supplemented by nocturnal PSG—to screen for other sleep disorders that may cause excessive sleepiness—and daytime MSLT interpreted using pediatric norms.[22] Most children with narcolepsy demonstrated mean sleep latency of fewer than 7 min and multiple sleep-onset REM periods on their MSLT studies.[105]

Treatment of narcolepsy in children parallels that of adults in most respects. Although detailed practice parameters[106] and guidelines for treatment of narcolepsy[107] have been published, these do not specifically address drug treatment in children, which is undertaken on an off-label basis. Daytime sleepiness in narcoleptic children is treated using modafinil, stimulants, and other wake-promoting medications, sometimes supplemented by planned daytime naps. Cataplexy often responds to administration of tricyclic antidepressant agents or selective serotonin reuptake inhibitors. Sodium oxybate has been found to be effective in the treatment of sleepiness and cataplexy in adults with narcolepsy, and limited data suggest that this agent may be effective for affected children as well.[108]

Kleine-Levin syndrome, also known as recurrent hypersomnia, is a rare disorder characterized by recurrent episodes of excessive sleepiness, often accompanied by concurrent behavioral disturbances, which may include irritability, aggression, marked changes in appetite, and hypersexual behavior.[11] Episodes last from several days to several weeks and occur between once and 10 times yearly. Kleine-Levin syndrome most commonly affects adolescent males, and limited evidence suggests that the severity and duration of the condition may be worse for patients who are older at the age of onset.[109]

The pathophysiology of Kleine-Levin syndrome remains poorly understood, but SPECT studies suggest that intermittent disturbances of hypothalamic, thalamic, and fronto-temporal function may coincide with episodes.[110,111] Treatment of the condition is symptomatic and often includes mood stabilizers and wake-promoting medications such as modafinil.

Conflicts of interest

The author declares no conflicts of interest.

References

1. Coons, S., C. Guilleminault, S. Coons & C. Guilleminault. 1982. Development of sleep-wake patterns and non-rapid eye movement sleep stages during the first six months of life in normal infants. *Pediatrics* **69:** 793–798.

2. Guilleminault, C. & T.F. Anders. 1976. The pathophysiology of sleep disorders in pediatrics. Part II. Sleep disorders in children. *Adv. Pediatrics* **22:** 151–174.

3. Iglowstein, I., O.G. Jenni, L. Molinari & R.H. Largo. 2003. Sleep duration from infancy to adolescence: reference values and generational trends [see comment]. *Pediatrics* **111:** 302–307.

4. Anders, T.F. & C. Guilleminault. 1976. The pathophysiology of sleep disorders in pediatrics. Part I. Sleep in infancy. *Adv. Pediatrics* **22:** 137–150.

5. Ferber, R.. 1996. Childhood sleep disorders. *Neurol. Clin.* **14:** 493–511.

6. Sadeh, A., P. Lavie, A. Scher, *et al.* 1991. Actigraphic home monitoring of sleep-disturbed and control infants and young children: a new method for pediatric assessment of sleep-wake patterns. *Pediatrics* **87:** 494–499.

7. Sheldon, S.H. 2005. Disorders of initiating and maintaining sleep. In *Principles and Practice of Pediatric Sleep Medicine.* Sheldon, S.H., R. Ferber & M.H. Kryger, Eds.: 127–160. Philadelphia: Saunders.

8. Mosko, S., C. Richard & J. McKenna. 1997. Infant arousals during mother-infant bed sharing: implications for infant sleep and sudden infant death syndrome research. *Pediatrics* **100:** 841–849.

9. Ramchandani, P., L. Wiggs, V. Webb & G. Stores. 2000. A systematic review of treatments for settling problems and night waking in young children. *BMJ* **320:** 209–213.

10. Stores, G. 1999. Children's sleep disorders: modern approaches, developmental effects, and children at special risk. *Dev. Med. Child Neurol.* **41:** 568–573.

11. Anonymous. 2005. *The International Classification of Sleep Disorders,* 2nd edn. American Academy of Sleep Medicine. Westchester.

12. Kuhn, B.R. & A.J. Elliott. 2003. Treatment efficacy in behavioral pediatric sleep medicine. *J. Psychosom. Res.* **54:** 587–597.

13. Douglas, J & N. Richman. 1984. *My Child Won't Sleep.* Penguin Books. Harmondsworth.

14. Ferber, R. 1985. *Solve Your Child's Sleep Problems.* Simon & Schuster. New York.

15. Mindell, J.A., B. Kuhn, D.S. Lewin, *et al.* 2006. Behavioral treatment of bedtime problems and night wakings in infants and young children [erratum appears in Sleep. 2006 Nov 1;29(11):1380]. *Sleep* **29:** 1263–1276.

16. Morgenthaler, T.I., J. Owens, C. Alessi, *et al.* 2006. Practice parameters for behavioral treatment of bedtime problems and night wakings in infants and young children. *Sleep* **29:** 1277–1281.

17. Owens, J.A., C.L. Rosen & J.A. Mindell. 2003. Medication use in the treatment of pediatric insomnia: results of a survey of community-based pediatricians. *Pediatrics* **111**(5 Pt 1): e628–e635.

18. France, K.G., N.M. Blampied & P. Wilkinson. 1999. A multiple-baseline, double-blind evaluation of the effects of trimeprazine tartrate on infant sleep disturbance. *Exp. Clin. Psychopharmacol.* **7:** 502–513.

19. Simonoff, E.A. & G. Stores. 1987. Controlled trial of trimeprazine tartrate for night waking. *Arch. Dis. Child.* **62:** 253–257.

20. Merenstein, D., M. Diener-West, A.C. Halbower, *et al.* 2006. The trial of infant response to diphenhydramine: the TIRED study–a randomized, controlled, patient-oriented trial. *Arch. Pediatr. Adolesc. Med.* **160:** 707–712.

21. Pelayo, R. & M. Dubik. 2008. Pediatric sleep pharmacology. *Semin. Pediatr. Neurol.* **15:** 79–90.

22. Hoban, T.F. & R.D. Chervin. 2001. Assessment of sleepiness in children. *Semin. Pediatr. Neurol.* **8:** 216–228.

23. Carskadon, M.A. & W. Dement. 1987. Sleepiness in the normal adolescent. In *Sleep and Its Disorders in Children.* Guilleminault, C. Ed.: 53–66. Raven Press. New York.

24. Blader, J.C., H.S. Koplewicz, H. Abikoff & C. Foley. 1997. Sleep problems of elementary school children. *Arch. Pediatr. Adolesc. Med.* **151:** 473–480.

25. Saarenpaa-Heikkila, O., P. Laippala & M. Koivikko. 2000. Subjective daytime sleepiness in schoolchildren. *Family Pract.* **17:** 129–133.

26. Carskadon, M.A.. 1982. The second decade. In *Sleeping and Waking Disorders: Indications and Techniques.* Guilleminault, C. Ed.: 99–125. Addison Wesley. Menlo Park.

27. Van Den Bulck, J. 2004. Television viewing, computer game playing, and Internet use and self-reported time to bed and time out of bed in secondary-school children [see comment]. *Sleep* **27:** 101–104.

28. Owens, J., R Maxim, M. McGuinn, *et al.* 1999. Television-viewing habits and sleep disturbance in school children. *Pediatrics* **104:** e27.

29. Van Den Bulck, J. 2007. Adolescent use of mobile phones for calling and for sending text messages after lights out: results from a prospective cohort study with a one-year follow-up. *Sleep* **30:** 1220–1223.

30. Crowley, S.J., C. Acebo, M.A. Carskadon, *et al.* 2007. Sleep, circadian rhythms, and delayed phase in adolescence. *Sleep Med.* **8:** 602–612.

31. Czeisler, C., G. Richardson, R. Coleman, *et al.* 1981. Chronotherapy: resetting the circadian clocks of patients with delayed sleep phase insomnia. *Sleep* **4:** 1–21.

32. Guilleminault, C., C.C. McCann, M. Quera-Salva & M. Cetel. 1993. Light therapy as treatment of dyschronosis in brain impaired children. *Eur. J. Pediatr.* **152:** 754–759.

33. Okawa, M., M. Uchiyama, S. Ozaki, *et al.* 1998. Circadian rhythm sleep disorders in adolescents: clinical trials of combined treatments based on chronobiology. *Psychiatry Clin. Neurosc.* **52:** 483–490.

34. Patois, E., J. Valatx & A. Alperovitch. 1993. Prevalence of sleep and wakefulness disorders in high school students at the Academy of Lyon. *Rev. Epiedmiol. Sante Publique* **41:** 383–388.

35. Ledoux, S., M. Choquet & R. Manfredi. 1994. Self-reported use of drugs for sleep or distress among French adolescents. *J. Adolesc. Health* **15:** 495–502.

36. Ivanenko, A., V.M. Crabtree, R. Tauman & D. Gozal. 2003. Melatonin in children and adolescents with insomnia: a retrospective study. *Clin. Pediatr.* **42:** 51–58.

37. Szeinberg, A., K. Borodkin, Y. Dagan, *et al.* 2006. Melatonin treatment in adolescents with delayed sleep phase syndrome. *Clin. Pediatr. (Phila)* **45:** 809–818.

38. Smits, M., H. Van Stel, K. Van Der Heijen, *et al.* 2003. Melatonin improves health status and sleep in children with idiopathic chronic sleep-onset insomnia: a randomized, placebo-controlled trial. *J. Am. Acad. Child Adolesc. Psychiatry* **42:** 1286–1293.

39. Stores, G. 2003. Medication for sleep-wake disorders. *Arch. Dis. Child.* **88:** 899–903.

40. Hublin, C., J. Kaprio, M. Partinen & M. Koskenvu. 2001. Parasomnias: co-occurrence and genetics. *Psychiatr. Genet.* **11:** 65–70.

41. Lecendreux, M., C. Bassetti, Y. Dauvilliers, *et al.* 2003. HLA and genetic susceptibility to sleepwalking. *Mol. Psychiatry* **8:** 114–117.

42. Guilleminault, C., L. Palombini, R. Pelayo, *et al.* 2003. Sleepwalking and sleep terrors in prepubertal children: what triggers them? *Pediatrics* **111:** e17–e25.

43. Laberge, L., R.E. Tremblay, F. Vitaro & J. Montplaisir. 2000. Development of parasomnias from childhood to early adolescence. *Pediatrics* **106:** 67–74.

44. Klackenberg, G. 1982. Somnambulism in childhood–prevalence, course and behavioral correlations. A prospective longitudinal study (6–16 years). *Acta Paediatrica Scandinavica* **71:** 495–499.

45. Frank, N.C., A. Spirito, L. Stark & J. Owens-Stively. 1997. The use of scheduled awakenings to eliminate childhood sleepwalking. *J. Pediatr. Psychol.* **22:** 345–353.

46. Durand, V.M. & J.A. Mindell. 1999. Intervention for childhood sleep terrors. *Behav. Ther.* **30:** 705–715.

47. Remulla, A., C. Guilleminault, A. Remulla & C. Guilleminault. 2004. Somnambulism (sleepwalking). *Expert Opin. Pharmacother.* **5:** 2069–2074.

48. Pesikoff, R. & P. Davis. 1971. Treatment of pavor nocturnus and somnambulism in children. *Am. J. Psychiatry* **128:** 778–781.

49. Smedje, H., J.E. Broman, J. Hetta, *et al.* 1999. Parents' reports of disturbed sleep in 5–7-year-old Swedish children. *Acta Paediatrica* **88:** 858–865.

50. Butler, R.J., P. Holland, S. Gasson, *et al.* 2007. Exploring potential mechanisms in alarm treatment for primary nocturnal enuresis. *Scand. J. Urol. Nephrol.* **41:** 407–413.

51. Lottmann, H.B. & I. Alova. 2007. Primary monosymptomatic nocturnal enuresis in children and adolescents. *Int. J. Clin. Pract.* **Supplement**(155): 8–16.

52. Ferrara, P., G. Marrone, V. Emmanuele, *et al.* 2008. Homotoxicological remedies versus desmopressin versus placebo in the treatment of enuresis: a randomised, double-blind, controlled trial [see comment]. *Pediatr. Nephrol.* **23:** 269–274.

53. Neveus, T., K. Tullus, T. Neveus & K. Tullus. 2008. Tolterodine and imipramine in refractory enuresis; a placebo-controlled crossover study. *Pediatr. Nephrol.* **23:** 263–267.

54. Larney, V. & R. Dwyer. 2006. Hyponatraemic convulsions and fatal head injury secondary to desmopressin treatment for enuresis. *Eur. J. Anaesthesiol.* **23:** 895–897.

55. Stone, J., P.S. Malone, D. Atwill, *et al.* 2008. Symptoms of sleep-disordered breathing in children with nocturnal enuresis. *J. Pediatr. Urol.* **4:** 197–202.

56. Weider, D.J. & P.J. Hauri. 1985. Nocturnal enuresis in children with upper airway obstruction. *Int. J. Pediatr. Otorhinolaryngol.* **9:** 173–182.

57. Weissbach, A., A. Leiberman, A. Tarasiuk, *et al.* 2006. Adenotonsilectomy improves enuresis in children with obstructive sleep apnea syndrome. *Int. J. Pediatr. Otorhinolaryngol.* **70:** 1351–1356.

58. Rajaram, S.S., A.S. Walters, S.J. England, *et al.* 2004. Some children with growing pains may actually have restless legs syndrome. *Sleep* **27:** 767–773.

59. Chervin, R.D., K.H. Archbold, J.E. Dillon, *et al.* 2002. Associations between symptoms of inattention, hyperactivity, restless legs, and periodic leg movements. *Sleep* **25:** 213–218.

60. Picchietti, D., R.P. Allen, A.S. Walters, *et al.* 2007. Restless legs syndrome: prevalence and impact in children and adolescents–the Peds REST study [see comment]. *Pediatrics* **120:** 253–266.

61. Cortese, S., E. Konofal, M. Lecendreux, *et al.* 2005. Restless legs syndrome and attention-deficit/hyperactivity disorder: a review of the literature. *Sleep* **28:** 1007–1013.

62. Picchietti, D.L., D.J. Underwood, W.A. Farris, *et al.* 1999. Further studies on periodic limb movement disorder and restless legs syndrome in children with attention-deficit hyperactivity disorder. *Mov. Disord.* **14:** 1000–1007.

63. Picchietti, D.L., S.J. England, A.S. Walters, *et al.* 1998. Periodic limb movement disorder and restless legs syndrome in children with attention-deficit hyperactivity disorder. *J. Child Neurol.* **13:** 588–594.

64. Muhle, H., A. Neumann, K. Lohmann-Hedrich, *et al.* 2008. Childhood-onset restless legs syndrome: clinical and genetic features of 22 families. *Mov. Disord.* **23:** 1113–1121; quiz 203.

65. Oner, P., E.B. Dirik, Y. Taner, *et al.* 2007. Association between low serum ferritin and restless legs syndrome in patients with attention deficit hyperactivity disorder. *Tohoku J. Exp. Med.* **213:** 269–276.

66. Picchietti, M.A., D.L. Picchietti, M.A. Picchietti & D.L. Picchietti. 2008. Restless legs syndrome and periodic limb movement disorder in children and adolescents. *Semin. Pediatr. Neurol.* **15:** 91–99.

67. Kryger, M.H., K. Otake & J. Foerster. 2002. Low body stores of iron and restless legs syndrome: a correctable cause of insomnia in adolescents and teenagers. *Sleep Med.* **3:** 127–132.

68. Konofal, E., I. Arnulf, M. Lecendreux, *et al.* 2005. Ropinirole in a child with attention-deficit hyperactivity disorder and restless legs syndrome. *Pediatr. Neurol.* **32:** 350–351.

69. Walters, A.S., D.E. Mandelbaum, D.S. Lewin, *et al.* 2000. Dopaminergic therapy in children with restless legs/periodic limb movements in sleep and ADHD.

Dopaminergic Therapy Study Group. *Pediatr. Neurol.* **22:** 182–186.

70. Hoban, T.F. 2003. Rhythmic movement disorder in children. *Cns Spectrums* **8:** 135–138.

71. Klackenberg, G. 1971. Rhythmic movements in infancy and early childhood. *Acta Paediatrica Scandinavica* **224**(suppl): 74–82.

72. Hoban, T.F. Sleep related rhythmic movement disorder. In *The Parasomnias and Other Sleep-related Movement Disorders.* Thorpy, M. & G. Plazzi, Eds. Cambridge University Press. Cambridge. In Press.

73. Guilleminault, C., F.L. Eldridge, F.B. Simmons & W.C. Dement. 1976. Sleep apnea in eight children. *Pediatrics* **58:** 23–30.

74. Iber, C., S. Ancoli-Israel, A. Chesson & S.F. Quan. 2007. *The AASM Manual for the Scoring of Sleep and Associated Events.* American Academy of Sleep Medicine. Westchester.

75. Guilleminault, C., R. Pelayo, D. Leger, *et al.* 1996. Recognition of sleep-disordered breathing in children. *Pediatrics* **98:** 871–882.

76. Marcus, C.L. 2001. Sleep-disordered breathing in children. *Am. J. Respir. Crit. Care Med.* **164:** 16–30.

77. Shott, S.R., R. Amin, B. Chini, *et al.* 2006. Obstructive sleep apnea: Should all children with Down syndrome be tested? *Arch. Otolaryngol. – Head Neck Surg.* **132:** 432–436.

78. Ng, D.K., H.N. Hui, C.H. Chan, *et al.* 2006. Obstructive sleep apnoea in children with Down syndrome. *Singapore Med. J.* **47:** 774–779.

79. Gozal, D. 1998. Sleep-disordered breathing and school performance in children. *Pediatrics* **102:** 616–620.

80. Chervin, R.D., D.L. Ruzicka, B.J. Giordani, *et al.* 2006. Sleep-disordered breathing, behavior, and cognition in children before and after adenotonsillectomy. *Pediatrics* **117:** e769–e778.

81. Li, A.M., C.T. Au, R.Y. Sung, *et al.* 2008. Ambulatory blood pressure in children with obstructive sleep apnoea: a community based study. *Thorax* **63:** 803–809.

82. Leung, L.C., D.K. Ng, M.W. Lau, *et al.* 2006. Twenty-four-hour ambulatory BP in snoring children with obstructive sleep apnea syndrome. *Chest* **130:** 1009–1017.

83. Cox, M.A., G.L. Schiebler, W.J. Taylor, *et al.* 1965. Reversible pulmonary hypertension in a child with respiratory obstruction and cor pulmonale. *J. Pediatr.* **67:** 192–197.

84. Sofer, S., E. Weinhouse, A. Tal, *et al.* 1988. Cor pulmonale due to adenoidal or tonsillar hypertrophy or both in children. Noninvasive diagnosis and follow-up. *Chest* **93:** 119–122.

85. Marcus, C.L., S. Curtis, C.B. Koerner, *et al.* 1996. Evaluation of pulmonary function and polysomnography in obese children and adolescents. *Pediatr. Pulmonol.* **21:** 176–183.

86. Kalra, M., T. Inge, V. Garcia, *et al.* 2005. Obstructive sleep apnea in extremely overweight adolescents undergoing bariatric surgery. *Obes. Res.* **13:** 1175–1179.

87. Marcus, C.L. & C.L. Marcus. 2002. Total energy expenditure in children with obstructive sleep apnoea syndrome [comment]. *Eur. Respir. J.* **19:** 1215–1216.

88. Grigg-Damberger, M., D. Gozal, C.L. Marcus, *et al.* 2007. The visual scoring of sleep and arousal in infants and children. *J. Clin. Sleep. Med.* **3:** 201–240.

89. Rosen, C.L., L. D'Andrea & G.G. Haddad. 1992. Adult criteria for obstructive sleep apnea do not identify children with serious obstruction. *Am. Rev. Respir. Dis.* **146**(5 Pt 1): 1231–1234.

90. Zaremba, E.K., M.E. Barkey, C. Mesa, *et al.* 2005. Making polysomnography more "child friendly:" a family-centered care approach. *J. Clin. Sleep. Med.* **1:** 189–198.

91. Mangat, D., W.C. Orr & R.O. Smith. 1977. Sleep apnea, hypersomnolence, and upper airway obstruction secondary to adenotonsillar enlargement. *Arch. Otolaryngol.* **103:** 383–386.

92. Section on Pediatric Pulmonology SoOSASAAoP. 2002. Clinical practice guideline: diagnosis and management of childhood obstructive sleep apnea syndrome [see comment]. *Pediatrics* **109:** 704–712.

93. Brietzke, S.E. & D. Gallagher. 2006. The effectiveness of tonsillectomy and adenoidectomy in the treatment of pediatric obstructive sleep apnea/hypopnea syndrome: a meta-analysis. *Otolaryngol. Head Neck Surg.* **134:** 979–984.

94. Tauman, R., T.E. Gulliver, J. Krishna, *et al.* 2006. Persistence of obstructive sleep apnea syndrome in children after adenotonsillectomy. *J. Pediatr.* **149:** 803–808.

95. Guilleminault, C., Y.S. Huang, C. Glamann, *et al.* 2007. Adenotonsillectomy and obstructive sleep apnea in children: a prospective survey. *Otolaryngol. Head Neck Surg.* **136:** 169–175.

96. Guilleminault, C., M. Partinen, J.P. Praud, *et al.* 1989. Morphometric facial changes and obstructive sleep apnea in adolescents. *J. Pediatr.* **114:** 997–999.

97. Amin, R., L. Anthony, V. Somers, *et al.* 2008. Growth velocity predicts recurrence of sleep-disordered breathing 1 year after adenotonsillectomy. *Am. J. Respir. Crit. Care Med.* **177:** 654–659.

98. O'Donnell, A.R., C.L. Bjornson, S.G. Bohn & V.G. Kirk. 2006. Compliance rates in children using noninvasive

continuous positive airway pressure. *Sleep* **29:** 651–658.

99. Massa, F., S. Gonsalez, A. Laverty, *et al.* 2002. The use of nasal continuous positive airway pressure to treat obstructive sleep apnoea. *Arch. Dis. Child.* **87:** 438–443.

100. Kheirandish-Gozal, L., D. Gozal, L. Kheirandish-Gozal & D. Gozal. 2008. Intranasal budesonide treatment for children with mild obstructive sleep apnea syndrome. *Pediatrics* **122:** e149–e155.

101. Mansfield, L.E., G. Diaz, C.R. Posey & J. Flores-Neder. 2004. Sleep disordered breathing and daytime quality of life in children with allergic rhinitis during treatment with intranasal budesonide. *Ann. Allergy Asthma Immunol.* **92:** 240–244.

102. Kotagal, S. 1996. Narcolepsy in children. *Semin. Pediatr. Neurol.* **3:** 36–43.

103. Smit, L.S., G.J. Lammers & C.E. Catsman-Berrevoets. 2006. Cataplexy leading to the diagnosis of Niemann-Pick disease type C. *Pediatr. Neurol.* **35:** 82–84.

104. Tobias, E.S., J.L. Tolmie & J.B. Stephenson. 2002. Cataplexy in the Prader-Willi syndrome. *Arch. Dis. Child.* **87:** 170.

105. Vendrame, M., N. Havaligi, C. Matadeen-Ali, *et al.* 2008. Narcolepsy in children: a single-center clinical experience. *Pediatr. Neurol.* **38:** 314–320.

106. Morgenthaler, T.I., V.K. Kapur, T. Brown, *et al.* 2007. Practice parameters for the treatment of narcolepsy and other hypersomnias of central origin. *Sleep* **30:** 1705–1711.

107. Wise, M.S., D.L. Arand, R.R. Auger, *et al.* 2007. Treatment of narcolepsy and other hypersomnias of central origin. *Sleep* **30:** 1712–1727.

108. Murali, H. & S. Kotagal. 2006. Off-label treatment of severe childhood narcolepsy-cataplexy with sodium oxybate. *Sleep* **29:** 1025–1029.

109. Arnulf, I., L. Lin, N. Gadoth, *et al.* 2008. Kleine-Levin syndrome: a systematic study of 108 patients. *Ann. Neurol.* **63:** 482–493.

110. Arnulf, I., M. Lecendreux, P. Franco & Y. Dauvilliers. 2008. [Kleine-Levin syndrome: state of the art]. *Rev. Neurol. (Paris)* **164:** 658–668.

111. Portilla, P., E. Durand, A. Chalvon, *et al.* 2002. [SPECT-identified hypoperfusion of the left temporomesial structures in a Kleine-Levin syndrome]. *Rev. Neurol. (Paris)* **158**(5 Pt 1): 593–595.

Ann. N.Y. Acad. Sci. ISSN 0077-8923

ANNALS OF THE NEW YORK ACADEMY OF SCIENCES

REM sleep behavior disorder

Updated review of the core features, the REM sleep behavior disorder-neurodegenerative disease association, evolving concepts, controversies, and future directions

Bradley F. Boeve

Department of Neurology and Center for Sleep Medicine, Mayo Clinic, Rochester, Minnesota, USA

Address for correspondence: Bradley F. Boeve, M.D., Mayo Clinic, 200 First Street SW, Rochester, Minnesota 55905. Voice: 507-538-1038; fax: 507-538-6012. bboeve@mayo.edu

Rapid eye movement (REM) sleep behavior disorder (RBD) is a parasomnia manifested by vivid, often frightening dreams associated with simple or complex motor behavior during REM sleep. The polysomnographic features of RBD include increased electromyographic tone +/− dream enactment behavior during REM sleep. Management with counseling and pharmacologic measures is usually straightforward and effective. In this review, the terminology, clinical and polysomnographic features, demographic and epidemiologic features, diagnostic criteria, differential diagnosis, and management strategies are discussed. Recent data on the suspected pathophysiologic mechanisms of RBD are also reviewed. The literature and our institutional experience on RBD are next discussed, with an emphasis on the RBD–neurodegenerative disease association and particularly the RBD-synucleinopathy association. Several issues relating to evolving concepts, controversies, and future directions are then reviewed, with an emphasis on idiopathic RBD representing an early feature of a neurodegenerative disease and particularly an evolving synucleinopathy. Planning for future therapies that impact patients with idiopathic RBD is reviewed in detail.

Keywords: REM sleep behavior disorder; parasomnia; synucleinopathy; neurodegenerative disease

Overview

Rapid eye movement sleep behavior disorder (RBD) is characterized by loss of normal skeletal muscle atonia during rapid eye movement (REM) sleep with prominent motor activity and dreaming. In this article, the clinical, epidemiologic, and polysomnographic (PSG) features of RBD will be reviewed, followed by discussions of the criteria for diagnosis of RBD and the management of this disorder. Recent data on the pathophysiologic underpinnings of RBD are next discussed. RBD associated with neurodegenerative disorders will then be discussed, with a particular emphasis on the RBD-synucleinopathy association. The concept of "idiopathic" RBD (iRBD) and the multitude of findings on ancillary studies in those labeled with iRBD will next be reviewed. Discussions on the evolving concepts and controversies will then follow. Finally, several issues pertaining to planning for fu-

ture therapeutic trials in those with iRBD due to an underlying and evolving neurodegenerative disorder will be presented. Readers are directed to some key recent reviews on the fascinating parasomnia of RBD.[1-3]

The core aspects of rapid eye movement sleep behavior disorder

Terminology

Some of the terms relating to REM sleep and RBD are confusing, and many reviews of RBD have not tended to elaborate on the ever-important issue of terminology.

Stage R—the new nomenclature proposed by the American Academy of Sleep Medicine has changed the term *Stage REM* to *Stage R*.[4] For historical and other reasons, the term *REM sleep* will be used throughout most of this article.

Dream enactment behavior (DEB)—this is a term that many investigators use to describe a history of recurrent nocturnal dream enactment behavior (abbreviated DEB). While almost all patients with RBD have a history of DEB (the few that do not are diagnosed purely on PSG; see below), not all patients with a history of DEB have RBD; similar behavior can also occur in untreated obstructive sleep apnea,[5] as well as in sleepwalking and sleep terrors in adults, epilepsy, post-traumatic stress disorder, or as an effect of alcohol or drug administration or withdrawal.[1,6] Thus, most experts consider that PSG confirmation of RBD is essential to make the diagnosis, since DEB is not specific for RBD.

REM sleep without atonia (RSWA)—this is the PSG-defined finding of increased electromyographic (EMG) tone during REM sleep (Stage R). Normally during REM sleep, there is active inhibition of EMG activity leading to complete or near complete atonia on the EMG derivations, but REM sleep without atonia (often abbreviated RSWA) represents the abnormal state of increased EMG tone. A major issue in PSG methodology currently is to establish what degree of EMG activity is considered within normal limits and what exceeds this and should be considered abnormal. This issue will be discussed further in the sections that follow.

REM sleep behavior disorder (RBD)—REM sleep behavior disorder (abbreviated RBD) is a distinct parasomnia characterized by both abnormal REM sleep electrophysiology—RSWA—and abnormal REM sleep behavior—a history of recurrent nocturnal DEB. Most experts consider that the diagnosis of RBD cannot be applied unless both DEB and RSWA are present, and hence a polysomnogram is required to make the diagnosis. The shortened term *REM behavior disorder* is incomplete—it is the abnormal behaviors during REM sleep that the disorder of RBD represents (rapid eye movements or REMs occur during wakefulness are not relevant to the subject of RBD).

Subclinical RBD—some authors have equated the PSG finding of RSWA with subclinical RBD,[7,8] implying that such patients with increased EMG tone during REM sleep (Stage R) will subsequently develop clinical RBD. While we have certainly evaluated patients with RSWA who develop not only clinical RBD, but also a neurodegenerative disorder, this author would argue that there has not been a sufficient number of prospectively followed subjects

with RSWA who subsequently develop clinical RBD to justify use of the term *subclinical RBD*. Hence, the PSG finding of RSWA should be applied, and longitudinal data will justify or refute equating RSWA with subclinical RBD.

Clinically probable RBD or *probable RBD (pRBD)*—this term is synonymous with recurrent nocturnal DEB and is being used more frequently at present in epidemiologic studies when PSG confirmation of RBD is not feasible in all cases and by investigators who are not able to perform sleep studies due to lack of availability of sleep centers and/or lack of reimbursement for PSGs.

Idiopathic RBD (iRBD)—this term refers to RBD occurring in the absence of any other obvious associated neurologic disorder. There is a large amount of recent data suggesting that many patients with iRBD actually represent an evolving neurodegenerative disorder (discussed in detail later in this review), which has fostered many authors to qualify the term idiopathic RBD with surrounding quotation markers ("idiopathic" RBD).

Secondary or *symptomatic RBD*—these terms refer to the combination of RBD plus another neurologic disorder, such as narcolepsy or a neurodegenerative disease.

Considering some of these issues relating to terminology, one could propose some minor changes to some key terms as is shown in Table 1. These are merely suggestions based on this author's experience and opinions.

Illustrative case

There are many illustrative examples in the literature. One patient evaluated at our institution fell asleep as a passenger on a transatlantic commercial flight and then exhibited punching and kicking behavior (months later the patient still recalled the dream of fighting animals in a cave). The behavior was interpreted as a seizure, and the pilot urgently redirected the airliner back to the United States mainland for emergency medical care, resulting in tens of thousands of dollars being spent on the emergency landing, thousands more during the inpatient work-up of a suspected seizure, and requiring hundreds of passengers to change their travel plans. The initial inpatient evaluation was unrevealing, but the patient was prescribed phenytoin, which he continued to use up to his initial evaluation at

Table 1. Proposed minor changes to the definitions and diagnostic criteria for REM sleep without atonia and REM sleep behavior disorder

---

REM sleep without atonia (RSWA)

Abnormal EMG tone during REM sleep

- the electrophysiologic finding of excessive amounts of sustained or intermittent elevation of submental EMG tone and/or excessive transient muscle activity on the submental or limb derivations

Probable RBD

Abnormal behaviors during REM sleep

- a history of recurrent abnormal and disruptive sleep behavior with injuries or the potential for injury
- the behaviors are usually (but not necessarily) associated with dream mentation
- the behaviors are usually (but not necessarily) associated with dreams involving a chasing or attacking theme

Definite RBD

Abnormal sleep behavior and abnormal EMG tone during REM sleep. Items A + B + C must be present for the diagnosis of definite RBD

A. Presence of RSWA
- the electrophysiologic finding of excessive amounts of sustained or intermittent elevation of submental EMG tone and/or excessive transient muscle activity on the submental or limb derivations (the specifics of which require further study)

B. Presence of abnormal REM sleep behavior by history and/or on PSG
- a history of recurrent abnormal and disruptive sleep behavior with injuries or the potential for injury (fulfills criteria for probable RBD) and/or
- documentation of abnormal REM sleep behaviors during polysomnographic monitoring (i.e., prominent limb or truncal jerking; complex, vigorous, or violent behaviors)

C. Absence of EEG epileptiform activity during REM sleep
- unless RBD can be clearly distinguished from any concurrent REM sleep-related seizure disorder

---

our institution several weeks after the plane incident. Periodic nocturnal dream enactment behavior had continued. The description of the prior spell and many other episodes of nocturnal dream enactment behavior over the preceding years, as described by the patient himself (he was a widower), were classic for RBD, and the diagnosis was confirmed on polysomnography. Phenytoin was discontinued, and low-dose clonazepam proved to provide complete control of his nightmares and behaviors. Upon reevaluation 2 years later for a newly developed rest tremor in one limb, shuffling gait, slowness of movement, and other symptoms, he had developed the cardinal features of Parkinson's disease.

Clinical features

The demographic and clinical phenomenologies of RBD are summarized in Table 2; examples of specific features and examples of behaviors can be found in numerous references.[1–3,9–27] One can characterize the three primary aspects of RBD as abnormal vocalizations, abnormal motor behavior, and altered dream mentation.

Abnormal vocalizations

While individuals may grunt, speak, laugh, or vocalize in a variety of ways during non-REM (NREM) and REM sleep, and such vocalizations are not necessarily "abnormal," the vocalizations in RBD tend to be loud and suggest unpleasant dream mentation. Shouting, screaming, and swearing are common and are often described as being very unlike the typical soft-spoken nature of the person's tendency to speak during wakefulness.

Abnormal motor behavior

Infrequent limb jerks are also common during sleep in individuals without RBD, but in those with RBD, the motor activity often begins with some repetitive jerking or movements, followed seconds later by more dramatic and seemingly purposeful activity such as punching, flailing as if to protect oneself, running, jumping out of bed, and so forth. It is during these behaviors that injuries to patients and their bed partners can occur. Some bed partners have attempted to awaken patients during an episode, and their comments and gestures become interwoven into the dream, sometimes resulting in injury. One spouse would keep a broom under her side of the bed and use it as her "wake-up poker" to abort her

Table 2. Demographics and clinical phenomenology of REM sleep behavior disorder

Demographics
  Male gender predilection
  Age of onset typically 40–70 years (range 15–80
    years)
Clinical Phenomenology
  Abnormal vocalizations—orating, yelling, swearing,
    screaming
  Abnormal motor behavior—limb flailing, punching,
    kicking, lurching out of bed
  Altered dream mentation—typically involve a
    chasing/attacking theme, with the insects, animals,
    or other humans being the aggressors and the
    patient being the defender
  Exhibited behaviors mirror dream content
Behaviors tend to occur in the latter half of the sleep
  period.

husband's RBD episode while she stood 4 feet away, yet on occasion it would be grabbed by her husband and used as a sword to fend off his attackers. Bruises, pulled hair, limb fractures, and subdural hematomas have all been reported.

Altered dream mentation

Most patients view their dreams as nightmares, and the dream content often involves insects, animals, or people chasing or attacking them or their relatives or friends; the patient is almost always the defender and not the attacker. Many patients are able to recount the content of their dreams upon being awakened at the time of the behavior. Unlike most pleasant dreams and nightmares, after which most individuals typically recall the details of dreams vividly upon awakening but seemingly forget almost all details by noon the following day, those with RBD can often recall vivid details of the nightmares for days, and sometimes for weeks or years. Those with significant dementia may not be able to recall and/or describe their dreams; in such cases, bed partner observations of the abnormal behaviors are helpful.

The vocalizations and behaviors that are exhibited are strikingly consistent with the content of the dreams later reported by the patient—the behaviors mirror the dream content. Bed partners are often very accurate at predicting what the patient had just dreamed about based on their observations of the dream enactment behavior. One vivid example involved a man who held his wife's head in a headlock while moving his legs as if running while both were attempting to sleep in bed, then exclaimed, "I'm gonna make that touchdown!" and then attempted to forcefully throw her head down toward the foot of the bed. When awakened, he recalled a dream in which he was running for a touchdown and he spiked the "football" in the end zone. His wife knew precisely what he had been dreaming about.[17]

The timing of RBD episodes reflects when the patient is in REM sleep, and since the majority of REM sleep occurs during the latter half of the sleep period (particularly latter third of the sleep period, which for most individuals is after 3 am), RBD tends to be exhibited in the few hours prior to wake onset. There are exceptions to this, however, primarily in those who have narcolepsy (and thus enter REM sleep frequently within an hour of sleep onset) or who have an increased REM sleep drive due to sleep deprivation or untreated obstructive sleep apnea.

We have heard numerous descriptions from wives who experienced their first instance of being struck on their wedding night, thereby indicating that RBD can present in one's late teens or twenties. Many of these patients did not begin exhibiting features of a neurodegenerative disorder until 3–6 decades later. The frequency of DEB also varies widely—without treatment, some exhibit DEB every night, sometimes several times each night (presumably during most or all episodes of REM sleep), while others exhibit it no more than one night per month. Still others appear to exhibit clustering, with RBD occurring nightly for a week and then going months with little or no RBD, and then RBD occurring frequently some time later. Such patients are rarely able to identify an obvious trigger for the flurry of RBD. It is not known why the frequency varies so widely in patients with RBD.

Demographic and epidemiologic features

Most patients with RBD are male. Onset of symptoms varies widely, although most develop symptoms in the 40–70 age range. Those with RBD evolving before age 40 typically have narcolepsy (RBD and narcolepsy often coexist), although in some cases RBD that begins early in life can evolve into a neurodegenerative disorder decades later.[28,29] In one series, the percentage of males who have RBD associated with presumed Lewy body pathology

Table 3. Clinical features/diagnoses in residents of Olmsted County, Minnesota, who are participants in an aging and dementia research program and had PSG-proven RBD on January 1, 2008*

Primary clinical diagnoses	N
Normal neurologic functioning (idiopathic RBD)	8
Mild cognitive impairment (MCI)	2
MCI plus mild parkinsonian signs	2
Parkinson's disease with MCI	1
Dementia with Lewy bodies (DLB)	7
TOTAL	20

Population of Olmsted County, Minnesota on 1/1/08—approximately 100,000
20/100,000 = 0.02% = absolute minimum point prevalence of PSG-proven RBD
*3 additional participants (2 with Parkinson's disease and 1 with DLB) have classic features of RBD but no REM sleep was attained on PSG; thus RBD is suspected (i.e., probable RBD) but was not confirmed on PSG

[Parkinson's disease (209/255 = 82%) plus dementia with Lewy bodies (184/224 = 82%) equals 393/479 = 82%] is greater than the percentage of males who have RBD associated with multiple system atrophy (48/75 = 64%) [$P = 0.0003$], suggesting factors related to sex may impact the RBD–neurodegenerative disease association.[30] This is a topic clearly worthy of further study if indeed there are sex differences in the specific type of neurodegenerative disease associated with RBD. Other published data on the frequency of RBD associated with neurodegenerative disease are largely based on convenience samples and cannot be considered truly representative of the frequency of RBD associated with other neurodegenerative disorders.

The only published epidemiologic data on parasomnias in the population with relevance to RBD were based on telephone interviews in the United Kingdom. Ohayon and colleagues conducted interviews using the Sleep-EVAL system in 4,972 individuals aged 15–100 years and found 106 (2%) reported violent behaviors during sleep, most of whom were male.[31] Twenty-five of these participants (0.5% of the sample) reported features highly suggestive of RBD. This single study has thus formed the basis for the estimated prevalence of RBD to be 0.5%.

An investigation of all patients residing in Olmsted County, Minnesota, who carried the diagnosis of PSG-confirmed RBD on April 1, 2008, found a prevalence of 0.02% (Table 3) (Boeve *et al.*, unpublished data). This is by no means a sound epidemiologic study of the prevalence of RBD in a population, but the frequency of 20/100,000 could at least be considered a minimum estimate of the frequency of cases of RBD that have come to medical attention, undergone a PSG, and had the diagnosis confirmed in one county. This is also clearly a gross underestimate when one considers that the sample from which these subjects were derived includes only participants in an aging and dementia research program, and while many residents of Olmsted County with PD also have probable RBD, they either do not have RBD confirmed by PSG or do have PSG-confirmed RBD but are not participating in this particular research program.

Another study using the Mayo Sleep Questionnaire (MSQ) (discussed in more detail below) as a screening measure for probable RBD concluded that 79 (8.9%) of the 892 participants in the Mayo Clinic Study of Aging (MCSA) screened positive for RBD.[32] The MCSA is a population-based study assessing cognition, functional status, laboratory markers, neuroimaging markers, among other factors, in 70–89-year-old community-dwelling residents of Olmsted County, Minnesota. While the RBD questions on the MSQ are not 100% specific for RBD (specificity is around 70% based on one validation study),[33] our prior findings of increased frequency of parkinsonism,[34] apathy and anxiety,[35] and lower scores on measures of attention/executive functioning[36] associated with positive screening for RBD on the MSQ in the MCSA, do suggest a large proportion of those who screen positive likely do have RBD.

Considering the growing data that "idiopathic" RBD may actually represent an evolving neurodegenerative disorder in a sizable proportion (to be discussed in more detail below), a well-designed epidemiologic study of the prevalence of RBD is clearly warranted.

Diagnostic criteria

The second edition of the *International Classification of Sleep Disorders* requires the following for the clinical diagnosis of RBD:[37]

A. Presence of RSWA on PSG
B. At least one of the following:
   1. sleep-related, injurious, potentially injurious, or disruptive behaviors by history (i.e., dream enactment behavior)

2. abnormal REM sleep behavior documented during polysomnographic monitoring

C. Absence of EEG epileptiform activity during REM sleep unless RBD can be clearly distinguished from any concurrent REM sleep related seizure disorder

D. The sleep disorder is not better explained by another sleep disorder, medical or neurological disorder, mental disorder, medication use, or substance use disorder.

The American Academy of Sleep Medicine has critically evaluated the scoring methods of PSGs, and the formal diagnosis of RBD has changed slightly[4] and will likely change further as refinement occurs—this is discussed in more detail in the Polysomnographic Features section below.

Differential diagnosis

The differential diagnosis of recurrent DEB includes the NREM parasomnias (somnambulism, night terrors, confusional arousals), nocturnal panic attacks, nocturnal seizures, nightmares, nocturnal wandering associated with dementia, and obstructive sleep apnea (OSA). The history usually allows differentiation of these disorders from RBD. When diagnostic clarification is necessary, particularly when the risk for injury is high, the behaviors occur at any time of the night, other features suggesting an evolving neurodegenerative are present, or loud snoring and observed apnea suggestive of OSA are present, PSG with simultaneous video monitoring is warranted.

Polysomnographic features

Those unfamiliar with the updated sleep-stage characterization and scoring of PSGs should review the references that were authored by key authorities in the field of sleep medicine.[38,39] The new American Academy of Sleep Medicine Manual for the Scoring of Sleep and Related Events[4] has maintained many of the criteria and definitions for REM sleep (Stage R), primarily low-amplitude mixed-frequency EEG background, REMs, and low chin EMG tone. RSWA can be applied when there is (1) sustained muscle activity in REM sleep with 50% of the epoch having increased chin EMG amplitude, and/or (2) excessive transient muscle activity, defined by the presence of five or more miniepochs (a 30 second epoch is divided into 10 3-second mini-epochs) in

an epoch having transient muscle activity lasting at least 0.5 seconds. There was no minimum number of epochs showing abnormal muscle activity required for the RSWA designation—this was purposely not stated as there are few good normative data.[4]

One can appreciate normal REM sleep/Stage R as characterized by REMs, minimal to no EMG tone, and mixed alpha and theta activity on electroencephalography (EEG) as shown in Figure 1A. The characteristic electrophysiologic finding in patients with RBD is RSWA. This usually takes the form of a pathologic accentuation of transient muscle activity as shown in Figure 1B. Simultaneous video/PSG recording is essential for evaluating patients with suspected RBD, so that vocalizations and limb movements can be captured and viewed concurrently with PSG data. When vocalizations and/or limb movements emerge during REM sleep, without associated epileptiform activity on the EEG derivations (as in Fig. 1B), the diagnosis of RBD is established. In our experience, violent and complex dream enactment behavior is relatively uncommon during single-night PSG recordings; rather, increased EMG tone during REM sleep and sparse limb jerks are the norm.

Due to scheduling challenges and logistical issues, in which PSGs for evaluation of suspected RBD cannot be arranged in a timely manner at sleep disorder centers with procedures in place for assessing parasomnias, the sleep clinicians knowledgeable in the parasomnias attempt to work with local sleep clinicians to encourage them to perform PSGs with extrasurface EMG leads on the limbs and to have all video/PSG data time-locked or even more simply unsynchronized to simultaneous video/PSG recording. The local sleep clinician is also requested to scrutinize the degree to which EMG tone is increased during REM sleep, whereas there should be essentially complete atonia. Frustratingly, this is very rarely accomplished, and thus the question of whether individual patients have REM sleep without atonia or overt RBD captured on PSG remains unanswered. This lack of consistency has many root causes, not the least of which being inadequate training of sleep fellows in the assessment and management of parasomnias, as well as the variable views of how to operationalize the assessment of what truly constitutes REM sleep without atonia versus normal EMG atonia during REM sleep. This issue

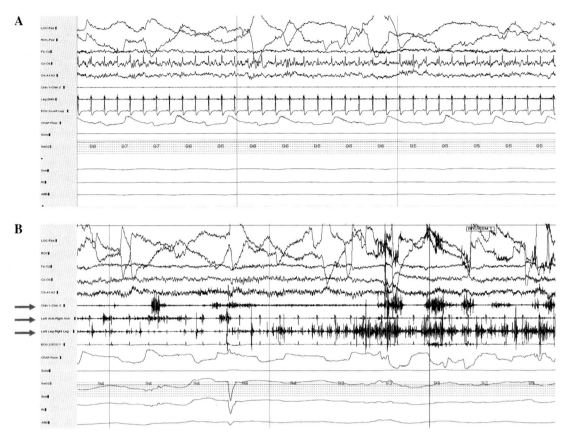

Figure 1. Thirty-second epoch polysomnograms showing normal REM sleep (A) and REM sleep without atonia—the electrophysiologic substrate for RBD (B). In A, note the absence of electromyographic (EMG) activity in the submental (Chin 1-Chin 2), and limb (Leg EMG) derivations, whereas increased EMG tone is present in the submental (Chin 1-Chin 3), upper limb (Left Arm-Right Arm), and lower limb (Left Leg-Right Leg) derivations in B (denoted by red arrows).

Management

The goals of therapy are to minimize the three cardinal features of the disorder—decrease the frequency and severity of the abnormal vocalizations (thereby reducing the embarrassing nature of screams and swearing with guests in the home, when traveling and sleeping in hotels, and when fishing/hunting/camping and sleeping in tents), decrease the frequency and severity of the abnormal behaviors (thereby reducing the risk of injury to the patient and bed partner), and decrease the unpleasant dreams (thereby reducing the anticipatory concerns about nightmares which sometimes re-

will be discussed further in the section on Evolving Concepts, Controversies, and Future Directions.

sults in overt "sleep phobia"). All patients and their bed partners should be counseled on simple steps to minimize injury, such as moving sharp and edged objects out of harm's way and placing a mattress or cushion of some type on the floor adjacent to the bed (many patients use foam rubber mattresses). Protective barriers placed on the side of the bed, such as those designed for infants to decrease the risk from falling off the bed, are variably effective.

Since most patients with RBD are male, it may be "male pride" that keeps them from using barriers designed for infants, and other techniques have been used. Some have constructed plywood barriers placed alongside the bed and on the bed in between the patient and spouse, with padding affixed to the sides of the plywood facing the patient. Others use a small mattress and place it on its side adjacent to the bed, with chairs leaning against the mattress to keep it in place. Some sleep in a sleeping bag in the bed in a cocoon-like fashion, with the open end of the sleeping bag toward the head tied as snuggly as possible. Some go to bed with oven mitts on their hands, with shoestrings tied around the wrists to keep the mitts in place. One man has used a rope with one end tied around him and the other end tied around the bedpost to alter his tendency to lurch and run out of bed. These and other colorful examples of safety ingenuity are described in other informative and entertaining sources[1]—Carlos Schenck's text on parasomnias is a must read for anyone interested in the RBD field.[2]

Clonazepam has been the drug of choice in those without significant cognitive impairment or OSA, and it is usually effective at 0.25–0.5 mg/night, though doses above 1 mg nightly are necessary in some patients.[12,22] Recent experience with melatonin shows that doses ranging from 3–12 mg/night can be effective, either as sole therapy or in conjunction with clonazepam when either melatonin or clonazepam alone is ineffective.[40,41] As noted in an excellent recent review on the subject of treatment,[42] other drugs reported to improve RBD include pramipexole,[43] donepezil,[44] levodopa,[45] carbamazepine,[46] triazolam,[22] and clozapine.[22] We have also found quetiapine to be quite effective for managing RBD in many patients.

For unmarried couples who are dating, intimacy invitations to women by males with RBD are made only after considerable planning. Many married couples choose to sleep in separate bedrooms, with the resulting loss of intimacy. All of these accounts described above may sound somewhat comical to those unfamiliar with the disorder of RBD, but for those with frequent and severe episodes, preparing for sleep requires completing a nightly routine with potentially disastrous consequences when the drug and nondrug aspects of management are not followed.

As noted above, most patients experience a marked improvement in the frequency and severity of RBD features with medical therapy. Yet there are rare individuals whose RBD continues despite using clonazepam in excess of 3 mg/night plus melatonin in excess of 12 mg/night. The addition of quetiapine, levodopa, or a dopamine agonist sometimes provides benefit, other times not. We are aware of one patient whose RBD continued with nightly nightmares, screaming, and occasional injuries to himself despite clonazepam 4 mg/night, melatonin 12 mg/night, and quetiapine 100 mg/night, but with the addition of sodium oxybate at 3 g at bedtime and 3 g taken 3 hours later, his RBD was essentially completely controlled. He was later able to control RBD entirely with sodium oxybate monotherapy, yet if he forgot to take a dose, RBD would invariably occur. This author views sodium oxybate as a last resort, but for the very rare individuals with otherwise medically refractory RBD, the benefit of markedly reduced risk of injury could be considered to outweigh the risks.

It is not clear why clonazepam, melatonin, and other agents improve RBD. Clonazepam reduces phasic activity in REM sleep, and while this agent clearly improves the three cardinal features in most patients, RSWA is still evident in those who undergo PSG while taking the drug. Melatonin has been shown to decrease the percentage of REM sleep epochs without muscle atonia and decrease the number of stage shifts in REM sleep, suggesting it has a more direct mode of action on REM sleep pathophysiology. One hypothesis is that it restores circadian modulation of REM sleep.[40] Most sleep experts are frankly puzzled why melatonin has any effect on RBD.

Some recent data suggest that some agents, particularly within the selective serotonin reuptake inhibitor (SSRI) and selective norepinephrine reuptake inhibitor (SNRI) classes, can precipitate or aggravate RBD in some individuals.[47,48] One interpretation is that these drugs sufficiently alter REM sleep physiology to seemingly induce RBD. Another interpretation is that in such patients, REM sleep control has already become dysregulated—perhaps due to an early evolving neurodegenerative disorder—and the SSRI or SNRI unmasks RBD which would have manifested months or years later (see section on Evolving Concepts and Controversies). In patients with both RBD and depression, which also often coexist, it may be best to favor an agent such as bupropion over the SSRI and SNRI agents due to its different pharmacologic properties.[1]

Pathophysiology

A comprehensive review of the known pathophysiology of RBD in animal models and the hypothesized pathophysiology in humans can be found

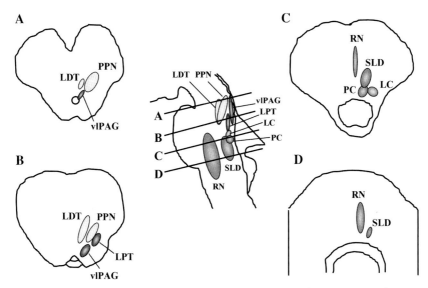

Figure 2. Proposed nuclei involved in REM sleep control as shown on human brain-stem templates. Letters represent cross-sectional views through the brain stem, with (A) corresponding to the pontomesencephalic junction, (B) to the upper/mid pons, (C) to lower/mid pons, and (D) just rostral to the pontomedullary junction. The REM-off region is represented by the vlPAG and LPT in red, and the REM-on region is represented by the PC and SLD in green. eVLPO, extended part of the ventrolateral preoptic nucleus; LC, locus coeruleus; LDTN, laterodorsal tegmental nucleus; LPT, lateral pontine tegmentum; PC, precoeruleus; PPN, pedunculopontine nucleus; REM, rapid eye movement; RN, raphe nucleus; SLD, sublaterodorsal nucleus; vlPAG, ventrolateral part of the periaqueductal gray matter. See text for details. From Ref. 3. Reprinted with permission from Oxford University Press.

elsewhere;[3] in this review, concepts and data pertaining to human RBD will be emphasized.

The proposed anatomic substrate for REM sleep control in humans is shown in Figure 2, and the proposed pathophysiology of human RBD is shown in Figure 3. The critical structures in the brain stem include the "REM-off" region consisting of the ventrolateral part of the periaqueductal gray matter (vlPAG) and lateral pontine tegmentum (LPT), the "REM-on" region consisting of the precoeruleus (PC) and sublaterodorsal nucleus (SLD), as well as the extended part of the ventrolateral preoptic nucleus (eVLPO), locus coeruleus (LC), laterodorsal tegmental nucleus (LDTN), pedunculopontine nucleus (PPN), and raphe nucleus (RN).

Studies in the cat and rat models suggested that there are two motor systems involved in normal REM sleep: one for generating muscle atonia and one for suppressing locomotor activity.[49–57] The absence of motor activity in normal REM sleep occurs via active inhibition of spinal motoneurons plus reduced drive within locomotor generators. While phasic oculomotor and locomotor activity such as rapid eye movements and brief and low-amplitude muscle twitches occur as normal phenomena in REM sleep, more elaborate motoric activity is directly or indirectly suppressed.[18,58] The final common pathway of spinal motor neuron inhibition was inferred to be via the medullary magnocellular reticular formation (MCRF); this inhibitory nucleus is known to suppress anterior horn cell activity via projections of the ventrolateral reticulospinal tract (VLST). The pontine nuclei described above are known to influence the REM and NREM sleep circuits. In addition, midbrain and forebrain structures have been tied into these circuits: substantia nigra, hypothalamus, thalamus, basal forebrain, and frontal cortex.

The brain-stem regions that have classically been considered in RBD pathophysiology based on lesion studies in cat include the MCRF, locus coeruleus/subcoeruleus complex, PPN, LDTN, and possibly substantia nigra (SN).[49–57] Although these studies have identified components of REM sleep

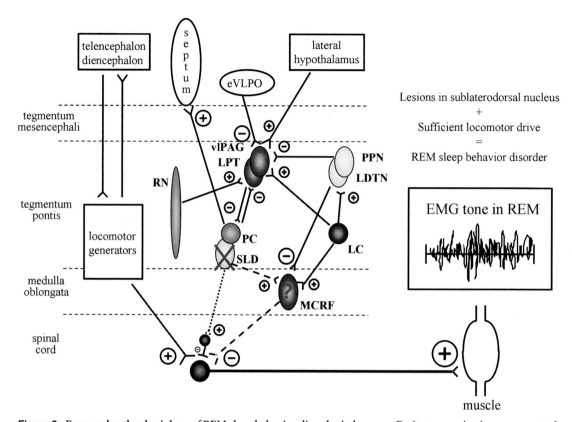

Figure 3. Proposed pathophysiology of REM sleep behavior disorder in humans. Excitatory projections represented by (+), inhibitory projections represented by (−), with the size of these symbols representing the relative effect of each projection on the synapsing nuclei. Nuclei are represented by circles or ovals, with solid colored circles and ovals reflecting those with normal populations of neurons, and speckled circles and ovals reflecting those with significantly reduced populations of neurons. An X reflects ablation of a nucleus. The relative tonic influences of each projection are represented by line thickness, with thicker lines depicting stronger influences, thinner lines depicting weaker influences, and dashed and dotted lines depicting weak influences due to damage to neurons in the respective nuclei. The REM-off region is represented by the vlPAG and LPT in red, and the REM-on region is represented by the PC and SLD in green. The SLD (or analogous nucleus in humans) projects to spinal interneurons ("direct route," denoted by the dotted line from SLD to spinal interneurons) and likely represents the final common pathway that causes active inhibition of skeletal muscle activity in REM sleep. The "indirect route," denoted by the dashed line from SLD to the MCRF to the spinal interneurons, may also contribute to EMG atonia. However, in humans, it is not yet known whether lesions in structures that project to and from the MCRF, and lesioning the MCRF itself, are critical in affecting EMG atonia during REM sleep. EMG, electromyographic; eVLPO, extended part of the ventrolateral preoptic nucleus; LC, locus coeruleus; LDTN, laterodorsal tegmental nucleus; LPT, lateral pontine tegmentum; MCRF, magnocellular reticular formation; PC, pre-coeruleus; PPN, pedunculopontine nucleus; REM, rapid eye movement; RN, raphe nucleus; SLD, sublaterodorsal nucleus; vlPAG, ventrolateral part of the periaqueductal gray matter. See text for details. From Ref. 3. Reprinted with permission from Oxford University Press.

circuits, the primary sites and interactions have been debated. Lesions in the MCRF release the tonic inhibition on spinal motoneurons, leading to RSWA, but these lesions also destroy fibers of passage. Lesions in the coeruleus/subcoeruleus complex cause RSWA, and the site and size of the lesion determines whether simple or complex behaviors are exhibited.[49] There is also debate whether lesions in the PPN cause RSWA.[45,55,56] The substantia nigra and the dopaminergic system have been proposed as components of this REM sleep system, but there is minimal direct evidence to implicate the substantia nigra or dopaminergic dysfunction in RBD pathophysiology. Similarly, no convincing examples of RSWA or RBD have resulted from lesions in the diencephalon or telencephalon. Most evidence now suggests that populations of neurons that are considered "REM-on" cells in the subcoeruleus region are central to REM sleep and the associated EMG atonia.[59,60]

The sublaterodorsal nucleus (SLD) identified by Boissard and coworkers, which is equivalent to the subcoeruleus or peri-locus coeruleus in the cat, is the major structure responsible for REM sleep.[61,62] More recent work has led to the concept of a putative on/off switch for control of REM sleep.[60]

We have hypothesized that the structures and networks in humans are similar to the animal models,[3] with the SLD or analogous nucleus with projections to spinal interneurons ("direct route," denoted by the dotted line from SLD to spinal interneurons in Fig. 3) being the final common pathway that causes active inhibition of skeletal muscle activity in REM sleep. The "indirect route" (denoted by the dashed line from SLD to spinal interneurons in Fig. 3) can also contribute, with SLD lesioning causing reduced excitation of the MCRF, thereby causing a net reduced inhibition of spinal motoneurons (either directly or via spinal interneurons). It is not clear yet if lesioning or degeneration of the MCRF is sufficient to cause RBD in humans.

The locomotor generators, which are presumed to project to the spinal motoneurons either directly or indirectly via other brain-stem nuclei, have yet to be identified and characterized. The neuronal circuitry for this process is poorly understood, and supratentorial influences on both the locomotor generators and the muscle atonia system are likely. One could predict that a variety of stimuli could alter locomotor drive and/or muscle atonia, such as other primary sleep disorders (e.g., obstructive sleep apnea), structural lesions in the brain stem, neurodegeneration, medications, illicit drugs, and head trauma.

This schema will require careful scrutiny based on meticulous histopathologic studies—this issue is discussed further in the concluding section.

The RBD–neurodegenerative disease association

Analyses in patients with RBD plus parkinsonism and/or dementia

The major clinical syndromes and histopathologic disorders that cause dementia and/or parkinsonism are shown in Figure 4. As shown in this figure, numerous cases of RBD have been reported in association with certain neurodegenerative disorders but not reported to date in association with most others. RBD is frequently associated with clinically diagnosed Parkinson's disease,[3,9,20–23,25,26,40,43,47,63–80] dementia with Lewy bodies,[3,17,26,27,41,80–87] and multiple system atrophy.[9,10,20,22,25,26,88–98] Pure autonomic failure has also been reported.[20,99] RBD was identified in several members of a kindred with a parkin mutation,[100] and Lewy body disease pathology has been reported in a different large kindred with parkin mutations.[101] Many of the cases described in the reports noted above have had postmortem examination, and all such cases have had Lewy body disease or MSA confirmed at autopsy.

RBD has also been associated with other neurodegenerative disorders, albeit far less frequently. Spinocerebellar atrophy–type 3 (SCA-3) has been reported associated with dream enactment behavior (although few have had PSG confirmation).[102–104] Three (12%) of the 25 patients with Huntington's disease studied by Arnulf and colleagues had evidence of RBD.[105] RSWA has been reported in a single case of sporadic corticobasal degeneration (CBD),[7] but this patient did not have clinical RBD features. RBD has been reported in two cases of clinically suspected sporadic progressive supranuclear palsy (PSP)[20,22] and in 2/15 (13%) of a group of PSP subjects.[106] We recently reported on a case who had the DLB phenotype including RBD, but had PSP pathology.[3] One case of RBD with amyotrophic lateral sclerosis has also been identified.[20] Guadeloupean parkinsonism (a tauopathy) has also been associated with RBD (7/9 patients studied), with three of these exhibiting RBD features many years prior to the onset of parkinsonism.[107]

One case of clinically diagnosed Alzheimer's disease (AD) was associated with RBD,[108] and neuropathologic analysis identified both AD and Lewy body disease.[109] We (Boeve et al., unpublished data) and others[80,110,111] have observed sparse cases of

Synucleinopathy
Lewy body disease (LBD)
   Incidental LBD
   Parkinson's disease (PD)
   PD with dementia (PDD)
   Dementia with Lewy bodies (DLB)
   Pure autonomic failure (PAF)
Multiple system atrophy (MSA)

Trinucleotide Repeat Disorders
Spinocerebellar Atrophy-3 (SCA-3)
Huntington's Disease (HD)

Prionopathy
Creutzfeldt-Jakob disease (CJD)
Fatal familial insomnia (FFI)
Gerstmann-Straussler-Scheinker (GSS)

Amyloidopathy
Alzheimer's disease (AD)

Tauopathy
Pick's disease
Corticobasal degeneration (CBD)
Progressive supranuclear palsy (PSP)
Argyrophilic grain disease (AGD)
Frontotemporal dementia with
   parkinsonism linked to chromosome
   17 (FTDP-17*MAPT*)
Guadeloupean parkinsonism

TDP-43opathy
Frontotemporal lobar degeneration (FTLD) with
   TDP-43-positive inclusions
FTLD with motor neuron disease (FTLD-MND)
Hippocampal sclerosis (HS)
Amyotrophic lateral sclerosis (ALS)
Frontotemporal dementia with parkinsonism
   linked to chromosome 17 (FTDP-17*PGRN*)

Figure 4. The clinical syndromes and histopathologic disorders associated with each proteinopathy in the major neurodegenerative disorders that cause dementia and/or parkinsonism. Those syndromes and disorders that are commonly associated with REM sleep behavior disorder (RBD) are shown in red, and those that have been rarely associated with RBD are shown in blue. Those syndromes and disorders associated with RBD in which at least one pathologically verified case has been identified are in italics. Those in black print have not been reported in association with RBD.

RBD associated with clinically probable AD. In the study by Postuma and coworkers,[80] the neuropsychological profile of probable AD cases was indistinguishable from those with probable DLB, which suggests such cases have underlying Lewy body disease (LBD); these data are consistent with other data showing RBD associated with dementia but not visual hallucinations or parkinsonism likely reflects underlying LBD.[83]

Our updated clinicopathologic experience involving patients evaluated at Mayo Clinic Rochester and Mayo Clinic Jacksonville who had RBD associated with cognitive impairment/dementia and/or parkinsonism is shown in Table 4, which demonstrates the preponderance of LBD and MSA in this series (41/43 = 95%). The patient described above with PSP pathology and a recently identified case with PSG-confirmed RBD who had atypical DLB clinical features yet AD pathology (Boeve *et al.*, unpublished data) are the exceptions.

These data include several hundred autopsy-proven cases of AD in the Mayo Alzheimer's Disease Research Center/Alzheimer's Disease Patient Registry and also several hundreds of autopsy-proven cases of PSP in the Society for PSP Brain Bank. Therefore, the vast majority of cases with RBD—with or without coexisting cognitive impairment and/or parkinsonism—represent an underlying synucleinopathy.

There are no published reports of RBD associated with Pick's disease, frontotemporal dementia, progressive nonfluent aphasia syndrome, semantic dementia, progressive subcortical gliosis, argyrophilic grain disease, frontotemporal lobar degeneration with ubiquitin- and TDP-43-positive inclusions, or dementia lacking distinctive histopathology.[82] No evidence of RSWA or RBD was found in a recent study of 11 members of the pallido-ponto-nigral degeneration kindred who have the N279K mutation in the microtubule-associated protein tau (*MAPT*), which represents a primary tauopathy.[112] We have also not encountered RBD in any of our families with familial frontotemporal dementia (FTD) +/− parkinsonism associated with other mutations in *MAPT* or with mutations in progranulin.[113]

Table 4. Updated clinicopathologic experience at Mayo Clinic from January 1990 to April 2009 of REM sleep behavior disorder associated with dementia and/or parkinsonism

Primary pathologic diagnoses	N
Lewy body disease	36
Multiple system atrophy	5
Progressive supranuclear palsy	1
Alzheimer's disease	1
TOTAL	43

Synucleinopathy pathology associated with RBD in this series: 41/43 = 95%.

Analyses in patients with idiopathic RBD

There are few studies published to date that involved patients with iRBD who have been followed prospectively. The seminal paper by Schenck and collaborators, which launched the interest in the RBD-neurodegenerative disease association, showed that among 29 iRBD patients followed longitudinally, 11 (38%) developed a parkinsonian disorder at a mean interval of 3.7 years after the diagnosis of RBD, and at a mean interval of 12.7 years after the onset of RBD.[114] As of 2005, over 65% of their original group has developed parkinsonism and/or cognitive impairment.[29] Four of these patients with iRBD plus cognitive impairment are currently being followed in the Mayo Alzheimer's Disease Research Center (kindly referred by Drs. Schenck and Mahowald), of whom one has nonamnestic mild cognitive impairment and the three others have classic DLB features.

Iranzo and colleagues reported on a series of 44 patients with iRBD with at least 2 years of clinical follow-up, of whom 20 (45%) developed a neurological disorder after a mean of 11.5 years from the reported onset of RBD.[26] The newly emerged disorders included PD ($n = 9$), DLB ($n = 6$), MSA ($n = 1$), and mild cognitive impairment ($n = 4$) in whom visuospatial dysfunction was prominent.[26]

Postuma and coworkers recently reported on a series of 93 patients with iRBD whom they followed longitudinally, of whom 26 patients developed a neurodegenerative disorder: PD in 14, DLB in 7, probable AD in 4, and MSA in 1.[80] The estimated 5-year risk for neurodegenerative disease was 17.7%,

the 10-year risk was 40.6%, and the 12-year risk was 52.4%.[80]

Two cases with iRBD have had LBD pathology identified (termed "incidental LBD"). Uchiyama and colleagues reported on a patient with a 20-year history of RBD who had no cognitive or motor findings throughout his clinical course. At autopsy, Lewy bodies were identified, particularly in the brain stem.[115] We reported on a surgeon with PSG-proven RBD (onset age 57 years) and no other neurologic signs or symptoms who underwent neuropathologic examination upon his death at age 72.[116] Histopathologic analysis showed LBD, with interestingly no significant neuronal loss or gliosis present in the substantia nigra or locus ceruleus.[116]

RBD and the synucleinopathies

The disorders of LBD and MSA, which have prominent α-synuclein-positive pathology, are collectively termed "synucleinopathies." Therefore, the clinical and pathologic data strongly support the association of RBD with the synucleinopathies, and most experts in the field now believe that patients with RBD plus cognitive impairment and/or parkinsonism likely have an underlying synucleinopathy.[3,26,27,76,80,82,84,110,117–119] Furthermore, among the nonsynucleinopathy disorders associated with RBD (e.g., PSP, SCA-3, and AD), patients have tended to have RBD evolve concurrently with or after the onset of parkinsonism, whereas RBD typically begins years or decades before the onset of cognitive and motor features of PD, DLB, MSA, and pure autonomic failure (PAF). Hence, RBD preceding the motor and cognitive features of a neurodegenerative disorder may be particularly common in the synucleinopathies, and there is considerable interest to study patients with "idiopathic" RBD (discussed in much more detail in the sections that follow).

RBD, the synucleinopathies, and selective vulnerability

The tendency of RBD to occur frequently in the synucleinopathies and rarely in the tauopathies and other neurodegenerative disorders supports the concept of selective vulnerability occurring in key brain-stem neuronal networks in the synucleinopathies, and such neuronal networks are likely to be less dysfunctional or normal in the tauopathies and other neurodegenerative disorders.[3,26,27,80,82,84,110,117,118] PD, DLB, MSA, the few other nonsynucleinopathy disorders associated with RBD, and the rare RBD cases with structural brainstem lesions may provide particular insights into RBD pathophysiology by demonstrating which neuronal networks are dysfunctional compared to the many disorders and cases that are not associated with RBD. Comparing the neuropathological findings (especially if neuronal quantification of key brain-stem structures can be performed) in the rare cases of RBD associated with nonsynucleinopathy disorders with the more common cases of nonsynucleinopathy disorders not associated with RBD may be particularly enlightening.

RBD in the context of the Braak staging system for Parkinson's disease

Braak and colleagues have proposed a staging system for the neuropathologic characterization of the phenotype of PD, and this system may be applicable to the timing of the evolution of RBD in the context of evolving LBD regardless if the clinical phenotype evolves as PD or DLB.[3,26,76,80,84,110,117,119–121] This staging system posits a temporal sequence of α-synuclein pathology in the brain beginning mainly in the medulla (and olfactory bulb) and gradually ascending to more rostral structures.[120,121] Dysfunction in the SLD +/− MCRF and peri-LC structures (Stage 2) could lead to RSWA and RBD, and more specifically, prominent degeneration in the SLD could be the critical nucleus involved. This temporal sequence of pathology could explain why RBD precedes parkinsonism and cognitive decline (Stages 3 and 4) and dementia (Stages 4–6) in many patients with Lewy body pathology. A schematic representation of this evolution through Stages 2 and 3 are shown in Figure 5.

Over the few years since Braak and colleagues presented their staging scheme for PD, they and others have provided evidence that LBD is a more systemic process that clearly affects the peripheral autonomic nervous system, and in some cases actually may begin in the spinal cord prior to the brain, and the peripheral autonomic system even before the central nervous system.[122–126] Lewy bodies and Lewy neurites have been found in the enteric nervous system, cardiac sympathetic system, and spinal cord (particularly intermediolateral cell col-

umn).[122–126] A schematic representation of this and the likely structures and associated clinical features are shown in Figure 6. This schematic is admittedly overly simplistic, and the actual contributions to the clinical features associated with LBD are surely more varied and complex than is depicted here. Yet the implications of this widespread pathology and possible evolution of LBD pathology from the periphery to the spinal cord and then ascending rostrally, consistent with the Braak scheme, provide a framework of testable hypotheses. The analyses addressing this framework are the focus of the next section.

Characterization of patients with "idiopathic" RBD

"Idiopathic" RBD—a potential early manifestation of a neurodegenerative disease

The retrospective and prospective data as reviewed above convincingly suggest that a significant proportion of individuals with iRBD represent an early manifestation of an evolving neurodegenerative disease (which underscores why some authors qualify the term *idiopathic* with quotation marks). Many recent studies have used cross-sectional analyses with iRBD as the central feature and a variety of other clinical, neuropsychological, electrophysiological, and imaging modalities to test hypotheses, and almost all have supported the concept that most cases of iRBD likely reflect an evolving neurodegenerative disorder, which in most instances is LBD. The clinical and ancillary test findings associated with iRBD published to date are reviewed below.

Clinical findings in "idiopathic" REM sleep behavior disorder

Anosmia/dysosmia

Several studies have found impaired olfactory functioning in patients with iRBD. Stiasny-Kolster and coworkers studied 30 patients with clinical (idiopathic [$n = 6$]; symptomatic [$n = 13$], mostly associated with narcolepsy; or subclinical [$n = 11$], associated with narcolepsy) RBD according to standard criteria and 30 age- and gender-matched healthy control subjects using "Sniffin' Sticks."[119] RBD patients had a significantly higher olfactory threshold, lower discrimination score, and lower identification score. Compared with normative data,

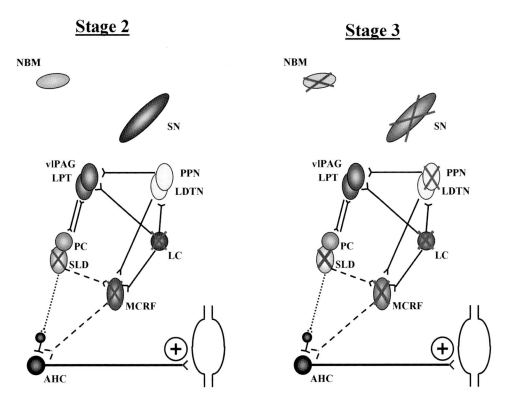

Figure 5. Schematic of brain-stem nuclei and connections pertinent to REM sleep, movement, and cognition. As per the Braak staging scheme, the temporal sequence of α-synuclein pathology begins mainly in the medulla and then ascends to the cortex (6 stages). In Stage 1 (not shown), the dorsal IX/X motor nucleus, intermediate reticular zone, and olfactory bulb are affected, with presumably coexisting degenerative changes in these structures. In Stage 2, there is progression in the structures involved in Stage 1, plus the caudal raphe nuclei, MCRF, peri-LC structures, and possibly SLD. RBD may evolve when sufficient degenerative changes have occurred in the SLD, peri-LC structures, and MCRF (denoted by red Xs within nuclei). In Stage 3, there is progression in the structures involved in Stage 2, plus the PPN, SN, and NBM (denoted by red Xs within nuclei). When sufficient degeneration occurs in the SN, then parkinsonism becomes manifest. When sufficient degeneration occurs in the NBM, then cognitive changes may become manifest. Additional α-synuclein pathology and neurodegeneration evolves in limbic and neocortical structures over Stages 4–6 (not shown). This temporal sequence of pathology could explain why RBD precedes parkinsonism and dementia in many patients with Lewy body pathology. Abbreviations: AHC, anterior horn cell; LC, locus coeruleus; LDTN, laterodorsal tegmental nucleus; LPT, lateral pontine tegmentum; MCRF, magnocellular reticular formation; NBM, nucleus basalis of Meynert; PC, precoeruleus; PPN, pedunculopontine nucleus; SLD, sublaterodorsal nucleus; SN, substantia nigra; vlPAG, ventrolateral part of the periaqueductal gray matter.

97% of the iRBD patients had a pathologically increased olfactory threshold, 63% an impaired odor discrimination score, and 63% a decreased identification score. The authors concluded that iRBD patients with olfactory impairment might represent Stage 2 preclinical α-synucleinopathy.[119]

Fantini and colleagues studied 54 consecutive PSG-confirmed iRBD patients and 54 age- and gender-matched control subjects with the Brief University of Pennsylvania Smell Identification Test (B-

UPSIT).[127] They found 33 (61.1%) RBD patients, versus 9 (16.6%) controls, to have abnormal olfactory function ($P < 0.0001$). Difficulties in recognize paint thinner odorant showed the highest positive predictive value (0.95) for identifying iRBD. They interpreted these findings as showing that the olfactory deficits found in most iRBD patients are similar to those described in PD, and that dysosmia may be a sign of a widespread neurodegenerative process. They also felt that its detection might help

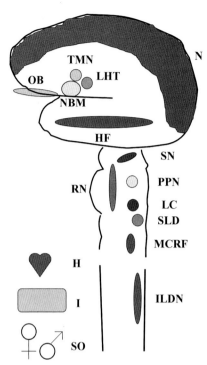

Dysfunction of structure and associated clinical feature

OB = anosmia
TMN = altered arousal/sleep
LHT = hypersomnia
NBM = cognitive impairment
HF = cognitive impairment
N = cognitive impairment
SN = parkinsonism
PPN = altered arousal/attention
RN = depression
LC = depression
SLD = ? RBD
MCRF = ? RBD
ILDN = orthostatism
H = cardiac dysfunction
I = constipation
SO = impotence

Figure 6. Schematic representation of the brain, spinal cord, and key peripheral and autonomic structures which can be affected by Lewy body disease pathology, and the clinical features associated with dysfunction of each structure. The structures (abbreviations) and likely associated clinical features are as follows: olfactory bulb (OB) = anosmia; tuberomamillary nucleus (TMN) = altered arousal/sleep; lateral hypothalamus (LHT) = hypersomnia; nucleus basalis of Meynert (NBM) = cognitive impairment; hippocampal formation (HF) = cognitive impairment; neocortex (N) = cognitive impairment; substantia nigra (SN) = parkinsonism; pedunculopontine nucleus (PPN) = altered arousal/attention; raphe nucleus (RN) = depression; locus coeruleus (LC) = depression; sublaterodorsal nucleus (SLD) = ? RBD; magnocellular reticular formation (MCRF) = ? RBD; intermediolateral cell column (ILDN) = orthostatism; sympathetic innervation of the heart (H) = cardiac dysfunction; enteric innervation of the intestines (I) = constipation; and autonomic innervation of the sex organs (SO) = impotence.

in identifying subjects at higher risk for developing an α-synucleinopathy disorder.[127]

Postuma and colleagues compared 25 patients with PSG-confirmed RBD without PD with age- and sex-matched controls.[76] Olfaction was assessed using the B-UPSIT. When results were compared with age- and sex-adjusted normative values, 14 out of 25 patients with iRBD but only 2 of 25 controls scored below the 25th percentile. The authors concluded that olfactory dysfunction, like many other potential early markers of Parkinson's disease, are significantly abnormal in iRBD.[76]

Subtle parkinsonism

In the same study by Postuma and colleagues, the 25 subjects and 25 controls were assessed by the alternate tap test, Purdue Peg Board, and a timed up and go test measure of standing and walking. The results showed that many subjects exhibited subtle abnormalities on quantitative testing of motor and gait speed.[76]

Mihci and coworkers analyzed sleep and motor data among normal control participants (n = 765) aged 70–89 in the Mayo Clinic Study of Aging—a population-based study of aging and cognition in Olmsted County, Minnesota.[34] All participants who had a bed partner completed the MSQ, with an affirmative response to one question on RBD (and hence considered probable RBD) being 98% sensitive for definite RBD based on a PSG-validation analysis (Boeve and colleagues, submitted). The motor subtest of the

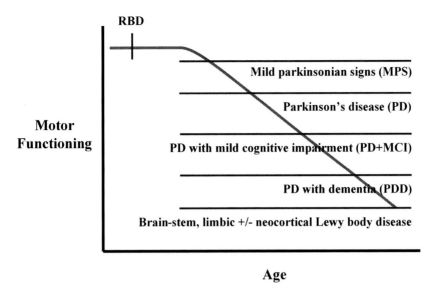

Figure 7. Schematic representation of the hypothesized progression in motor functioning with increasing age and disease severity in evolving Lewy body disease in the Parkinson's disease–predominant phenotype. The onset of RBD typically begins years or decades prior to the onset of subtle motor signs (mild parkinsonian signs or MPS); such motor signs may be asymptomatic and only detectable on clinical examination. Typical features of Parkinson's disease (PD) evolve months or years later. Over time, PD with mild cognitive impairment (PD+MCI) evolves, followed some time thereafter by parkinsonism, which is less levodopa-responsive, and a full dementia syndrome (PD with dementia, or PDD) becomes manifest.

Unified Parkinson's Disease Rating Scale (UPDRS) was completed on all subjects, and parkinsonism was considered present if any subject had a score of 2 or greater in at least two of the core features: rigidity, bradykinesia, rest tremor, and postural instability. Data were analyzed for subjects who underwent the key assessments and were considered cognitively normal. The investigators found that 71 (9.3%) had parkinsonism alone, 46 (6.0%) had probable RBD alone, 14 (1.8%) had both parkinsonism and probable RBD, and 632 (82.6%) had neither. Parkinsonism was indeed significantly associated with probable RBD ($P = 0.002$). The authors concluded that parkinsonism is associated with probable RBD among cognitively normal subjects in this population-based study, and longitudinal characterization and eventual neuropathologic examinations will be needed to determine which clinical phenotypes will evolve and whether LBD and MSA will be the primary underlying pathologies.[34]

These findings and perspectives can be viewed conceptually as shown in Figure 7, which depicts the hypothesized progression in motor functioning with increasing age and disease severity in evolving LBD in the Parkinson's disease–predominant phenotype. The onset of RBD typically begins years or decades prior to the onset of subtle motor signs—these subtle signs are also termed "mild parkinsonian signs" and abbreviated as "MPS."[128] MPS may be asymptomatic and only detectable on clinical examination, or may be minimally symptomatic and not functionally disabling. Typical features of PD evolve months or years later. Over time, PD with mild cognitive impairment (PD+MCI) evolves, followed some time thereafter by progressive parkinsonism, which is progressively less levodopa-responsive despite aggressive dosing, and a full dementia syndrome (PD with dementia, or PDD) becomes manifest.[129,130]

Inherent in any schema such as this is the known individual variability, with some patients with PD living for more than 20 or 30 years with relatively preserved cognitive functioning, and some patients with PD never exhibiting RBD at all. However, most patients with "idiopathic" RBD who later develop typical features of PD and subsequent cognitive changes evolve in the manner depicted in Figure 7.

Other

Additional findings on clinical measures in patients with iRBD include impairment of color discrimination[76] and more frequent reports of autonomic dysfunction (urinary dyscontrol, erectile function, and constipation).[76] Depression and personality traits have also been studied, but no difference has been found between iRBD patients and controls.[76] Apathy and anxiety have also been associated with probable RBD.[35] Investigators with the Honolulu-Asia Aging Study found that subjective hypersomnolence was associated with increased incidence of subsequent Parkinson's disease.[131] Although objective evidence of hypersomnolence was not found in patients with iRBD,[1] this issue may be worthy of further study.

Cognitive and neuropsychological features/findings in "idiopathic" REM sleep behavior disorder

Ferini-Strambi and coworkers evaluated 17 consecutive patients with iRBD and 17 matched controls on a battery of neuropsychological measures that assessed verbal and spatial memory, visual selective attention, cognitive set shifting, visuoconstructional abilities, visuospatial learning, verbal fluency, semantic fluency, and executive functions.[132] The exclusion criteria included abnormalities on neurologic examination and a Mini-Mental State Exam score below 24. Results showed that the iRBD patients had lower scores on visuoconstructional abilities and visuospatial learning. Because deficits in these domains have been demonstrated in patients with DLB,[17,81,83,133] the authors interpreted their results as possibly reflecting early DLB in these patients.[132]

In a study by Massicotte-Marque and collaborators, 14 patients with iRBD and 14 healthy control subjects underwent neuropsychological evaluation.[134] Compared with controls, patients with iRBD showed lower performance on neuropsychological tests measuring attention, executive functions, and learning, but not on tasks measuring delayed recall or visuospatial functioning. The authors concluded that the impaired cognitive profile in patients with iRBD is similar to that observed in early stages of some synucleinopathies.[134]

Terzaghi and colleagues compared the neuropsychological functions in 23 iRBD subjects with a group of healthy controls.[135] Considering mean values, poorer performances were observed in the iRBD subjects on Word Span, Rey–Osterrieth's complex figure recall, Digit Span, and Logic Memory tests. On the basis of equivalent scores, the iRBD subjects performed significantly more poorly on tests of visuoconstructional learning abilities. They interpreted their data as showing the possible presence of cognitive deficits in iRBD sharing common features with LBD.[135]

Mild cognitive impairment (MCI) refers to the intermediate state between normal aging and dementia.[136] Most individuals with prominent memory impairment but preserved functioning in the other nonmemory domains (often termed "amnestic MCI" and abbreviated aMCI) subsequently develop the typical clinical, neuropsychological, neuroimaging, and neuropathological features of AD.[137] Other degenerative conditions such as dementia with Lewy bodies, frontotemporal dementia, primary progressive aphasia, corticobasal syndrome, and posterior cortical atrophy, as well as other etiologic categories of disease such as depression, cerebrovascular disease, and metabolic disorders, likely also evolve through an MCI intermediate state, but little data have been published to support this view. The concept of MCI has therefore been further subtyped such that the clinical and neuropsychological profile of impairment can be extended beyond single-domain MCI with amnesia (i.e., aMCI) to also include multiple-domain MCI with amnesia, single-domain nonamnestic MCI, and multiple-domain nonamnestic MCI.[137] This conceptual framework allows one to test hypotheses, and a few key questions pertaining to RBD and the synucleinopathies have recently been studied.

Based on the data accumulated thus far in RBD as well as DLB, one could hypothesize that (1) those individuals with RBD plus MCI likely reflect evolving LBD and (2) the MCI subtypes with impairment maximal in the attention/executive and visuospatial functioning domains would be most likely to reflect evolving LBD. Molano *et al.* recently analyzed the clinical and neuropsychological data on all patients who were diagnosed with MCI, prospectively followed, and eventually underwent neuropathologic examination and had limbic +/− neocortical LBD.[138] Eight subjects were identified, of whom 6 were male. Seven developed DLB prior to death; 1 died characterized as MCI. RBD preceded cognitive symptom onset in 6 cases by a median of 10 years (range 2–47 years). Each of the MCI subtypes were represented, with 7 of the 8 patients having impairment in the attention/executive functioning and/or visuospatial functioning domains. These authors concluded that LBD can pass through an MCI intermediate state, with any MCI subtype can potentially evolve into DLB. Furthermore, since all cases with RBD and MCI eventually were shown to have autopsy-proven LBD, these data suggest that RBD plus MCI likely reflects brain-stem and cerebral LBD.[138]

Molano and colleagues also compared the neuropsychological profiles among the same cohort described above in the analysis by Michi and colleagues, in which normal control participants ($n = 765$) aged 70–89 in the Mayo Clinic Study of Aging were the focus of analysis.[36] All participants who had a bed partner had the MSQ completed. The neuropsychological battery assessed performance in the attention/executive, memory, language, and visuospatial domains. A domain score was computed and transformed to a z-scale to allow comparisons. The frequency of probable RBD was 8.0%. Those with probable RBD had significantly lower median scores (25th–75th percentile scores) for the attention/executive domain. Scores were also lower in subjects with probable RBD compared with those without RBD across the other domains, although none reached statistical significance. The authors interpreted these findings to be consistent with very mild neuropsychological changes that may reflect evolving LBD in most subjects, although clearly longitudinal follow-up will be necessary to substantiate this hypothesis.[36]

While at first glance some of these studies appear to show inconsistent results, when one considers the domains that are most consistently impaired in PD and particularly DLB patients—attention/executive functions, learning, and visuospatial functioning, with relative preservation in delayed recall and confrontation naming measures—the data could still be interpreted as reflecting the pattern of impairment that is often seen in the phenotypes most commonly associated with synucleinopathy pathology. This pattern of impairment is not typical of AD or many of the tauopathies and TDP-43opathies. Furthermore, even though patients with PD and mild cognitive impairment or dementia, and those with

DLB, tend to show abnormalities on measures of attention/executive functioning, learning, and visuospatial/visuoconstructive functioning, there is considerable variability between individuals. Hence one would expect to see variability across measures in individuals with iRBD. Some individuals with iRBD surely do not reflect an evolving synucleinopathy, or are so early in the disorder that only the brain stem and not the cerebrum is significantly affected by synucleinopathy pathology, neuronal loss, and neurochemical dysfunction. Investigators seeking to study neuropsychological functioning in iRBD patients should utilize measures that assess all cognitive domains, with several focused on attention/concentration, executive functioning, learning, and visuospatial/visuoconstructive functioning.

This author has also evaluated numerous patients with iRBD who have clear cognitive complaints, particularly problems with multitasking and anterograde memory processing that are impacting their ability to perform at their prior baseline at work and keep up with the daily tasks at home. To a seasoned clinician, these complaints sound neurologically based, yet in many of these patients there is no obvious impairment on detailed neuropsychological testing. Many who have been followed longitudinally subsequently develop more obvious MCI or frank DLB. One must therefore conclude that many of the standard neuropsychological tests do not adequately capture the essence of what these patients are experiencing. We need measures that more adequately reflect their symptoms! This is an obvious area warranting further research.

Similar to the concept of iRBD evolving into a PD-predominant phenotype as discussed above, one could hypothesize a similar progression in cognitive functioning with increasing age and disease severity in evolving LBD in the DLB-predominant phenotype (Fig. 8). The onset of RBD typically begins years or decades prior to the onset of cognitive decline and a diagnosis of MCI, with subtle and often asymptomatic motor signs (i.e., MPS, represented by the area shaded in light yellow) evolving concurrently or after the onset of cognitive decline. More obvious features of parkinsonism (represented by the area shaded in dark yellow) evolves no earlier than 1 year prior to the onset of dementia, thereby fulfilling the "one-year rule" for the diagnosis of DLB.[139] Over time, dementia, parkinsonism, and

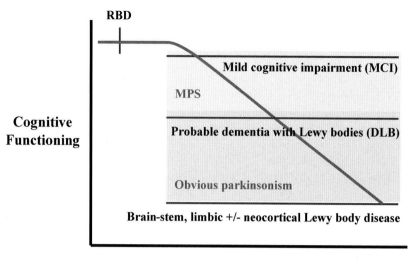

Figure 8. Schematic representation of the hypothesized progression in cognitive functioning with increasing age and disease severity in evolving Lewy body disease in the dementia with Lewy bodies (DLB)–predominant phenotype. The onset of RBD typically begins years or decades prior to the onset of cognitive decline and a diagnosis of mild cognitive impairment (MCI), with subtle and often asymptomatic motor signs (mild parkinsonian signs or MPS—represented by the area shaded in light yellow) evolving concurrently or after the onset of cognitive decline. More obvious features of parkinsonism (represented by the area shaded in dark yellow) evolves no earlier than 1 year prior to the onset of dementia to warrant the DLB diagnosis. Over time, dementia, parkinsonism, and problematic neuropsychiatric features such as visual hallucinations and delusions tend to progress.

problematic neuropsychiatric features such as visual hallucinations and delusions tend to progress.

As in the PD-predominant phenotype, inherent in any schema such as this is the known individual variability, with some patients with MCI not progressing to dementia even after 10 years, or some with autopsy-proven LBD never exhibiting significant parkinsonism, and still others with DLB never exhibiting RBD at all. However, most patients with iRBD who later develop typical features of DLB evolve in the manner that is depicted here.

Electroencephalographic findings in "idiopathic" REM sleep behavior disorder

Fantini and coworkers performed quantitative analyses of waking and REM sleep EEG in 15 patients with idiopathic RBD and in 15 matched controls.[140] The exclusion criteria included abnormalities on neurologic examination and presence of affective disorders or dementia. EEG slowing was demonstrated in the RBD group, thus suggesting impaired cortical activity during both wakefulness and REM sleep. The authors interpreted these findings as pos-

sibly reflecting a very early sign of central nervous system dysfunction.[140]

In a study by Massicotte-Marque and colleagues, 14 patients with iRBD and 14 healthy control subjects underwent waking EEG recordings.[141] Compared with controls, patients with iRBD showed EEG slowing (higher delta and theta power) during wakefulness in all brain areas. The authors concluded that waking EEG slowing in patients with iRBD is similar to that observed in early stages of some synucleinopathies.[141]

Neuroimaging findings in "idiopathic" REM sleep behavior disorder

Structural magnetic resonance imaging
Culebras and Moore reported on T2 signal changes on magnetic resonance imaging (MRI) in six patients with RBD and suggested vascular changes in the brain stem could disrupt REM sleep networks and result in RBD.[142] However, the vast majority of patients with RBD in whom MRI has been performed have not corroborated this finding.[12,17,22]

Magnetic resonance spectroscopy

Miyamoto and colleagues detected an increase (compared with reference values from another institution) in the choline/creatine ratio on proton magnetic resonance spectroscopy (^{1}H-MRS) in the pons of a 69-year-old man with idiopathic RBD.[143] Since other ratios were normal, the investigators interpreted these findings as demonstrating functional impairment at the cell membrane level.[143]

Iranzo and coworkers performed ^{1}H-MRS in a larger sample of patients with idiopathic RBD ($n = 15$) to determine if midbrain or pontine tegmentum abnormalities could be detected compared with matched controls ($n = 15$).[144] No significant differences in N-acetylaspartate/creatine, choline/creatine, and myoinosito/creatine ratios were found between patients and controls, which they interpreted as suggesting that marked mesopontine neuronal loss or ^{1}H-MRS-detectable metabolic disturbances do not occur in idiopathic RBD.[144]

The discrepant findings between these two studies could be due in part to methodologic issues (location of regions of interest, reference values for determining abnormal results, and others). No ^{1}H-MRS study with the medulla as the region of interest has been reported as yet in patients with idiopathic RBD; the Braak staging system of Parkinson's disease suggests that this region of interest may be worth investigating.[120,121]

Single photon emission computed tomography

IPT-SPECT and IBZM-SPECT. Eisensehr and collaborators used (N)-(3-iodopropene-2-yl)-2beta-carbomethoxy-3beta-(4-chlorophenyl) tropane labeled with iodine 123 (IPT) single-photon emission computed tomography (SPECT), which reflects presynaptic dopaminergic transporter integrity, and (S)-2hydroxy-3iodo-6-methoxy-([1-ethyl-2-pyrrolidinyl]methyl) benzamide labeled with iodine 123 (IBZM-SPECT), which reflects postsynaptic dopaminergic D2 receptor integrity, to investigate dopaminergic parameters in patients with RBD, PD, and controls.[145] RBD cases had reduced striatal IPT uptake compared with controls, yet uptake was more similar (albeit symmetric) to PD cases. Furthermore, there was no significant difference in postsynaptic dopaminergic D2 receptors between RBD patients and controls. The reduction in dopaminergic transporters was thought either to be directly involved in RBD pathogenesis, or that RBD is the initial manifestation of PD.[145] In a subsequent study, these investigators compared muscle activity in REM sleep on PSG and IPT-SPECT and IBZM-SPECT in normal controls ($n = 11$), patients with idiopathic "subclinical" RBD ($n = 8$), patients with idiopathic RBD ($n = 8$), and patients with early Parkinson's disease ($n = 8$).[70] They found that IPT uptake was highest in controls, lower for patients with "subclinical" RBD, still lower for patients with clinically manifest RBD, and lowest in patients with PD. Muscle activity during REM sleep was independently associated with reduction of striatal dopamine transporters. IBZM uptake was not significantly different between the groups. The investigators interpreted their findings as suggesting that there is a continuum of reduced striatal dopamine transporters involved in the pathophysiologic mechanisms causing increased muscle activity during REM sleep in patients with "subclinical" RBD.[70]

ECD-SPECT. Mazza and colleagues investigated the regional cerebral perfusion in patients with idiopathic REM behavior disorder (iRBD) by using (99m)Tc-Ethylene Cysteinate Dimer (ECD) SPECT on eight patients with PSG-confirmed RBD and nine age-matched controls.[146] They found increased perfusion in the pons and putamen bilaterally and in the right hippocampus, and decreased perfusion in frontal and temporoparietal cortices. The authors concluded that perfusional abnormalities in patients with iRBD were located in the brain stem, striatum, and cortex, and that such findings are consistent with the anatomic metabolic profile of Parkinson's disease.[146]

I-123-FP-CIT-SPECT. In a study focused on olfactory function in patients with RBD, Stiasny-Kolner and colleagues performed [I-123] N-ω-fluoropropyl-2β- carbomethoxy-3β-(4-iodophenyl) nortropane (I-123-FP-CIT, also known as Ioflupane and marketed in Europe as DaTSCAN) SPECT in several of their patients with RBD, and found three patients with reduced nigrostriatal uptake: one with newly identified parkinsonism on clinical examination, and two with idiopathic RBD.[119] The authors interpreted their findings as suggesting that iRBD patients with olfactory impairment might represent a preclinical α-synucleinopathy.[119]

Positron emission tomography

DTBZ-PET. Using dihydrotetrabenazine (DTBZ) positron emission tomography (PET), Albin and coworkers compared findings in elderly subjects with iRBD with those in similarly aged controls.[147] Striatal binding of DTBZ was reduced in the iRBD subjects compared with controls, suggesting reduced dopaminergic substantia nigra neuron number. The authors concluded that this reduction is consistent with the hypothesis that RBD reflects an evolving degenerative parkinsonian disorder and suggested that RBD either reflects dysfunction of the PPN secondary to basal ganglia dysfunction or primary dysfunction of the PPN or other brain-stem structures that is temporally associated with basal ganglia dysfunction.[147]

FDG-PET. Caselli and colleagues sought to determine if healthy adults reporting dream-enactment behavior (DEB+) have a reduced cerebral metabolic rate for glucose (CMRgl) on fluorodeoxyglucose (FDG) PET in regions preferentially affected in patients with DLB.[148] Among 17 cognitively normal patients with DEB+ and 17 control subjects (DEB–), the DEB+ group was associated with significantly lower CMRgl in several brain regions known to be preferentially affected in both DLB and AD (parietal, temporal, and posterior cingulate cortexes) and in several other regions, including the anterior cingulate cortex. The authors interpreted these findings as supporting further study of DEB as a possible risk factor for the development of DLB.[148]

PiB-PET. One of the most important advances in imaging in the aging and dementia field was the advent of Pittsburgh-compound B (PiB) PET, in which the PiB ligand binds to amyloid and allows visualization of cerebral amyloid in plaques and vessels in patients with AD.[149,150] PiB-PET imaging findings in patients with RBD have not yet been published, but this imaging modality warrants a few words of caution for researchers in the RBD field. While some degree of controversy exists on the interpretation on PiB-positive PET scans, particularly in cognitively normal individuals, the use of PiB-PET imaging in DLB and PDD has recently begun[151] and may have some applicability to imaging subjects with iRBD. On the one hand, it may seem reasonable to consider PiB-positive scans in those with iRBD as indicative of evolving AD pathology. The facts that (1) some cognitively normal subjects have PiB-positive scans

and (2) most DLB patients have some degree of co-existing AD pathology and hence would likely have PiB-positive scans make the use of PiB-PET imaging less than ideal as a "rule-out AD" biomarker for iRBD research purposes.

Cardiac metaiodobenzylguanidine imaging

Recent evidence supports the notion that cardiac sympathetic involvement is a very early event in the evolution of LBD in humans, occurring prior to the deposition of α-synuclein pathology in the central nervous system in many patients.[126] Cardiac (123)I-metaiodobenzylguanidine (MIBG) reflects cardiac sympathetic integrity, and reduced uptake on MIBG imaging is consistent with the loss of sympathetic terminals in the heart. Ample data now exist on reduced cardiac MIBG uptake being present in patients with LBD regardless whether the disorder is exhibited as PD, DLB, PD with dementia, or pure autonomic failure (PAF).[152–154] Several investigators have therefore suggested that MIBG could be used to identify who has underlying LBD regardless of the other clinical features being exhibited.

Further support for this hypothesis has come from cardiac MIBG imaging in patients with idiopathic RBD, in which uptake is reduced.[155–157] In contrast, cardiac MIBG uptake in MSA—another synucleinopathy often associated with RBD—is typically within normal limits.[156,158] Since the topography of degeneration in MSA is almost exclusively the central nervous system,[159–161] while LBD involves the peripheral autonomic and sensorimotor systems and multiple networks in the central nervous system, the evidence accumulated thus far suggests that reduced cardiac MIBG uptake may be one of the most specific biomarkers for underlying LBD. The sensitivity of cardiac MIBG imaging for LBD is not yet known, and this technique does have several limitations such as questionable validity in those with other medical disorders that affect cardiac sympathetic integrity (such as diabetes mellitus), high cost, and limited availability. Yet additional work with cardiac MIBG imaging in idiopathic RBD, particularly in countries outside of Japan (all MIBG publications on RBD have emanated from the excellent work from several centers in Japan), is clearly warranted.

Evolving concepts, controversies, and future directions

Does the RBD diagnosis require polysomnography?

The simple answer to this question is "yes." If a patient is exhibiting recurrent dream enactment behavior, the dreams are viewed as unpleasant, and the potential for injury to the patient or bed partner is high, PSG with synchronous video monitoring is essential. Given the implications of a formal PSG-confirmed diagnosis of RBD and the known tendency for some patients with moderate to severe obstructive sleep apnea (OSA)[5] to have a history of recurrent dream enactment behavior associated with dreams involving a chasing or attacking theme (which is essentially identical to that of RBD), a PSG is imperative. This author has evaluated numerous middle-aged males with concerns about RBD and the future implications thereof, but rather minimal historical and examination findings to suggest clinically significant OSA, yet on PSG moderate to severe OSA is found, EMG atonia during REM sleep is normal, and nasal continuous positive airway pressure (CPAP) subsequently eliminates the unpleasant dreams and recurrent dream enactment behavior completely. A PSG should be strongly considered in each and every patient with suspected RBD and should be performed whenever feasible particularly if the potential for injury is high.

However, there are many circumstances when PSG confirmation of RBD is not feasible or possible (see below). Yet there is growing appreciation of the importance of identifying patients with RBD for clinical and particularly research purposes. PSG confirmation of RBD is mandatory in the current diagnostic criteria schemes.

When is a diagnosis of "probable RBD" justified?

In the instances when (1) PSG cannot be performed for whatever reason, (2) PSG is performed and little or no apparent REM sleep is present, or (3) the EMG tone during REM sleep is equivocally elevated, this author would suggest the use of the term *probable RBD* for those who otherwise have a classic history of recurrent dream enactment behavior associated with dreams involving a chasing or attacking theme; the confidence in this diagnosis is heightened

further if there are no historical features (loud disruptive snoring, observed choking/gasping/apnea during sleep) or anatomic findings (narrow oropharynx, large neck circumference, obesity) to suggest OSA, nor any features to strongly suspect nocturnal seizures or sleepwalking. The diagnosis of "probable RBD" could also be justified if questionnaires are shown to be adequately sensitive and specific for RBD based on PSG validation (see below).

How accurate are screening measures for RBD?

PSG is essential to establish the diagnosis of RBD, but the procedure does require appropriate monitoring equipment, including synchronized video recordings, specially trained technologists, bed availability in a sleep laboratory, and clinicians who can interpret the data. The procedure is costly (>$1000 per study at most centers for a clinical PSG), especially for patients with limited insurance coverage. Subjects must be willing and able to sleep in a sleep laboratory and undergo monitoring. Some patients with coexisting neurologic disorders are too cognitively or physically impaired to tolerate and undergo an adequate study, are too uncooperative to permit all monitoring equipment to remain in place, have a risk for falls during the night, or are institutionalized. Since the background EEG is often so abnormal in those with moderate to severe dementia, determining which epochs represent REM sleep on PSG can be difficult if not impossible. Some even with only mild cognitive impairment have features of status dissociatus, in which an experienced sleep clinician cannot determine a sleeping versus a waking EEG with certainty even when viewing the synchronous video. Some patients have no REM sleep on a PSG. Due to the limited number of sleep disorders centers in many countries, PSG is not possible even when clearly medically warranted. In some patients, the dream enactment behavior is so infrequent and mild that a clinical PSG is difficult to justify. Reimbursement for PSG is not always covered by insurance and federal healthcare plans. Especially for research purposes, it could be useful to use a validated measure to screen for RBD by querying the bed partners of patients who are cognitively impaired, severely disabled, or deceased. It is also impractical to perform PSGs in large numbers of subjects in epidemiologic studies of sleep disorders. Therefore, questionnaires that adequately screen for RBD could be useful for clinical and research purposes.

Mayo Sleep Questionnaire

Our group developed the MSQ, a 16-item measure that poses questions about RBD, periodic limb movements during sleep, restless legs syndrome, sleepwalking, obstructive sleep apnea, and sleep-related leg cramps. There were two versions initially developed—one completed by the patient and one completed by his/her bed partner/informant. Our early pilot data using the MSQ through 2002,[162,163] in which responses on the MSQ were compared with the findings on PSG, indicated that the sensitivity and specificity were higher for the bed partner/informant version compared with the patient version, regardless of whether the patient was cognitively impaired or not. Since 2002, we have therefore only used the bed partner/informant version of the MSQ. The measure is free and available to anyone to use—one can access the MSQ at this website: http://www.mayoclinic.org/sleep-disorders/research.html. Our updated validation data in two groups of subjects who have had the MSQ completed by their bed partner and undergone PSG—an aging and dementia cohort ($n = 159$) and a population-based cohort of community-dwelling elderly subjects ($n = 70$)—indicate that an affirmative response to one question was $\geq 98\%$ sensitive and $\geq 69\%$ specific for PSG-confirmed RBD; specificity increased depending on the responses to additional questions on RBD particularly if there was no history to suggest OSA (Boeve and colleagues., submitted).

Semistructured questionnaire based on International Classification of Sleep Disorders, revised, diagnostic criteria for RBD

The Bologna, Genova, Parma, and Pisa Universities group for the study of REM Sleep Behavior Disorder (RBD) in Parkinson's Disease used a questionnaire-based method to study RBD in PD patients.[73] Six trained neurologists used a semistructured questionnaire based on *International Classification of Sleep Disorders*, 2nd ed. (ICSD-2) diagnostic criteria for RBD to evaluate 200 PD patients and their caregivers. RBD was defined according to clinical ICSD-R minimal diagnostic criteria: Limb or body

movements associated with dream mentation (criterion B) in the presence of at least one of the following: harmful or potentially harmful sleep behaviors (criterion C1); dreams appear to be "acted out" (criterion C2); sleep behaviors disrupt sleep continuity (criterion C3). They found that 34% of their PD patients had a history suggestive of RBD.[73]

REM Sleep Behavior Disorder Screening Questionnaire

Stiasny-Kolster and colleagues developed the REM Sleep Behavior Disorder Screening Questionnaire (RBDSQ), which is a 10-item patient self-rating questionnaire (maximum total score of 13 points) covering the clinical features of RBD.[164] They studied 54 patients with PSG-confirmed RBD, 160 control subjects in whom RBD was excluded by history and PSG, and 133 unselected healthy subjects who did not undergo PSG. The found that the mean RBDSQ score in the RBD group was 9.5 points compared with 4.6 points in control group, and using an RBDSQ score of 5 points as a positive test result, the results yielded a sensitivity of 96% and a specificity of 56%.[164]

The high sensitivity and ease of use for the MSQ and RBDSQ questionnaires make either measure appealing as a screening tool for RBD, with the MSQ likely more appropriate for use in those with cognitive impairment/dementia since the responses are provided by bed partners. In those who screen positive using either measure but are unable or unwilling to undergo PSG, or who have little or no apparent REM sleep during a PSG, then a diagnosis of "probable RBD" would be justified.

Does REM sleep without atonia represent subclinical RBD?

There is debate as to the terminology and clinical significance of increased EMG tone during REM sleep (that is, REM sleep without atonia or RSWA) in patients who have never exhibited dream enactment behavior. Such patients have been classified as having "preclinical" or "subclinical" RBD. While (at least in our experience) some patients with RSWA subsequently develop clinical RBD, and a few of these patients have subsequently developed PD or DLB, not all patients with RSWA have developed clinical RBD. No prospective systematic study of patients with RSWA has been carried out to clarify this issue. Thus, based on the available data, RSWA appears to be the more appropriate terminology rather than preclinical or subclinical RBD, and future research can involve patients with RSWA and follow them longitudinally to determine outcome and predictors of outcome.

How does one assess electromyographic tone during REM sleep on polysomnographic?

Most individuals who undergo PSG have unequivocal findings in REM sleep, with either essentially complete EMG atonia during REM sleep (as shown in Fig. 3A) or clearly increased EMG tone during REM sleep (as shown in Fig. 3B) +/− obvious vocalizations and motor activity such as limb flailing or punching. When sleep clinicians view the PSG, it is rather straightforward, and comments such as "clearly normal EMG atonia" or "clearly increased EMG tone" (also with comments on the observed abnormal behaviors) are made in the results or interpretation of the PSG. Yet some have equivocal findings, with occasional periods of increased EMG tone during tonic and (more often) phasic REM sleep while normal EMG atonia exists over most of the REM sleep epochs. These findings pose challenges for the clinician interpreting the PSG, particularly if one of the indications for PSG was "rule in" or "rule out" RBD; the "rule out" determination is made even more difficult when no apparent dream enactment behavior occurred on the synchronous video during the periods of increased EMG tone.

Frauscher and coworkers framed the current state of affairs in assessing EMG tone during REM sleep very well:[165]

> The *International Classification of Sleep Disorders*-2 defined REM sleep without atonia as the "electromyographic (EMG) finding of excessive amounts of sustained or intermittent elevation of submental EMG tone or excessive phasic submental or (upper or lower) limb EMG twitching." This definition has several limitations. First, a precise definition of "excessive amounts of tonic and phasic EMG activity" was not provided, since normal values of these measures are unknown. Second, it is not stated how the tonic and phasic EMG activity have to be measured. Third, it is unclear which

muscle or combination of muscles of the body (either axial or extremity muscles, lower or upper extremity muscles, or proximal or distal extremity muscles) provides the highest rates of abnormal REM sleep EMG activity in RBD.

These concerns have led several groups to study this issue further, and some have developed scoring systems to not only qualify the EMG tone as normal or abnormal, but also to quantify the degree to which EMG tone is abnormal.[165–169] There are pros and cons with each of the proposed systems, with the main drawback of manual systems being the time and effort required to assess the miniepochs of REM sleep. The automated systems are more appealing for obvious reasons; whether any become standard practice—even among academic centers interested in this issue—remains to be seen.

Does idiopathic RBD represent an early neurodegenerative disease in all patients?

The answer to this question is certainly "no." There are many other medical conditions that have been associated with RBD, and some of these may be etiologically related. Certain medications, particularly some of the selective serotonin reuptake inhibitors (SSRIs) and selective noradrenergic reuptake inhibitors (SNRIs) appear to increase EMG tone during REM sleep and may also precipitate or aggravate RBD.[47,48] While it may seem reasonable to presume that anyone with RBD who has no other known medical condition associated with RBD and does not take SSRIs or SNRIs is most likely to have an underlying evolving neurodegenerative disorder, this is purely speculative at this point. It is also important to again note that a 10–20 year history of RBD has been associated with otherwise asymptomatic LBD,[115,116] so even in the setting of RBD representing a manifestation of an early neurodegenerative disorder, not all such patients will experience changes in motor or cognitive functioning during their lifetime.

The RBD–SSRI/SNRI association raises other questions. Why do some individuals using a medication in either of these classes appear to develop RBD features, while millions of individuals take one of these medications and do not develop RBD features? Are some of the SSRI and SNRI medications actually "unmasking" RBD that would have evolved months or years later had they not used these medications? This issue is worthy of further study.

How should clinicians discuss the RBD-neurodegenerative disease association with iRBD patients?

Some experts believe there is insufficient evidence to conclude that most individuals with iRBD have an evolving neurodegenerative disorder, and even among those who are exhibiting RBD due to underlying LBD, not all such patients subsequently exhibit parkinsonism or dementia despite 10–20 years of RBD features.[115,116] Thus, the feeling is that discussing iRBD as a possible risk factor for a neurodegenerative disorder, particularly in an era when no therapy exists, is not appropriate and no discussion is warranted, as only undue anxiety would result.

Other experts feel that there is sufficient evidence to warrant discussion with iRBD patients (and sometimes with their spouses) about the RBD–neurodegenerative disease association, with the timing of such a discussion dependent on the circumstances of the situation—if the patient resides near the center where the diagnosis was made and longitudinal follow-up is planned, then this discussion can occur at some point along the course of follow-up. This author views the RBD–neurodegenerative disease association similar to an autosomal dominant mutation with incomplete penetrance, with the big unknowns being if and when any other signs of a neurodegenerative disorder could become manifest.

Clinicians should also be mindful of the internet-savvy nature of most of the public, whereby newly-diagnosed patients with iRBD are very likely to search on "RBD," "REM behavior disorder," or "REM sleep behavior disorder," leading to acute anxiety about the information on various websites concerning increased future risk of PD or dementia. Such individuals may become angry with their physician for not sharing this information with them at the time of diagnosis. Moreover, many highly educated middle-aged males read about this association and attempt to contact experts in the RBD field, which is certainly understandable as they are seeking medication and nonmedication approaches to stave off parkinsonism and dementia.

This author tends to discuss this issue briefly at the time of diagnosis, and in more detail over subsequent visits, again depending on the circumstances with each individual patient. It may be prudent for sleep medicine clinicians, neurologists, and psychiatrists to consult with their medical genetics colleagues for further advice on discussing this important issue with patients.

What is the specificity of RBD for the synucleinopathies?

Whenever a hypothesis is proposed, it warrants scientific scrutiny from several groups of investigators to test the hypothesis and ultimately support it, refute it, or refine/qualify it. This has appropriately occurred in the RBD field, particularly testing the hypothesis that RBD associated with neurodegenerative disease usually reflects an underlying synucleinopathy.[82] The roots of this hypothesis were based on the wealth of clinical and clinicopathologic studies available as of 2001 and continued observation of how frequently RBD has been associated with PD, DLB, and MSA particularly and the more rare association of RBD with AD, PSP, SCA-3, Guadeloupean parkinsonism, and Huntington's disease. RBD has not been reported in association with several other neurodegenerative disorders. Most of the studies published since the original hypothesis have involved clinically and/or genetically diagnosed patients, and the gold standard for almost any study in neurodegenerative disease research requires gross and microscopic analyses of tissue, with the latter analyses being done using appropriate routine and immunocytochemical staining techniques. This latter point has been emphasized in the setting of parkinsonism-associated mutations in the leucine-rich repeat kinase 2 (*LRRK2*) gene, in which pleomorphic pathology has been found: Lewy body Parkinson's disease, diffuse LBD, nigral degeneration without distinctive histopathology, and PSP-like pathology.[170] In other words, analyses involving patients with RBD during life are clearly important, but neuropathologic examination is crucial to assessing the RBD-proteinopathy and RBD-pathophysiology mechanisms.

While our own ongoing clinicopathologic experience as reviewed above has shown an overwhelming tendency for RBD to be associated with the disorders collectively termed the synucleinopathies, our own data have also revealed one case of PSP and one case of AD with RBD. Thus, RBD is not 100% specific for the synucleinopathies, nor did we ever expect it to be, given the known variability in humans. Yet the tendency for RBD to occur frequently in the synucleinopathies and infrequently in the non-synucleinopathies suggests that the selective vulnerability of key brain-stem networks involved in RBD pathophysiology in the synucleinopathies is relatively consistent, and these same brain-stem networks tend not to be similarly affected in the non-synucleinopathies. Furthermore, when RBD precedes the onset of parkinsonism and/or cognitive impairment by several years, the literature would suggest that such cases are much more likely to represent an evolving synucleinopathy, whereas RBD evolving concurrently with or after the onset of parkinsonism and/or cognitive impairment has occurred more frequently in the nonsynucleinopathy disorders. Moreover, some of these nonsynucleinopathy cases appeared to have been diagnosed more on the basis of the PSG, with a rather minimal history of dream enactment behavior. Hence, not only may the presence of RBD be important to the specificity of RBD to which neurodegenerative disease process is at play, but the timing of RBD onset as well as frequency and severity of dream enactment behavior also appear to have relevance. These issues should be studied with more rigor.

What are the implications of the evolution of RBD and other clinical features in the PD- and Dementia with Lewy bodies-predominant phenotypes on the topography of degeneration in Lewy body disease?

A clinical feature or sign in neurodegenerative disease reflects sufficient neuronal/glial/neurotransmitter dysfunction in a critical neuronal network. While some of these features or signs have known or suspected networks of dysfunction, the underlying substrate for other features or signs is less clear. Parkinsonism most likely is associated with dopaminergic depletion due to sufficient degeneration in the nigrostriatal system, and cognitive impairment is likely associated, at least in part, with cholinergic depletion due to basal forebrain/limbic system/neocortex degeneration. It is highly likely that RBD reflects sufficient degeneration in brain-stem networks as described above. The underlying

pathobiology of visual hallucinations in DLB and PDD and fluctuations in cognition/arousal in DLB is not well understood, but these tend to be features that evolve well after the onset of cognitive impairment and parkinsonism in DLB and PDD.[80,171]

Along this same line of reasoning, the evolution of clinical features must reflect the topography of degeneration over time. Many patients with DLB tend to experience RBD prior to cognitive impairment, with subsequent development of parkinsonism. This evolution suggests that dysfunction in the pontomedullary circuitry precedes dysfunction in the basal forebrain, limbic system, and neocortical circuitry as well dysfunction in the nigrostratial circuitry. One could argue, as others recently have,[172] that this evolution of features and presumed pathophysiologic basis does not support the Braak staging scheme of PD, yet it may provide some clues into LBD pathoanatomy of the DLB phenotype.

There are several aspects to consider. The Braak staging system was indeed proposed for LBD as it relates to the phenotype and evolution of signs in PD and not DLB.[120,121] Many investigators have viewed this staging system to be quite consistent with the usual evolution of features in PD, where RBD and anosmia occur prior to parkinsonism with subsequent development of dementia, visual hallucinations, and delusions. In other words, a "bottom-to-top" or ascending progression of Lewy neurites, Lewy bodies, and neuronal degeneration as proposed in Stages 1–6 of the Braak scheme explains the evolution of features in typical PD quite well.[120,121] A similar evolution of degenerative changes may occur in both PD and DLB, and the timing of clinical features may reflect when the critical thresholds of neuronal network degeneration are reached. Neurons with Lewy bodies and/or Lewy neurites may reflect diseased/dysfunctional neurons, but clinical manifestations do not evolve until a sufficient threshold of degeneration has occurred. For example, if an 80% depletion of dopaminergic neurons is needed to manifest parkinsonism, and a 50% depletion of cholinergic neurons is needed to manifest cognitive impairment, it would be reasonable to suggest a "bottom-to-top" progression of LBD pathology could still explain the onset of cognitive symptoms prior to parkinsonism if both systems are affected gradually over years but the thresholds for the expression of clinical deficits are different such that cognitive impairment becomes evident prior to parkinsonism. In other words, the evolution of features in the DLB phenotype does not necessarily refute the Braak staging system for LBD progression.

Another explanation is that, at least in some cases, a "top-to-bottom" or descending progression of degenerative changes from the neocortex/limbic system to the nigrostriatal system may better explain the onset of cognitive impairment prior to parkinsonism in many DLB cases. Or a more patchy and discontinuous evolution of progression could evolve. Most cases of evolving AD develop amnestic MCI with subsequent development of language, attention/executive, and visuospatial dysfunction tend to follow the Braak stages of neurofibrillary tangle deposition, but there are certainly cases of atypical AD (which tend to have "hippocampal sparing AD" pathology) that have presented as focal cortical syndromes such as progressive aphasia,[173] corticobasal syndrome,[174] or posterior cortical atrophy[175] with relative preservation of memory and who clearly did not have neurofibrillary tangle deposition evolve in the typical manner of AD. Therefore, there will always be exceptions to any model of neurodegenerative disease progression, and surely LBD will evolve in more than one manner.

Yet if the majority of cases in any disease evolve in a relatively consistent fashion, this suggests common dysfunctional mechanisms of system biology. RBD may present years or decades prior to the onset of cognitive impairment in patients diagnosed with DLB or PD. This finding supports the bottom-to-top progression with variations in the relative degree of degeneration in critical structures. One therefore could predict that in DLB and PDD, visual hallucinations, and fluctuations would be caused by sufficient degeneration and/or neurochemical dysfunction in the diencephalon and telencephalon, or at least a diffuse topography of degeneration/dysfunction. More work in understanding the hallucinatory and fluctuating phenomenology as well as sleep–wake mechanisms is necessary before the underlying substrates of visual hallucinations and fluctuations are known.

How should clinicopathologic studies be performed in patients with RBD?

It is imperative to plan for autopsy in any willing individual with iRBD as well as those with RBD associated with any neurodegenerative disease. Ide-

ally, performing detailed histologic examinations in those who had PSG-proven RBD and those who had no history of RBD-like behavior and had PSG confirming normal EMG atonia during REM sleep will be most informative.

There are many challenges to studying tissue to determine which populations of neurons and/or glia are critical to RBD pathophysiology. Whether the brain-stem networks involve the nuclei proposed in the RBD pathophysiology scheme as shown in Figures 2 and 3, or others in combination with these nuclei, or other nuclei completely different from those proposed, needs to be examined. Stereologic studies involving neuronal count quantification, while certainly very laborious, are likely to be informative. Yet some of the brain-stem nuclei have unclear borders, or they span a convoluted area of tissue, which complicates the technical aspects of quantifying multiple nuclei.

Implications of "idiopathic" RBD for future drug trials in the synucleinopathies

As noted above, RBD tends to precede the onset of parkinsonism or dementia in patients with MSA, PD, and DLB by years or decades.[1,17,22,63,65,81,82,84,91,92,109,114,176,177] Almost 40% of patients with iRBD in one series were subsequently found to have developed a parkinsonian disorder,[114] and continued follow-up of this cohort has shown approximately 65% have now developed parkinsonism and/or cognitive impairment.[29] RBD preceded dementia and/or parkinsonism in 67% of another series,[84] and preceded the onset of cognitive impairment in autopsy-proven LBD by a median of 10 years.[138] The prospectively followed cohorts by Iranzo and colleagues and Postuma and colleagues are particularly important.[26,80] Therefore, iRBD may represent the harbinger of an evolving neurodegenerative disorder, which in most cases may be a synucleinopathy.[1,3,24,26,76,80,84,110,117–119]

Thus, if iRBD is the earliest clinical manifestation of an evolving neurodegenerative disorder, the presence of RBD may be particularly relevant early in the course of a neurodegenerative disease when intervention may be most critical. Agents that may positively affect synucleinopathy pathophysiology could be instituted in patients with appropriately identified iRBD and potentially delay or prevent the development of cognitive impairment or

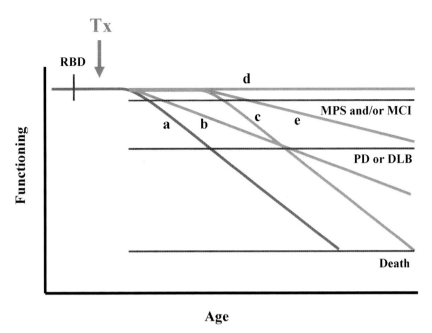

Figure 9. Schematic representation of the hypothesized progression in functioning with increasing age and disease severity in evolving Lewy body disease (LBD) in the Parkinson's disease (PD)– and dementia with Lewy bodies (DLB)–predominant phenotypes, and the potential effect of therapy. The onset of REM sleep behavior disorder (RBD) typically begins many years prior to the onset of cognitive decline and a diagnosis of mild cognitive impairment (MCI) and/or many years prior to the onset of motor decline and detectable mild parkinsonian signs (MPS). Progression typically continues over subsequent years to either PD or DLB, and ultimately on to death. This evolution of progression in the current era of primarily symptomatic treatments, with no agent convincingly showing altered progression in the underlying disease process of LBD, is depicted by the red line marked "a." One could envision at least four potential effects of a synucleinopathy-active therapy (labeled "Tx" and instituted along the time course as shown by the orange arrow) in patients with appropriately identified "idiopathic" RBD. The agent could slow down the rate of progression (as shown by the green line marked "b"), delay the onset of cognitive and/or motor decline (as shown by the green line marked "c"), or prevent progression to cognitive and motor decline altogether (as shown by the green line marked "d"). Or, perhaps a synucleinopathy-active therapy could delay the onset of symptoms and slow down the rate of progression (as shown by the green line marked "e").

parkinsonism (see Fig. 9 and accompanying legend). This is an exciting avenue for future drug therapy, but considerable work is still necessary to identify patients with iRBD, develop biomarkers and predictors of those with an underlying synucleinopathy, and study the natural history of patients with iRBD so that eventual clinical trials can be powered to the estimated effect sizes of therapies.

A proposed decision tree

A proposed decision tree for assessing patients with iRBD could be formulated somewhat like that presented in Figure 10. One would first seek to determine in individual patients who is manifesting features of an early neurodegenerative disor-

der and who is not (Step 1). Perhaps many of the clinical features and ancillary test findings discussed in this review, and hopefully many others yet to be identified and developed, will function as accurate biomarkers. Next, if the biomarkers are sufficiently specific to pinpoint the underlying proteinopathy (i.e., synucleinopathy versus non-synucleinopathy), then such biomarkers will function in Steps 1 and 2; if not, new biomarkers with adequate sensitivity and specificity for proteinopathies and particularly synucleinopathies will need to be developed. Finally, it remains to be seen if agents that ultimately affect synucleinopathy pathophysiology will be safe and efficacious in all of the synucleinopathies regardless of whether

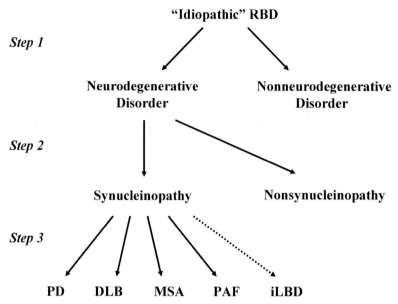

Figure 10. Proposed decision tree for assessing patients with "idiopathic" RBD for research and ultimately treatment purposes. Presuming that one of the ultimate goals of identifying patients with apparently "idiopathic" RBD is to commence one or more therapies that could delay the onset of cognitive impairment and/or parkinsonism or slow down the course or halt progression of an underlying neurodegenerative disorder altogether, one would first seek to determine in individual patients who is manifesting features of an early neurodegenerative disorder and who is not (Step 1). Perhaps many of the clinical features and ancillary test findings covered in this review, and hopefully many others yet to be developed, will function as accurate biomarkers. Next, if the biomarkers are sufficiently specific to pinpoint the underlying proteinopathy (i.e., synucleinopathy vs. nonsynucleinopathy), then such biomarkers will function in Steps 1 and 2; if not, new biomarkers with adequate sensitivity and specificity for proteinopathies and particularly synucleinopathies will need to be developed. Finally, it remains to be seen if agents that ultimately affect synucleinopathy pathophysiology will be safe and efficacious in all of the synucleinopathies regardless of whether the pathologic process is LBD or MSA, or the phenotype is PD-predominant, DLB-predominant, MSA-predominant, or PAF-predominant. Incidental LBD (iLBD) will be impossible to predict without pathology. The challenge for investigators at present is to study adequate numbers of patients with "idiopathic" RBD with a spectrum of clinical tests and potential biomarkers longitudinally to assess the natural history and prepare for future clinical trials. Abbreviations: DLB, dementia with Lewy bodies; MSA, multiple system atrophy; PAF, pure autonomic failure; PD, Parkinson's disease; RBD, REM sleep behavior disorder.

the pathologic process is LBD or MSA, or the phenotype is PD-predominant, DLB-predominant, MSA-predominant, or PAF-predominant.

Biomarkers

The term *biomarker* is used very loosely in this context and is meant to include any clinical feature or finding and any finding on a diagnostic test that may indicate a particular disorder or disease state. A list of potential biomarkers that have been or could be studied in patients with iRBD is shown in Figure 11. (Note that this author emphasizes the many esteemed members of the International RBD Study Group [Chair: Prof. Dr. med. Wolfgang Oer-tel], who have used and studied many of these biomarkers or are proposing to use and study these biomarkers, deserve the credit for moving the RBD field forward on biomarker research.) This is clearly a partial list of potential biomarkers, which will surely be expanded upon over the years to come.

Based on the published data for certain biomarkers in specific phenotypes and disorders, as well as the findings that are suspected despite the lack of published data, one could propose a profile of abnormalities on various biomarkers in patients with iRBD resulting from an underlying synucleinopathy (Fig. 12). The phenotypes and diseases include PD, DLB, MSA, PAF, and incidental LBD

Clinical
Mini-Mental State Exam (MMSE)
Unified Parkinson's Disease Rating
    Scale (UPDRS)
Other measures of motor functioning
Olfaction
Color vision
Epworth Sleepiness Scale (ESS)

Neuropsychological
Battery with core measures across
    all cognitive domains

Blood
Beta amyloid
Many other proteins
Genotyping

CSF
α-synuclein
Beta amyloid
Total tau and phospho-tau
Many other proteins

Electrophysiologic
EEG spectral analyses
PSG with EMG and EEG analyses
Multiple Sleep Latency Test (MSLT)
Maintenance of Wakefulness Test (MWT)

Autonomic
Autonomic reflex screen (ARS)
Thermoregulatory sweat test (TST)

Imaging
Magnetic resonance imaging (MRI)
Magnetic resonance spectroscopy (MRS)
Positron emission tomography (PET)
    - fluorodeoxyglucose (FDG)
    - many others focused on dopamine ligands
Single photon emission computed tomography (SPECT)
    - dopamine transporter (DaT or DaTSCAN)
Cardiac (123)I-metaiodobenzylguanidine (MIBG)

Figure 11. List of potential biomarkers to study in patients with idiopathic RBD.

Phenotype/ Disorder	Cog	Motor	Smell	Aut	MRI/MRS	DaT	PET	MIBG
iLBD	Nl	Nl	+/-	+/-	Nl	+/-	Nl	Abnl
PD	Nl	Abnl*	Abnl	Abnl	Nl	Abnl	Nl	Abnl
DLB	Abnl*	Abnl*	Abnl	Abnl	Abnl*	Abnl	Abnl*	Abnl
MSA	Nl	Abnl*	Nl	Abnl	Nl	Abnl	Nl	Nl
PAF	Nl	Nl	Nl	Abnl	Nl	Nl	Nl	Nl

Figure 12. Hypothesized profile of abnormalities on various biomarkers in patients with iRBD resulting from an underlying synucleinopathy. The phenotypes/diseases include incidental Lewy body disease (iLBD), Parkinson's disease (PD), dementia with Lewy bodies (DLB), multiple system atrophy (MSA), and pure autonomic failure (PAF). One would predict a different pattern of normal (Nl) and abnormal (Abnl) findings based on the biomarkers being performed, with some results more difficult to predict (represented by "+/−"). Some abnormal findings may be particularly suggestive of specific phenotypes/disorders (represented by an asterisk). Abbreviations: Cog, cognitive/neuropsychological testing; Aut, autonomic studies; MRI, magnetic resonance imaging; MRS, magnetic resonance spectroscopy; DaT, DaTSCAN; PET, positron emission tomography of the brain using various ligands; MIBG, Cardiac (123)I-metaiodobenzylguanidine imaging.

Phenotype/ Disorder	Cog	Motor	Smell	Aut	MRI/MRS	DaT	PET	MIBG
AD	Abnl*	Nl	+/-	Nl	Abnl-AD*	Nl	Abnl-AD*	Nl
Tauopathy	+/-	+/-	Nl	Nl	Abnl-FTLD*	+/-	Abnl-FTLD*	Nl
TDP-43opathy	Abnl	+/-	Nl	Nl	Abnl-FTLD*	+/-	Abnl-FTLD*	Nl
All others	+/-	+/-	Nl	Nl	Nl	+/-	+/-	Nl

Figure 13. Hypothesized profile of abnormalities on various biomarkers in patients with iRBD resulting from an underlying nonsynucleinopathy neurodegenerative disorder. The phenotypes/diseases include Alzheimer's disease (AD), one of the tauopathies (Pick's disease, corticobasal degeneration, progressive supranuclear palsy, multisystem tauopathy, or frontotemporal dementa with parkinsonism associated with a mutation in the microtubule associated protein tau), or one of the TDP-43-associated pathologies (frontotemporal lobar degeneration [FTLD] with TDP-43 positive inclusions, FTLD with motor neuron disease, or FTLD with a mutation in progranulin). One would predict a different pattern of normal (Nl) and abnormal (Abnl) findings based on the biomarkers being performed, with some results more difficult to predict (represented by "+/−"). Some abnormal findings may be particularly suggestive of specific phenotypes/disorders (represented by an asterisk). Abbreviations: Cog, cognitive/neuropsychological testing; Aut, autonomic studies; MRI, magnetic resonance imaging; MRS, magnetic resonance spectroscopy; DaT, DaTSCAN; PET, positron emission tomography of the brain using various ligands; MIBG, Cardiac (123)I-metaiodobenzylguanidine imaging.

(iLBD), which is the term applied to those individuals who have no obvious neurologic impairment but have LBD found at autopsy. One would predict a different pattern of normal (Nl) and abnormal (Abnl) findings based on the biomarkers being used. Some results are more difficult to predict, such as whether any abnormalities on smell testing, autonomic testing, and dopamine transporter scan using ioflupane (DaTSCAN) would occur in iLBD. Also, some abnormal findings may be particularly suggestive of specific phenotypes/disorders, such as the neuropsychological profile of impairment in DLB.

A different profile of abnormalities on various biomarkers in patients with iRBD resulting from an underlying nonsynucleinopathy degenerative disorder could also be predicted, as shown in Fig. 13. Normal findings would be expected on smell testing (despite the literature on olfaction being impaired early in AD, it now appears many of these patients have co-existing Lewy body disease).[178,179] The findings on neuropsychological testing, MRI, MRS, and FDG-PET are distinctly different between Alzheimer's disease, the tauopathies, and the TDP-43opathies, and these findings are also qualitatively

different from DLB and PDD. As described above, cardiac MIBG is typically normal in disorders outside of the PD-PDD-DLB-PAF spectrum. Findings on DaTSCAN tend to be normal in AD, but it remains to be seen if findings are typically abnormal in PSP and CBD, as few such cases with DaTSCAN performed antemortem have undergone autopsy.

The challenges

The challenge for basic scientists is to develop therapies that impact the cascade of events involved in synucleinopathy and other neurodegenerative disorder pathophysiologies. The challenge for clinical investigators at present is to study adequate numbers of patients with "idiopathic" RBD longitudinally with a spectrum of clinical tests and potential biomarkers to assess the natural history of the current state with no truly disease-altering therapies, and prepare for future clinical trials. The hurdles are even more challenging when one considers that the funding cycles for most federal and private funding institutions run over 5-year periods, while the unique work of Postuma and colleagues suggests that only 50% of those with iRBD develop parkinsonism and/or dementia within 12 years. This is a core "nature of the beast" in this line of research—LBD appears to evolve slowly over several decades in many individuals—but this cannot thwart our attempts to plan for disease-altering therapies. Yet it is extremely important to realize for therapeutic advances—a minor effect on pathophysiology early in the disease course in a process that evolves over decades could potentially delay or alter the clinical manifestations by many years such that morbidity or mortality could occur outside of the neurodegenerative realm. Securing funding to plan for future therapeutic trials will require ingenuity by investigators, a large investment in infrastructure and biomarker technologies, and frank optimism on the part of funding agencies, but surely most would agree that the literature amply suggests that the scientific basis for this line of future research is sound.

The optimism

It is difficult to envision the heightened optimism even a decade ago in the potential of impacting a neurodegenerative process early in its course. Idiopathic RBD is one of the more intriguing clinical curiosities in medicine, and certainly in sleep medicine and neurology. Idiopathic RBD likely represents a window of opportunity for impacting neurodegenerative disease like few other disorders, particularly among the apparent sporadic cases. The scientific community should educate the public on the importance of early diagnosis and treatment of RBD (being ever mindful of the anxiety over what the disorder may represent) and follow iRBD longitudinally with a battery of clinical assessments and potential biomarkers, while we await agents that impact neurodegenerative disease pathophysiology.

Acknowledgments

Supported by grants AG 15866, AG 16574, AG 06786, and P50 NS40256 and the Robert H. and Clarice Smith and Abigail Van Buren Alzheimer's Disease Research Program of the Mayo Foundation.

Conflicts of interest

My only disclosures are grant support from Myriad Pharmaceuticals for a clinical trial and an honorarium from GE Healthcare.

References

1. Schenck, C. & M. Mahowald. 2002. REM sleep behavior disorder: Clinical, developmental, and neuroscience perspectives 16 years after its formal identification in SLEEP. *Sleep* **25:** 120–138.

2. Schenck, C. 2005. Paradox Lost – Midnight in the Battleground of Sleep and Dreams – Violent Moving Nightmares, REM Sleep Behavior Disorder. Extreme-Nights, LLC.

3. Boeve, B., M. Silber, C. Saper, *et al.* 2007. Pathophysiology of REM sleep behaviour disorder and relevance to neurodegenerative disease. *Brain* **130:** 2770–2788.

4. Iber, C., S. Ancoli-Israel, A. Chesson, S. Quan for the for the American Academy of Sleep Medicine. 2007. The AASM manual for the scoring of sleep and associated events: rules, terminology and technical specifications. American Academy of Sleep Medicine. Chicago, IL.

5. Iranzo, A. & J. Santamaria. 2005. Severe obstructive sleep apnea/hypopnea mimicking REM sleep behavior disorder. *Sleep* **28:** 203–206.

6. Schenck, C., D. Milner, T. Hurwitz, *et al.* 1989. A polysomnographic and clinical report on sleep-related injury in 100 adult patients. *Amer. J. Psychiatr.* **146:** 1166–1173.

7. Kimura, K., N. Tachibana, A. Toshihiko, *et al.* 1997. Subclinical REM sleep behavior disorder in a patient with corticobasal degeneration. *Sleep* **20:** 891–894.

8. Pareja, J., A. Caminero, J. Masa & J. Dobato. 1996. A first case of progressive supranuclear pasy and pre-clinical REM sleep behavior disorder presenting as inhibition of speech during wakefulness and somniloquy with phasic muscle twitching during REM sleep. *Neurologia* **11:** 304–306.

9. Schenck, C.H., S.R. Bundlie, M.G. Ettinger & M.W. Mahowald. 1986. Chronic behavioral disorders of human REM sleep: a new category of parasomnia. *Sleep* **9:** 293–308.

10. Schenck, C.H., S.R. Bundlie, A.L. Patterson & M.W. Mahowald. 1987. Rapid eye movement sleep behavior disorder. A treatable parasomnia affecting older adults. *JAMA* **257:** 1786–1789.

11. Schenck, C.H., D.M. Milner, T.D. Hurwitz, *et al.* 1989. A polysomnographic and clinical report on sleep-related injury in 100 adult patients. *Amer. J. Psychiatry* **146:** 1166–1173.

12. Schenck, C. & M. Mahowald. 1990. A polysomnographic, neurologic, psychiatric and clinical outcome report on 70 consecutive cases with REM sleep behavior

disorder (RBD): sustained clonzepam efficacy in 89.5% of 57 treated patients. *Clev. Clin. J. Med.* **57**(suppl): 10–24.

13. Schenck, C., T. Hurwitz & M. Mahowald. 1993. REM sleep behaviour disorder: an update on a series of 96 patients and a review of the world literature. *J. Sleep Res.* **2:** 224–231.

14. Schenck, C.H. & M.W. Mahowald. 1996. Long-term, nightly benzodiazepine treatment of injurious parasomnias and other disorders of disrupted nocturnal sleep in 170 adults. *Amer. J. Med.* **100:** 333–337.

15. Schenck, C.H. & M.W. Mahowald. 1996. REM sleep parasomnias. *Neurologic Clinics* **14:** 697–720.

16. Gross, P. 1992. REM sleep behavior disorder causing bilateral subdural hematomas. *Sleep Res.* **21:** 204.

17. Boeve, B.F., M.H. Silber, T.J. Ferman, *et al.* 1998. REM sleep behavior disorder and degenerative dementia: an association likely reflecting Lewy body disease. *Neurology* **51:** 363–370.

18. Mahowald, M. & C. Schenck. 2000. REM sleep behavior disorder. In *Principles and Practice of Sleep Medicine.* Kryger, M., T. Roth & W. Dement, Eds.: 724–741. WB Saunders. Philadelphia.

19. Dyken, M., D. Lin-Dyken, P. Seaba & T. Yamada. 1995. Violent sleep-related behavior leading to subdural hemorrhage. *Arch. Neurol.* **52:** 318–321.

20. Sforza, E., J. Krieger & C. Petiau. 1997. REM sleep behavior disorder: clinical and physiopathological findings. *Sleep Med. Rev.* **1:** 57–69.

21. Comella, C., T. Nardine, N. Diederich & G. Stebbins. 1998. Sleep-related violence, injury, and REM sleep behavior disorder in Parkinson's disease. *Neurology* **51:** 526–529.

22. Olson, E., B. Boeve & M. Silber. 2000. Rapid eye movement sleep behavior disorder: demographic, clinical, and laboratory findings in 93 cases. *Brain* **123:** 331–339.

23. Gagnon, J.-F., M.-A. Medard, M. Fantini, *et al.* 2002. REM sleep behavior disorder and REM sleep without atonia in Parkinson's disease. *Neurology* **59:** 585–589.

24. Turner, R.S. 2002. Idiopathic rapid eye movement sleep behavior disorder is a harbinger of dementia with Lewy bodies. *J. Geriatr. Psychiatr. Neurol.* **15:** 195–199.

25. Iranzo, A., J. Santamaria, D.B. Rye, *et al.* 2005. Characteristics of idiopathic REM sleep behavior disorder and that associated with MSA and PD. *Neurology* **65:** 247–252.

26. Iranzo, A., J. Molinuevo, J. Santamaría, *et al.* 2006. Rapid-eye-movement sleep behaviour disorder as an early marker for a neurodegenerative disorder: a descriptive study. *Lancet Neurol.* **5:** 572–577.

27. Boeve, B., M. Silber, T. Ferman, *et al.* 2003. REM sleep behavior disorder in Parkinson's disease, dementia with lewy bodies, and multiple system atrophy. In *Mental and Behavioral Dysfunction in Movement Disorders.* Bedard, M., et al., Eds.: 383–397. Humana Press. Totowa.

28. Claassen, D., K. Josephs, J. Ahlskog, *et al.* 2009. REM sleep behavior disorder may precede PD, DLB, or MSA by up to half a century. *Neurology* **72**(Suppl 3): A324.

29. Schenck, C., S. Bundlie & M. Mahowald. 2003. REM behavior disorder (RBD): Delayed emergence of parkinsonism and/or dementia in 65% of older men initially diagnosed with idiopathic RBD, and an analysis of the minimum & maximum tonic and/or phasic electromyographic abnormalities found during REM sleep. *Sleep* **26:** A316.

30. Tang, J., B. Boeve, M. Tippmann-Peikert & M. Silber. 2009. Gender effect in patients with REM sleep behavior disorder associated with multiple system atrophy compared with Parkinson's disease and dementia with Lewy bodies. *Neurology* **72**(Suppl 3): A325.

31. Ohayon, M., M. Caulet & R. Priest. 1997. Violent behavior during sleep. *J. Clin. Psychiatr.* **58:** 369–376.

32. Molano, J., B. Boeve, R. Roberts, *et al.* 2009. Frequency of sleep disorders in the community-dwelling elderly: The Mayo Clinic Study of Aging. *Neurology* **72**(Suppl 3): A107.

33. Boeve, B., J. Molano, T. Ferman, *et al.* 2009. Screening for REM sleep behavior disorder in patients with cognitive impairment and/or parkinsonism: Updated validation data on the Mayo Sleep Questionnaire. *Neurology* **72:** A248.

34. Mihci, E., J. Molano, B. Boeve, *et al.* 2008. Parkinsonism is associated with probable REM sleep behavior disorder in cognitively normal elderly subjects: The Mayo Clinic Study of Aging. *Neurology* **70**(Suppl 1): A150.

35. Molano, J., E. Mihci, B. Boeve, *et al.* 2008. Anxiety and apathy are associated with probable REM sleep behavior disorder among cognitively normal elderly subjects: The Mayo Clinic Study of Aging. *Neurology* **70**(Suppl 1): A146.

36. Molano, J., E. Mihci, B. Boeve, *et al.* 2008. Lower scores in attention/executive functioning is associated with probable REM sleep behavior disorder among cognitively normal elderly subjects: The Mayo Clinic Study of Aging. *Neurology* **70**(Suppl 1): A66.

37. *International Classification of Sleep Disorders: Diagnostic and Coding Manual,* 2005, 2nd edn. American Academy of Sleep Medicine. Westchester, IL.

38. Silber, M., S. Ancoli-Israel, M. Bonnet, *et al*. 2007. The visual scoring of sleep in adults. *J. Clin. Sleep Med*. **15:** 121–131.

39. Redline, S., R. Budhiraja, V. Kapur, *et al*. 2007. The scoring of respiratory events in sleep: reliability and validity. *J. Clin. Sleep Med*. **15:** 169–200.

40. Kunz, D. & F. Bes. 1999. Melatonin as a therapy in REM sleep behavior disorder patients: An open-labeled pilot study on the possible influence of melatonin on REM-sleep regulation. *Mov. Disord*. **14:** 507–511.

41. Boeve, B., M. Silber & T. Ferman. 2003. Melatonin for treatment of REM sleep behavior disorder in neurologic disorders: results in 14 patients. *Sleep Med*. **4:** 281–284.

42. Gagnon, J., R. Postuma & J. Montplaisir. 2006. Update on the pharmacology of REM sleep behavior disorder. *Neurology* **67:** 742–747.

43. Fantini, M., J.-F. Gagnon, D. Filipini & J. Montplaisir. 2003. The effects of pramipexole in REM sleep behavior disorder. *Neurology* **61:** 1418–1420.

44. Ringman, J. & J. Simmons. 2000. Treatment of REM sleep behavior disorder with donepezil: a report of three cases. *Neurology* **55:** 870–871.

45. Rye, D. 1997. Contributions of the pedunculopontine region to normal and altered REM sleep. *Sleep* **20:** 757–788.

46. Bamford, C. 1993. Carbamazepine in REM sleep behavior disorder. *Sleep* **16:** 33–34.

47. Onofrj, M., A.L. Luciano, A. Thomas, *et al*. 2003. Mirtazapine induces REM sleep behavior disorder (RBD) in parkinsonism. *Neurology* **60:** 113–115.

48. Winkelman, J. & L. James. 2004. Serotonergic antidepressants are associated with REM sleep without atonia. *Sleep* **15:** 317–321.

49. Hendricks, J., A. Morrison & G. Mann. 1982. Different behaviors during paradoxical sleep without atonia depend on pontine lesion site. *Brain. Res*. **239:** 81–105.

50. Jouvet, M. & F. Delorme. 1965. Locus coeruleus et sommeil paradoxal. *C. R. Soc. Biol*. **159:** 895–899.

51. Lai, Y. & J. Siegel. 1988. Medullary regions mediating atonia. *J. Neurosci*. **8:** 4790–4796.

52. Lai, Y. & J. Siegel. 1990. Muscle tone suppression and stepping produced by stimulation of midbrain and rostral pontine reticular formation. *J. Neurosci*. **10:** 2727–2734.

53. Lai, Y. & J. Siegel. 1997. Brainstem-mediated locomotion and myoclonic jerks. I. Neural substrates. *Brain Res*. **745:** 257–264.

54. Lai, Y. & J. Siegel. 1997. Brainstem-mediated locomtion and myoclonic jerks. II. Pharmacological effects. *Brain Res*. **745:** 265–270.

55. Morrison, A. 1998. The pathophysiology of REM-sleep behavior disorder. *Sleep* **21:** 446.

56. Rye, D. 1998. The pathophysiology of REM-sleep behavior disorder. *Sleep* **21:** 446–449.

57. Shouse, M. & J. Siegel. 1992. Pontine regulation of REM sleep components in cats: integrity of the pedunculopontine tegmentum (PPT) is important for phasic events but unnecessary for atonia during REM sleep. *Brain Res*. **571:** 50–63.

58. Mahowald, M.W. & C.H. Schenck. 2004. Rem sleep without atonia–from cats to humans. *Arch. Ital. Biol*. **142:** 469–478.

59. Siegel, J. 2006. The stuff dreams are made of: anatomical substrates of REM sleep. *Nat. Neurosci*. **9:** 721–722.

60. Lu, J., D. Sherman, M. Devor & C. Saper. 2006. A putative flip-flop switch for control of REM sleep. *Nature* **441:** 589–594.

61. Boissard, R., D. Gervasoni, M. Schmidt, *et al*. 2002. The rat ponto-medullary network responsible for paradoxical sleep onset and maintenance: a combined microinjection and functional neuroanatomical study. *Eur. J. Neurosci*. **16:** 1959–1973.

62. Boissard, E., P. Fort, D. Gervasoni, *et al*. 2003. Localization of the GABAergic and non-GABAergic neurons projecting to the sublaterodorsal nucleus and potentially gating paradoxical sleep onset. *Eur. J. Neurosci*. **18:** 1627–1639.

63. Silber, M. & J. Ahlskog. 1992. REM sleep behavior disorder in parkinsonian syndromes. *Sleep Res*. **21:** 313.

64. Silber, M., D. Dexter, J. Ahlskog, *et al*. 1993. Abnormal REM sleep motor activity in untreated Parkinson's disease. *Sleep Res*. **22:** 274.

65. Tan, A., M. Salgado & S. Fahn. 1996. Rapid eye movement sleep behavior disorder preceding Parkinson's disease with therapeutic response to levodopa. *Mov. Disord*. **11:** 214–216.

66. Rye, D., L. Johnston, R. Watts & D. Bliwise. 1999. Juvenile Parkinson's disease with REM sleep behavior disorder, sleepiness, and daytime REM onset. *Neurology* **53:** 1868–1872.

67. Arnulf, I., A.M. Bonnet, P. Damier, *et al*. 2000. Hallucinations, REM sleep, and Parkinson's disease: a medical hypothesis. *Neurology* **55:** 281–288.

68. Onofrj, M., A. Thomas, G. D'Andreamatteo, *et al*. 2002. Incidence of RBD and hallucination in patients affected by Parkinson's disease: 8-year follow-up. *Neurol. Sci*. **23:** S91-S94.

69. Onofrj, M., A.L. Luciano, D. Iacono, *et al*. 2003. HLA typing does not predict REM sleep behaviour disorder

and hallucinations in Parkinson's disease. *Mov. Disord.* **18:** 337–340.

70. Eisensehr, I., R. Linke, K. Tatsch, *et al.* 2003. Increased muscle activity during rapid eye movement sleep correlates with decrease of striatal presynaptic dopamine transporters. IPT and IBZM SPECT imaging in subclinical and clinically manifest idiopathic REM sleep behavior disorder, Parkinson's disease, and controls. *Sleep* **26:** 507–512.

71. Ozekmekci, S., H. Apaydin & E. Kilic. 2005. Clinical features of 35 patients with Parkinson's disease displaying REM behavior disorder. *Clin. Neurol. Neurosurg.* **107:** 306–309.

72. Pacchetti, C., R. Manni, R. Zangaglia, *et al.* 2005. Relationship between hallucinations, delusions, and rapid eye movement sleep behavior disorder in Parkinson's disease. *Mov. Disord.* **20:** 1439–1448.

73. Scaglione, C., L. Vignatelli, G. Plazzi, *et al.* 2005. REM sleep behaviour disorder in Parkinson's disease: a questionnaire-based study. *Neurol. Sci.* **25:** 316–321.

74. Hanoglu, L., F. Ozer, H. Meral & A. Dincer. 2006. Brainstem 1H-MR spectroscopy in patients with Parkinson's disease with REM sleep behavior disorder and IPD patients without dream enactment behavior. *Clin. Neurol. Neurosurg.* **108:** 129–134.

75. Sinforiani, E., R. Zangaglia, R. Manni, *et al.* 2006. REM sleep behavior disorder, hallucinations, and cognitive impairment in Parkinson's disease. *Mov. Disord.* **21:** 462–466.

76. Postuma, R., A. Lang, J. Massicotte-Marquez & J. Montplaisir. 2006. Potential early markers of Parkinson disease in idiopathic REM sleep behavior disorder. *Neurology* **66:** 845–851.

77. Gjerstad, M., B. Boeve, T. Wentzel-Larsen, *et al.* 2008. Occurrence and clinical correlates of REM sleep behavior disorder in patients with Parkinson's disease over time. *J. Neurol. Neurosurg. Psychiatry* **79:** 387–391.

78. Postuma, R., J. Gagnon, M. Vendette, *et al.* 2008. Manifestations of Parkinson disease differ in association with REM sleep behavior disorder. *Mov. Disord.* **23:** 1665–1672.

79. Postuma, R., J. Gagnon, M. Vendette, *et al.* 2008. REM sleep behaviour disorder in Parkinson's disease is associated with specific motor features. *J. Neurol. Neurosurg. Psychiatry* **79:** 1117–1121.

80. Postuma, R., J. Gagnon, M. Vendette, *et al.* 2009. Quantifying the risk of neurodegenerative disease in idiopathic REM sleep behavior disorder. *Neurology* **72:** 1296–1300.

81. Ferman, T.J., B.F. Boeve, G.E. Smith, *et al.* 1999. REM sleep behavior disorder and dementia: cognitive differences when compared with AD. *Neurology* **52:** 951–957.

82. Boeve, B., M. Silber, T. Ferman, *et al.* 2001. Association of REM sleep behavior disorder and neurodegenerative disease may reflect an underlying synucleinopathy. *Mov. Disord.* **16:** 622–630.

83. Ferman, T., B. Boeve, G. Smith, *et al.* 2002. Dementia with Lewy bodies may present as dementia with REM sleep behavior disorder without parkinsonism or hallucinations. *J. Internat. Neuropsychol. Soc.* **8:** 907–914.

84. Boeve, B., M. Silber, J. Parisi, *et al.* 2003. Synucleinopathy pathology and REM sleep behavior disorder plus dementia or parkinsonism. *Neurology* **61:** 40–45.

85. Massironi, G., S. Galluzzi & G. Frisoni. 2003. Drug treatment of REM sleep behavior disorders in dementia with Lewy bodies. *Int. Psychogeriatr.* **15:** 377–383.

86. Ferman, T., G. Smith, B. Boeve, *et al.* 2004. DLB fluctuations: Specific features that reliably differentiate DLB from AD and normal aging. *Neurology* **62:** 181–187.

87. Ferman, T., G. Smith, B. Boeve, *et al.* 2006. Neuropsychological differentiation of dementia with Lewy bodies from normal aging and Alzheimer's disease. *Clin. Neuropsychol.* **20.**

88. Plazzi, G., R. Corsini, F. Provini, *et al.* 1997. REM sleep behavior disorder in multiple system atrophy. *Neurology* **48:** 1094–1097.

89. Tachibana, N., K. Kimura, K. Kitajima, *et al.* 1997. REM sleep motor dysfunction in multiple system atrophy: with special emphasis on sleep talk as its early clinical manifestation. *J. Neurol. Neurosurg. Psychiatry* **63:** 678–681.

90. Quera Salva, M. & C. Guilleminault. 1986. Olivopontocerebellar degeneration, abnormal sleep, and REM sleep without atonia. *Neurology* **36:** 576–577.

91. Tison, F., G. Wenning, N. Quinn & S. Smith. 1995. REM sleep behavior disorder as the presenting symptom of multiple system atrophy. *J. Neurol. Neurosurg. Psychiatry* **58:** 379–380.

92. Wright, B., J. Rosen, D. Buysse, *et al.* 1990. Shy-Drager syndrome presenting as a REM behavioral disorder. *J. Geriatr. Psychiatry Neurol.* **3:** 110–113.

93. Manni, R., R. Morini, E. Martignoni, *et al.* 1993. Nocturnal sleep in multisystem atrophy with autonomic failure: polygraphic findings in ten patients. *J. Neurol.* **240:** 247–250.

94. Coccagna, G., P. Martinelli, M. Zucconi, *et al.* 1985. Sleep-related respiratory and haemodynamic changes

in Shy-Drager syndrome: a case report. *J. Neurol.* **232:** 310–313.

95. Tachibana, N. & Y. Oka. 2004. Longitudinal change in REM sleep components in a patient with multiple system atrophy associated with REM sleep behavior disorder: paradoxical improvement of nocturnal behaviors in a progressive neurodegenerative disease. *Sleep Med.* **5:** 155–158.

96. Vetrugno, R., F. Provini, P. Cortelli, *et al.* 2004. Sleep disorders in multiple system atrophy: a correlative video-polysomnographic study. *Sleep Med.* **5:** 21–30.

97. Schmeichel, A., L. Buchhalter, P. Low, *et al.* 2008. Mesopontine cholinergic neuron involvement in Lewy body dementia and multiple system atrophy. *Neurology* **70:** 368–373.

98. Gaig, C., A. Iranzo, E. Tolosa, *et al.* 2008. Pathological description of a non-motor variant of multiple system atrophy. *J. Neurol. Neurosurg. Psychiatry* **79:** 1399–1400.

99. Weyer, A., M. Minnerop, M. Abele & T. Klockgether. 2006. REM sleep behavioral disorder in pure autonomic failure (PAF). *Neurology* **66:** 608–609.

100. Kumru, H., J. Santamaria, E. Tolosa, *et al.* 2004. Rapid eye movement sleep behavior disorder in parkinsonism with parkin mutations. *Ann. Neurol.* **56:** 599–603.

101. Pramstaller, P., M. Schlossmacher, T. Jacques, *et al.* 2005. Lewy body Parkinson's disease in a large pedigree with 77 Parkin mutation carriers. *Ann. Neurol.* **58:** 411–422.

102. Fukutake, T., H. Shinotoh, H. Nishino, *et al.* 2002. Homozygous Machado-Joseph disease presenting as REM sleep behavior disorder and prominent psychiatric symptoms. *Eur. J. Neurol.* **9:** 97–100.

103. Friedman, J. 2002. Presumed rapid eye movement behavior disorder in Machado-Joseph disease (spinocerebellar ataxia type 3. *Mov. Disord.* **17:** 1350–1353.

104. Iranzo, A., E. Muñoz, J. Santamaria, *et al.* 2003. REM sleep behavior disorder and vocal cord paralysis in Machado-Joseph disease. *Mov. Disord.* **18:** 1179–1183.

105. Arnulf, I., J. Nielsen, E. Lohmann, *et al.* 2008. Rapid eye movement sleep disturbances in Huntington disease. *Arch. Neurol.* **65:** 482–488.

106. Arnulf, I., M. Merino-Andreu, F. Bloch, *et al.* 2005. REM sleep behavior disorder and REM sleep without atonia in patients with progressive supranuclear palsy. *Sleep* **28:** 349–354.

107. De Cock, V., A. Lannuzel, S. Verhaeghe, *et al.* 2007. REM sleep behavior disorder in patients with guadeloupean parkinsonism, a tauopathy. *Sleep* **30:** 1026–1032.

108. Schenck, C.H., E. Garcia-Rill, R.D. Skinner, *et al.* 1996. A case of REM sleep behavior disorder with autopsy-confirmed Alzheimer's disease: postmortem brain stem histochemical analyses. *Biol. Psychiatry* **40:** 422–425.

109. Schenck, C.H., M.W. Mahowald, M.L. Anderson, *et al.* 1997. Lewy body variant of Alzheimer's disease (AD) identified by postmortem ubiquitin staining in a previously reported case of AD associated with REM sleep behavior disorder [letter]. *Biol. Psychiatry* **42:** 527–528.

110. Gagnon, J.-F., R. Postuma, S. Mazza, *et al.* 2006. Rapid-eye-movement sleep behaviour disorder and neurodegenerative diseases. *Lancet Neurol.* **5:** 424–432.

111. Gagnon, J., D. Petit, M. Fantini, *et al.* 2006. REM sleep behavior disorder and REM sleep without atonia in probable Alzheimer disease. *Sleep* **29:** 1321–1325.

112. Boeve, B., S.-C. Lin, A. Strongosky, *et al.* 2006. Absence of REM sleep behavior disorder in eleven members of the PPND kindred. *Arch. Neurol.* **63:** 268–272.

113. Kelley, B., W. Haidar, B. Boeve, *et al.* 2009 Prominent phenotypic variability associated with mutations in Progranulin. *Neurobiol. Aging* **30:** 387–391.

114. Schenck, C.H., S.R. Bundlie & M.W. Mahowald. 1996. Delayed emergence of a parkinsonian disorder in 38% of 29 older men initially diagnosed with idiopathic rapid eye movement sleep behaviour disorder. *Neurology* **46:** 388–393.

115. Uchiyama, M., K. Isse, K. Tanaka, *et al.* 1995. Incidental Lewy body disease in a patient with REM sleep behavior disorder. *Neurology* **45:** 709–712.

116. Boeve, B., D. Dickson, E. Olson, *et al.* 2007. Insights into REM sleep behavior disorder pathophysiology in brainstem-predominant Lewy body disease. *Sleep Med.* **8:** 60–64.

117. Boeve, B., M. Silber & T. Ferman. 2004. REM sleep behavior disorder in Parkinson's disease and dementia with Lewy bodies. *J. Ger. Psychiatry Neurol.* **17:** 146–157.

118. Boeve, B. & C. Saper. 2006. REM sleep behavior disorder: A possible early marker for synucleinopathies. *Neurology* **66:** 796–797.

119. Stiasny-Kolster, K., Y. Doerr, J. Möller, *et al.* 2005. Combination of 'idiopathic' REM sleep behaviour disorder and olfactory dysfunction as possible indicator for -synucleinopathy demonstrated by dopamine transporter FP-CIT-SPECT. *Brain* **128:** 126–137.

120. Braak, H., K. Del Tredici, U. Rub, *et al.* 2003. Staging of brain pathology related to sporadic Parkinson's disease. *Neurobiol. Aging* **24:** 197–211.

121. Braak, H., E. Ghebremedhin, U. Rub, *et al.* 2004. Stages in the development of Parkinson's disease-related pathology. *Cell Tissue Res.* **318:** 121–134.

122. Wakabayashi, K. & H. Takahashi. 1997. Neuropathology of autonomic nervous system in Parkinson's disease. *Eur. Neurol.* **38**(Suppl 2): 2–7.

123. Klos, K., J. Ahlskog, K. Josephs, *et al.* 2006. Alpha-synuclein pathology in the spinal cords of neurologically asymptomatic aged individuals. *Neurology* **66:** 1100–1102.

124. Fujishiro, H., R. Frigerio, M. Burnett, *et al.* 2008. Cardiac sympathetic denervation correlates with clinical and pathologic stages of Parkinson's disease. *Mov. Disord.* **23:** 1085–1092.

125. Dickson, D., H. Fujishiro, A. DelleDonne, *et al.* 2008. Evidence that incidental Lewy body disease is presymptomatic Parkinson's disease. *Acta Neuropathol.* **115:** 437–444.

126. Braak, H. & K. Del Tredici. 2009. Neuroanatomy and pathology of sporadic Parkinson's disease. *Adv. Anat. Embryol. Cell Biol.* **201:** 1–119.

127. Fantini, M., R. Postuma, J. Montplaisir & L. Ferini-Strambi. 2006. Olfactory deficit in idiopathic rapid eye movements sleep behavior disorder. *Brain Res. Bull.* **70:** 386–390.

128. Louis, E. & D. Bennett. 2007. Mild Parkinsonian signs: An overview of an emerging concept. *Mov. Disord.* **22:** 1681–1688.

129. Aarsland, D., K. Andersen, J. Larsen, *et al.* 2003. Prevalence and characteristics of dementia in Parkinson disease: an 8-year prospective study. *Arch. Neurol.* **60:** 387–392.

130. Emre, M., D. Aarsland, R. Brown, *et al.* 2007. Clinical diagnostic criteria for dementia associated with Parkinson's disease. *Mov. Disord.* **22:** 1689–1707.

131. Abbott, R., G. Ross, L. White, *et al.* 2005. Excessive daytime sleepiness and subsequent development of Parkinson disease. *Neurology* **65:** 1442–1446.

132. Ferini-Strambi, L., M. Di Gioia, V. Castronovo, *et al.* 2004. Neuropsychological assessment in idiopathic REM sleep behavior disorder (RBD): Does the idiopathic form of RBD really exist? *Neurology* **62:** 41–45.

133. Mori, E., T. Shimomura, M. Fujimori, *et al.* 2000. Visuoperceptual impairment in dementia with Lewy bodies. *Arch. Neurol.* **57:** 489–493.

134. Massicotte-Marquez, J., A. Décary, J. Gagnon, *et al.* 2008. Executive dysfunction and memory impairment in idiopathic REM sleep behavior disorder. *Neurology* **70:** 1250–1257.

135. Terzaghi, M., E. Sinforiani, C. Zucchella, *et al.* 2008. Cognitive performance in REM sleep behaviour disorder: a possible early marker of neurodegenerative disease? *Sleep Med.* **9:** 343–351.

136. Petersen, R., G. Smith, S. Waring, *et al.* 1999. Mild cognitive impairment: Clinical characterization and outcome. *Arch. Neurol.* **56:** 303–308.

137. Petersen, R. 2004. Mild cognitive impairment as a diagnostic entity. *J. Intern. Med.* **256:** 183–194.

138. Molano, J., B. Boeve, T. Ferman, *et al.* 2009. Mild cognitive impairment associated with Lewy body disease: a clinicopathologic study. *Brain* (in press).

139. McKeith, I., D. Dickson, J. Lowe, *et al.* 2005. Dementia with Lewy bodies: Diagnosis and management: Third report of the DLB Consortium. *Neurology* **65:** 1863–1872.

140. Fantini, M.L., J.F. Gagnon, D. Petit, *et al.* 2003. Slowing of electroencephalogram in rapid eye movement sleep behavior disorder. *Ann. Neurol.* **53:** 774–780.

141. Massicotte-Marquez, J., J. Carrier, A. Decary, *et al.* 2005. Slow-wave sleep and delta power in rapid eye movement sleep behavior disorder. *Ann. Neurol.* **57:** 277–282.

142. Culebras, A. & J. Moore. 1989. Magnetic resonance findings in REM sleep behavior disorder. *Neurology* **39:** 1519–1523.

143. Miyamoto, M., T. Miyamoto, J. Kubo, *et al.* 2000. Brainstem function in rapid eye movement sleep behavior disorder: the evaluation of brainstem function by proton MR spectroscopy (1H-MRS). *Psychiatr. Clin. Neurosci.* **54:** 350–351.

144. Iranzo, A., J. Santamaria, J. Pujol, *et al.* 2002. Brainstem proton magnetic resonance spectroscopy in idiopathic REM sleep behavior disorder. *Sleep* **25:** 867–870.

145. Eisensehr, I., R. Linke, S. Noachtar, *et al.* 2000. Reduced striatal dopamine transporters in idiopathic rapid eye movement sleep behaviour disorder: Comparison with Parkinson's disease and controls. *Brain* **123:** 1155–1160.

146. Mazza, S., J. Soucy, P. Gravel, *et al.* 2006. Assessing whole brain perfusion changes in REM sleep behavior disorder. *Neurology* **67:** 1618–1622.

147. Albin, R., R. Koeppe, R. Chervin, *et al.* 2000. Decreased striatal dopaminergic innervation in REM sleep behavior disorder. *Neurology* **55:** 1410–1412.

148. Caselli, R., K. Chen, D. Bandy, *et al.* 2006. A preliminary fluorodeoxyglucose positron emission tomography study in healthy adults reporting dream-enactment behavior. *Sleep* **29:** 927–933.

149. Klunk, W., H. Engler, A. Nordberg, *et al.* 2004. Imaging brain amyloid in Alzheimer's disease with Pittsburgh Compound-B. *Ann. Neurol.* **55:** 306–319.

150. Jack, C., Jr., V. Lowe, S. Weigand, *et al.* 2009. Serial PIB and MRI in normal, mild cognitive impairment and Alzheimer's disease: implications for sequence of pathological events in Alzheimer's disease. *Brain* **132:** 1355–1365.

151. Gomperts, S., D. Rentz, E. Moran, *et al.* 2008. Imaging amyloid deposition in Lewy body diseases. *Neurology* **71:** 903–910.

152. Taki, J., M. Yoshita, M. Yamada & N. Tonami. 2004. Significance of 123I-MIBG scintigraphy as a pathophysiological indicator in the assessment of Parkinson's disease and related disorders: it can be a specific marker for Lewy body disease. *Ann. Nucl. Med.* **18:** 453–461.

153. Orimo, S., T. Amino, Y. Itoh, *et al.* 2005. Cardiac sympathetic denervation precedes neuronal loss in the sympathetic ganglia in Lewy body disease. *Acta Neuropathol.* **109:** 583–588.

154. Oka, H., M. Yoshioka, M. Morita, *et al.* 2007. Reduced cardiac 123I-MIBG uptake reflects cardiac sympathetic dysfunction in Lewy body disease. *Neurology* **69:** 1460–1465.

155. Miyamoto, T., M. Miyamoto, Y. Inoue, *et al.* 2006. Reduced cardiac 123I-MIBG scintigraphy in idiopathic REM sleep behavior disorder. *Neurology* **67:** 2236–2238.

156. Miyamoto, T., M. Miyamoto, K. Suzuki, *et al.* 2008. 123I-MIBG cardiac scintigraphy provides clues to the underlying neurodegenerative disorder in idiopathic REM sleep behavior disorder. *Sleep* **31:** 717–723.

157. Oguri, T., N. Tachibana, S. Mitake, *et al.* 2008. Decrease in myocardial 123I-MIBG radioactivity in REM sleep behavior disorder: two patients with different clinical progression. *Sleep Med.* **9:** 583–585.

158. Braune, S., M. Reinhardt, R. Schnitzer, *et al.* 1999. Cardiac uptake of [123I]MIBG separates Parkinson's disease from multiple system atrophy. *Neurology* **53:** 1020–1025.

159. Benarroch, E.E. & A.M. Schmeichel. 2002. Depletion of cholinergic mesopontine neurons in multiple system atrophy: A substrate for REM behavior disorder? *Neurology* **58**(suppl 3): A345.

160. Benarroch, E., A. Schmeichel, P. Low, *et al.* 2005. Involvement of medullary regions controlling sympathetic output in Lewy body disease. *Brain* **128:** 338–344.

161. Benarroch, E.E., A.M. Schmeichel, P. Sandroni, *et al.* 2007. Brainstem respiratory control: Substrates of respiratory failure of multiple system atrophy. *Acta Neuropathol. (Berl.)* **113:** 75–80.

162. Boeve, B., M. Silber, T. Ferman & G. Smith. 2002. Validation of a questionnaire for the diagnosis of REM sleep behavior disorder. *Sleep* **25**(abstr suppl): A486.

163. Boeve, B., M. Silber, T. Ferman, *et al.* 2002. Validation of a questionnaire for the diagnosis of REM sleep behavior disorder. *Neurology* **58**(suppl 3): A509.

164. Stiasny-Kolster, K., G. Mayer, S. Schäfer, *et al.* 2007. The REM sleep behavior disorder screening questionnaire– a new diagnostic instrument. *Mov. Disord.* **22:** 2386–2393.

165. Frauscher, B., A. Iranzo, B. Högl, *et al.* 2008. Quantification of electromyographic activity during REM sleep in multiple muscles in REM sleep behavior disorder. *Sleep* **31:** 724–731.

166. Lapierre, O. & J. Montplaisir. 1992. Polysomnographic features of REM sleep behavior disorder: development of a scoring method. *Neurology* **42:** 1371–1374.

167. Ferri, R., C. Franceschini, M. Zucconi, *et al.* 2008. Searching for a marker of REM sleep behavior disorder: submentalis muscle EMG amplitude analysis during sleep in patients with narcolepsy/cataplexy. *Sleep* **31:** 1409–1417.

168. Mayer, G., K. Kesper, T. Ploch, *et al.* 2008. Quantification of tonic and phasic muscle activity in REM sleep behavior disorder. *J. Clin. Neurophysiol.* **25:** 48–55.

169. Bliwise, D. & D. Rye. 2008. Elevated PEM (phasic electromyographic metric) rates identify rapid eye movement behavior disorder patients on nights without behavioral abnormalities. *Sleep* **31:** 853–857.

170. Zimprich, A., S. Biskup, P. Leitner, *et al.* 2004. Mutations in LRRK2 cause autosomal-dominant parkinsonism with pleomorphic pathology. *Neuron* **44:** 601–607.

171. Smith, G., B. Boeve, V. Pankratz, *et al.* 2009. Time course of diagnostic features of Lewy body disease. *Neurology* **72**(Suppl 3): A246.

172. Burke, R., W. Dauer & J. Vonsattel. 2008. A critical evaluation of the Braak staging scheme for Parkinson's disease. *Ann. Neurol.* **64:** 485–491.

173. Josephs, K., J. Duffy, E. Strand, *et al.* 2006. Clinicopathological and imaging correlates of progressive aphasia and apraxia of speech. *Brain* **129:** 1385–1398.

174. Boeve, B.F., D.M. Maraganore, J.E. Parisi, *et al.* 1999. Pathologic heterogeneity in clinically diagnosed corticobasal degeneration. *Neurology* **53:** 795–800.

175. Tang-Wai, D., N. Graff-Radford, B. Boeve, *et al.* 2004. Clinical, genetic, and neuropathologic characteristics of posterior cortical atrophy. *Neurology* **63:** 1168–1174.

176. Turner, R.S., R.D. Chervin, K.A. Frey, *et al.* 1997. Probable diffuse Lewy body disease presenting as REM sleep behavior disorder. *Neurology* **49:** 523–527.

177. Turner, R., C. D'Amato, R. Chervin & M. Blaivas. 2000. The pathology of REM sleep behavior disorder with comorbid Lewy body dementia. *Neurology* **55:** 1730–1732.

178. McShane, R., Z. Nagy, M. Esiri, *et al.* 2001. Anosmia in dementia is associated with Lewy bodies rather than Alzheimer's pathology. *J. Neurol. Neurosurg. Psychiatry* **70:** 739–743.

179. Olichney, J., C. Murphy, C. Hofstetter, *et al.* 2005. Anosmia is very common in the Lewy body variant of Alzheimer's disease. *J. Neurol. Neurosurg. Psychiatry* **76:** 1342–1347.

Ann. N.Y. Acad. Sci. 1184 (2010) 15–54

Ann. N.Y. Acad. Sci. ISSN 0077-8923

ANNALS OF THE NEW YORK ACADEMY OF SCIENCES

Lewy body pathology in fetal grafts

Yaping Chu and Jeffrey H. Kordower

Department of Neurological Sciences, Rush University Medical Center, Chicago, Illinois, USA

Address for correspondence: Jeffrey Kordower, Department of Neurological Sciences, Rush University Medical Center, 1735 West Harrison Street, Chicago, IL 60612. Voice: 312-563-3570; fax: 312-563-3571. jkordowe@rush.edu

Although fetal nigral transplants have been shown to survive grafting into the striatum, increased [^{18}F]6-fluoro-L-3,4-dihydroxyphenylalanine (^{18}F-DOPA) uptake and improved motor function in open-label assessments have failed to establish any clinical benefits in double-blind, sham-controlled studies. To understand morphological and neurochemical alterations of grafted neurons, we performed postmortem analyses on six Parkinson's disease (PD) patients who had received fetal tissue transplantation 18–19 months, 4 years, and 14 years previously. These studies revealed robust neuronal survival with normal dopaminergic phenotypes in 18-month-old grafts and decreased dopamine transporter and increased cytoplasmic α-synuclein in 4-year-old grafts. We also found a decline of both dopamine transporter and tyrosine hydroxylase and the formation of Lewy body–like inclusions in 14-year-old grafts, which stained positive for α-synuclein and ubiquitin proteins. These pathological changes suggest that PD is an ongoing process that affects grafted cells in the striatum in a manner similar to how resident dopamine neurons are affected in the substantia nigra.

Keywords: fetal tissue transplantation; Parkinson's disease; dopaminergic phenotype; α-synuclein; ubiquitin; thioflavin-s

Introduction and background

Fetal nigral transplantation has been considered a viable therapeutic strategy for Parkinson's disease (PD) for over two decades. This strategy is based on the concept that new dopaminergic neurons can replace those that are lost in PD and, just as critically, replace dopaminergic innervation and dopaminergic synaptic connectivity to the denervated striatum. Several open-label reports indicate that patients experienced clinically meaningful benefits for a couple of years to a decade after transplatation.[1–7] Patients who exhibited significant improvements showed lowering of scores for the total Unified Parkinson Disease Rating Scale (UPDRS) during "off" state (off medication) and/or required substantially lower doses of antiparkinsonian medications.[3,6] These clinical changes have been associated with increased striatal [^{18}F]6-fluoro-L-3,4-dihydroxyphenylalanine (^{18}F-DOPA) uptake.[7,8] Several years after transplantation, patients experienced progressive worsening of PD features and experienced difficulty in gait, balance, and falling

that could not be controlled with medication.[9–11] To date, none of the positive outcomes has been replicated in a double-blinded trial of fetal nigral transplantation in PD.[12,13] In the course of both open-label and double-blinded trials, numerous patients have received fetal nigral transplants. These trials have employed a variety of parameters for tissue preparation, storage techniques, locus of implants, and others, and each case that ultimately comes to autopsy provides a rich reservoir of information that deserves careful examination. In the series of patients that have been part of a collaboration between Mt. Sinai, The University of South Florida at Tampa, and Rush University Medical Center, we have examined, using histochemical and immunohistochemical methods, six PD patients who received fetal tissue transplantation for 18–19 months ($n = 2$), 4 years ($n = 2$), and 14 years ($n = 2$). It has been 14 years since our original study demonstrating that fetal grafts can survive, innervate, and form synaptic contacts in PD patients that survived 18 months posttransplantation.[5] Since initial reporting, we[5] and others[14] have confirmed the robust

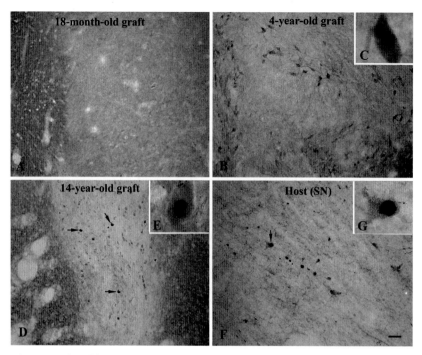

Figure 1. Low- (**A, B, D, F**) and high-power (**C, E, G**) photomicrographs from 18-month- (**A**), 4-year- (**B, C**), and 14-year-old (**D, E**) grafts and host nigra (SN; **F, G**) showing α-synuclein immunoreactivity (α-syn-ir; LB509). α-syn-ir was hardly detectable within 18-month-old grafted neurons (**A**). Conversely, cytoplasmic but not aggregative α-synuclein was distributed in perikarya and main processes in 4-year-old grafted neurons (**B, C**). Many α-syn-ir inclusions were observed within neuromelanin-laden neurons in 14-year-old graft (**D**, *arrows*). The inclusion with a lighter core surrounded dark staining was similar to the inclusion in host substantia nigra (**G**, SN). Scale bar = 80 μm in **F** (applies to **A, B, D**), 8 μm in **C, E, G**.

survival and innervation provided by grafted nigral neurons over longer periods of time. Recently, long-term transplants have come to autopsy in which the patients survived for more than 10 years after initial transplantation. Observations from both our lab[9,10] and from others[11] (Isacson, personal communication; Bill Langston, personal communication; and Kordower, unpublished observations) have shown that transplanted fetal nigral cells undergo pathological changes analogous to those seen in PD. Two types of findings have been observed; those involving graft phenotype and those involving structural changes and the formation of Lewy bodies. These changes provide insight into the understanding of disease pathogenesis and cell replacement therapy.

Pathological alteration of graft neurons

A subset of grafted neurons displayed a progressive dysfunction although grafted fetal nigral neu-

rons were aged only 14 years postnatally; which is far younger than the typical age at which PD affects nigral neurons. This dysfunction of grafts was not related to the shortage of blood supply, since most grafted neurons survived and functioned for several years. Whether the dysfunctional grafted neurons duplicate pathological alterations that occur in PD needs to be investigated. First, immunohistochemistry was employed to visualize α-synuclein (LB509) distribution and morphology in grafts. We found that α-synuclein was not detected at all in grafted neurons that survived for 18 months (Fig. 1A). Cytoplasmic, but not aggregated, α-synuclein immunoreactive (α-synuclein-ir) profiles were seen in 4-year-old grafts (Fig. 1B, C), and spherical α-synuclein-ir aggregated masses were deposited within neuromelanin laden neurons in 14-year-old grafts (Fig. 1D, E). Some of the spherical α-synuclein-ir masses displayed a lighter staining core surrounded by dark staining (Fig. 1E),

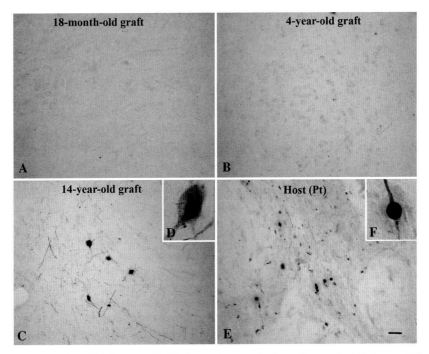

Figure 2. Low- (A, B, C, E) and high-power (D, F) photomicrographs from 18-month- (A), 4-year- (B), and 14-year-old (C, D) grafts and host putamen (Pt; E, F) illustrating S-129 α-synuclein immunoreactivity (α-syn-ir). S-129 α-syn-ir was hardly detectable within 18-month- and 4-year-old grafted neurons (A, B). Conversely, S-129 α-syn-ir perikarya, processes, and inclusions were observed in 14-year-old grafted neurons (C, D). Darkly stained swollen fibers were distributed in the host putamen (E, F; Pt). Scale bar = 35 μm in E (applies to A, B, C), 8 μm in D, F.

similar to Lewy bodies in the PD substantia nigra (Fig. 1F, G). In order to confirm that α-synuclein inclusions are a pathological feature, a second α-synuclein antibody that only detects α-synuclein phosphorylated on Ser-129 was employed to stain grafted tissue. This immunostaining demonstrated that α-synuclein inclusions in 14-year-old but not 18-month-old or 4-year-old grafts were phosphorylated at Ser-129 (Fig. 2). Phosphorylation at Ser-129 is a specific marker of α-synucleinopathies including PD.[15] The Ser-129 phosphorylation enhances α-synuclein toxicity, a fact verified in the *Drosophila* model of PD.[16] Ubiquitination of α-synuclein is another pathological event in PD,[17,18] and Lewy bodies are ubiquitin immunopositive. In this regard, we observed aggregated ubiquitin in 14-year-old but not in 18-month-old or 4-year-old grafts (Fig. 3). Some of the ubiquitin immunoreactive (ubiquitin-ir) inclusions in the grafts had the appearance of Lewy bodies similar to the PD substantia nigra (Fig. 3D, F). Finally, we confirmed that aggregates with α-synuclein and

ubiquitin staining in grafts were Lewy bodies by classic neuropathological stains such as thioflavin-S, the definitive light microscopic marker of Lewy bodies (Fig. 4). Several of the intracytoplasmic aggregates in the grafted neurons displayed a dense core surrounded by a lighter halo. This is the classic morphology of Lewy bodies found in catecholaminergic neurons in the substantia nigra and locus ceruleus, two regions that degenerate in PD, but distinct from the homogeneously stained Lewy bodies seen in the cerebral cortex in cortical Lewy body disease.

Another pathological feature within long-term fetal grafts is an increase in inflammatory cells within the grafted region. CD45 immunostaining revealed that every graft, from those with short survival times (18 months) to those with long survival times (14 years), was surrounded by activated microglia. CD45 (called the common leukocyte antigen) is a protein tyrosine phosphatase that has been shown to be an essential regulator of T and B cell antigen receptor signaling. It plays an important role in signal transduction and inhibition or

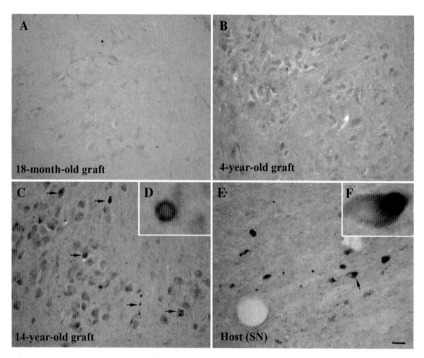

Figure 3. Low- (A, B, C, E) and high-power (D, F) photomicrographs from 18-month- (A), 4-year- (B), and 14-year-old (C, D) grafts and host substantia nigra (SN; E, F) illustrating ubiquitin (UB) immunoreactivity. The UB was hardly detectable within 18-month- and 4-year-old grafted neurons (A, B). In contrast, several UB immunoreactive inclusions (C, *arrows*) were observed in neuromelanin-laden neurons and fibers in 14-year-old grafts. The inclusion had a lighter core surrounded by dark staining (D), which was similar to the inclusion in host substantia nigra (F, SN). Scale bar = 35 μm in E (applies to A, B, C), 8 μm in D, F.

up-regulation of various immunological functions. The commercially available CD45 antibody recognizes a common epitope on all of the CD45 isoforms. CD45 immunoreactive cells were much denser around grafts than the host striatum in PD (Fig. 5). Activated microglial cells were also observed within the substantia nigra of patients with PD at postmortem and were identified by their immunoreactivity to human leucocyte antigen DR (HLA-DR), a cell-surface receptor belonging to the MHC class II.[19] This finding was confirmed by other investigators using additional markers, such as HLA-DP, HLA-DQ, HLADR, CD68, and ferritin.[20] However, microglial activation was not found in the putamen.[21] An increased expression of CD4[+] and CD45RO+ T cells (indicative of activated T cells) have been reported in the serum of patients with PD,[22,23] suggesting peripheral activation of lymphocytes. Although cellular and molecular studies indicate that there are neuro-inflammatory processes in the affected brain regions of patients with PD[24] and

in fetal tissue grafts,[10,11] these studies do not help determine whether such changes are involved in Lewy body formation or are merely a consequence of neuronal degeneration. In regard to this, a long-term Huntington's disease transplantation case (11 years posttransplant) had been examined. We found that there were clouded CD45 immunoreactive, activated microglia around the grafts but neither cytoplasmic α-synuclein-ir neurons nor Lewy bodies in the grafted cells (Fig. 6), indicating that Lewy body formation in grafts is not due to a generalized inflammatory response.

Alterations of dopaminergic phenotype in grafted neurons

To understand whether PD-like changes in dopaminergic phenotype were seen in grafted neurons, we studies neuromelanin, tyrosine hydroxylase (TH), dopamine transporter (DAT), and Vesicular

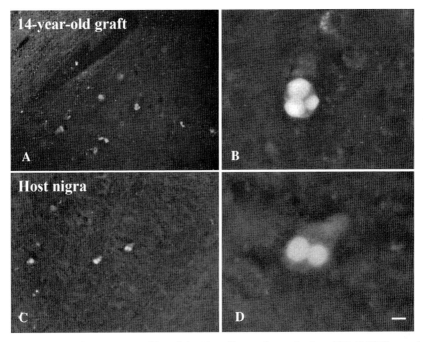

Figure 4. Photomicrographs from 14-year-old graft (A, B) and host substantia nigra (SN; C, D) illustrating thioflavin-S staining inclusions. Note that thioflavin-S-stained inclusions displayed a dense core surrounded by a lighter halo that is similar to host nigral thioflavin-S-stained inclusions. Scale bar = 4 μm in D (applies to B), 40 μm in A, C.

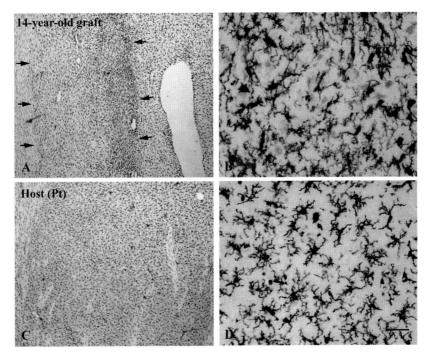

Figure 5. Low- (A, C) and high-power (B, D) photomicrographs from 14-year-old graft (A, B) and host putamen (Pt; C, D) illustrating CD45 immunoreactivity. Note that there were increased CD45 stained microglial cells in the graft (A, B) as compared with the host putamen (Pt; C, D) Scale bar = 35 μm in D (applies to B), 180 μm in A, C.

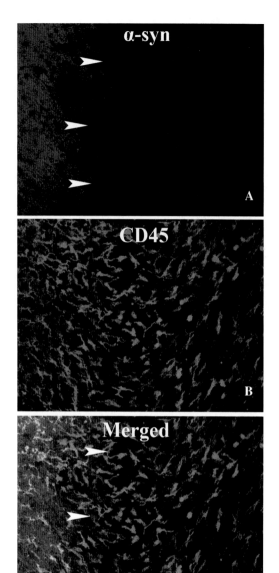

Figure 6. Laser confocal microscopic images from an 11-year posttransplant Huntington's disease case illustrating the absence of cytoplasmic α-synuclein cells and inclusions (A), but increased CD45 (B, C) (*arrowheads* point to graft). Scale bar = 60 μm in C (applies to all).

Monoamine Transporter 2 (VMAT2) expression in all cases.

Neuromelanin is an easily discernible endogenous marker for nigral dopaminergic neurons in the human brain, which appears after the first 2 to 3 years of life, accumulates during aging,[25,26] and

typically becomes extracellular following neural degeneration in PD. We tested whether neuromelanin accumulated in grafted cells at a rate similar to normal human nigral neurons. Neuromelanin was observed in 4-year-old grafts and 14-year-old grafts but not in 18-month-old grafts (Fig. 7). The density of neuromelanin was greater in 14-year-old grafts than in 4-year-old grafts. The majority of neuromelanin-laden neurons in grafts were immunopositive for Girk2, a marker of dopaminergic neurons in the substantia nigra pars compacta. To verify alteration of neuromelanin with age, the density of neuromelanin in grafted neurons was compared with normal aged nigral neurons. We found that the density of neuromelanin in 14-year-old grafted neurons appeared similar to 18-year-old nigral neurons (Fig. 7C, D) and interpret this expression of neuromelanin in grafted neurons as normal.

TH, the rate-limiting enzyme involved in the biosynthesis of the catecholamines dopamine and norepinephrine from tyrosine, is a useful marker for dopaminergic and noradrenergic neurons. To verify function of grafted neurons we first examined TH expression. Immunohistochemistry revealed that robust survival of TH immunoreative (TH-ir) neurons was observed in 18–19-month- and 4-year-old grafts placed in the postcommissural putamen (Fig. 8). TH-ir neurons in grafts in both groups appeared relatively normal with respect to morphological appearance. These neurons survived in an organotypic pattern and extended neurites, which extensively innervated the postcommissural putamen in a patch-matrix fashion. An electron microscopic analysis revealed that the graft and host made bidirectional synaptic contacts.[27] In the 4-year-old transplantation group, TH-ir neurons were present around the periphery but absent in center of grafts (Fig. 8C, E). In the 18-month and 4-year grafts, virtually all neuromelanin-positive cells expressed TH. In contrast, many neuromelanin-laden neurons displayed loss of TH immunoreactivity (Fig. 8F) in one of our two 14-year-old cases. That melanin-laden grafted neurons failed to express TH was similar to the alteration in PD nigral neurons.[28] For the most part, however, the grafted fetal mesencephalic tissue survived for a long period in the brain and restored dopaminergic innervation to the host putamen. This observation was associated with enhanced ^{18}F-DOPA uptake and clinical benefit.[5,7–9] Although there were robust TH-ir

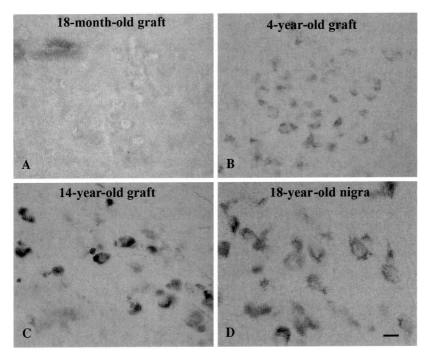

Figure 7. Photomicrographs of grafts (A–C) and nigra (D) illustrating alteration of neuromelanin (NM). NM was hardly detected in 18-month-old graft (A). As aging advanced, granular NM appeared in 4-year-old grafted neurons (B) and accumulated in 14-year-old grafted neurons (C). The density of NM in 14-year-old graft is similar to 18-year-old nigra (D). Scale bar = 18 μm in D (applies to all).

neurons in some grafts even after a decade, grafted fetal mesencephalic tissue became dysfunctional. Some neuronmelanin-laden neurons lost TH expression in 14-year-old grafts, indicating that there was a down-regulation of dopaminergic phenotype in implanted neurons. Therefore, it persuaded us to examine different dopaminergic phenotypes in grafted neurons.

Dopamine transporter is another dopaminergic neuronal marker, which mediates uptake of dopamine into neurons from the synapse and is a major target for various pharmacologically active drugs and environmental toxins. Dopamine nerve terminals and consequently DAT are reduced 30 to 50% in early PD[29] and to a greater extent in more severe PD.[30] To verify that alterations in DAT levels in grafted neurons resembles that seen in PD, DAT was examined using immunohistochemistry. DAT immunoreactive (DAT-ir) neurons were found in most of the grafts, but intensity of DAT-ir neurons declined with graft age (Fig. 9). In the 18-month-old grafts, dark DAT-stained neurons were distributed around grafts and DAT-ir neurites extensively in-

nervated the host putamen. The pattern of distribution of DAT-ir neurons was similar to that of TH-ir neurons. In the 4-year-old graft cases, some grafts contained dark DAT stained neurons while others enclosed few light DAT-ir neurons. In contrast, DAT staining revealed very light to no staining in neuromelanin-laden neurons in both of our 14-year-old graft cases (Fig. 9F), which is similar to what was observed in the PD nigra. One concern was that DAT severely declined, although there were robust TH-ir neurons in 14-year-old grafts. A decrease in DAT, although potentially serving as a compensatory mechanism in early disease, may ultimately result in increased dopamine turnover and higher oscillations in synaptic dopamine concentrations, thereby predisposing patients to motor complications during disease progression.

This morphological alteration of dopaminergic neurons in grafts from 18-month- to 14-year-old cases correlated with changes in motor function in the patients, although nondopaminergic and levodopa-unresponsive features emerge over this time. Although the grafted human ventral

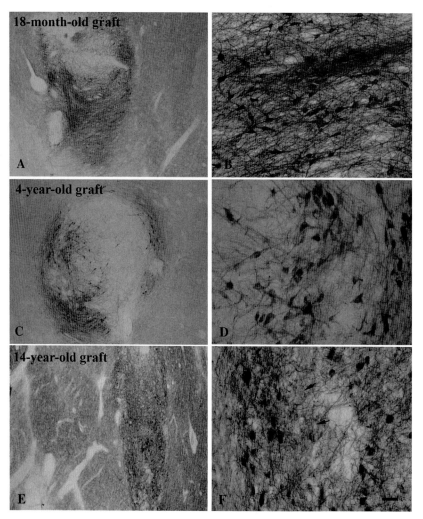

Figure 8. Low- (A, C, E) and high-power (A, D, F) photomicrographs from 18-month- (A, B), 4-year- (C, D), and 14-year-old (E, F) grafts illustrating alterations of tyrosine hydroxylase (TH) immunoreactivity. Note that TH immunostaining intensity was diminished (E) and some neuromelanin-laden neurons appeared TH immunonegative (F; *arrows*) in 14-year-old graft. Scale bar = 35 μm in F (applies to B, D), 180 μm in A, C, E.

mesencephalons were derived from different embryos, all the grafts underwent a process of being functional to becoming dysfunctional and showed decreases in dopaminergic phenotypes over time. The decline in DAT occurred much earlier and faster than the decrease in TH in grafted neurons. These features suggest that reduced dopaminergic transmission may occur over time, a compensatory response may occur, and an earlier manifestation of dopaminergic injury may be represented in the graft. As the level of dopaminergic transmission was much lower in the synapse, decrease of DAT in grafted neu-

rons may be a response intended to enhance functional dopamine at the synapse. Molecular imaging analysis revealed that higher DAT decrease in PD is in fact related to an advanced stage of neuronal loss. Loss of DAT observed in SPECT and PET can be seen even before the onset of symptoms, since clinical manifestations take place after more severe dopamine neuron deterioration.[31] Grafted cells also displayed diminished dopamine transporter, a PD-related pathogenesis. On the other hand, staining for VMAT2 was preserved in our cases, suggesting that it is a less sensitive index of cell injury than

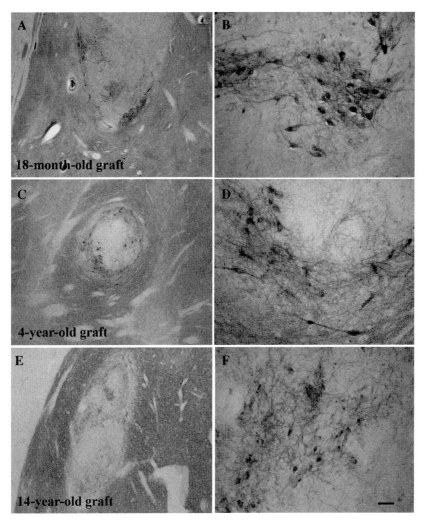

Figure 9. Low- (A, C, E) and high-power (B, D, F) photomicrographs from 18-month- (A, B), 4-year- (C, D), and 14-year-old (E, F) grafts illustrating alterations of dopamine transporter (DAT) immunoreactivity. Note that DAT immunostaining intensity was diminished in 4-year-old grafted neurons (C, D) and severely decreased in 14-year-old grafts (E, F). Scale bar = 35 μm in F (applies to B, D), 180 μm in A, C, E.

either TH or DAT.[9,10] DAT and VMAT2 are important implications for brain imaging of patients with PD and should be pursued.

Possible pathogenesis of Lewy body formation in grafts

Inflammation, oxidative stress and excitotoxity, loss of neurotrophic support, and prion disease–like mechanisms have all been proposed to explain the propagation of PD pathology from the host diseased brain to healthy transplanted neurons.[32] Our findings, accumulating cytoplasmic α-synclein in 4-year-old and aggregating α-synuclein in 14-year-old grafted neurons, support the concept that Lewy body formation is a chronic process and grafted nigral neurons can be attacked by PD even though they are placed in an ectopic location (putamen). Increase in cytoplasmic α-synuclein in grafted neurons is the basic condition required to form Lewy bodies. Phosphorylation and nitration of cytoplasmic α-synuclein are the processes involved in Lewy body formation.[33] Apparently these processes occur in the host and in the graft in a similar fashion.

It is known that the clinical manifestations of tremor, rigidity, and bradykinesia generally occur when there is a loss of 80% of striatal dopamine; this implies the existence of a relatively long preclinical period.[34,35] This latency between disease onset and appearance of clinical symptoms suggests that some of these changes may be of a compensatory nature, aimed at maintaining high enough synaptic dopamine levels to allow for relatively normal motor function. A critical site in the regulation of synaptic dopamine levels is DAT. Physiologically, DAT is a membrane-spanning protein that binds the neurotransmitter dopamine. DAT transports dopamine against a concentration gradient from the synapse into the intracellular space as the primary mechanism through which dopamine is cleared from synapses.[36,37] Under specific circumstances (e.g., exposure to amphetamines), DAT can reverse its normal functional role and mediate the transport of dopamine from the intracellular space into the synapse.[38,39] In PD pathophysiology, a decrease in DAT occurs early in the disease process, possibly providing compensation that ultimately results in enhanced dopamine function at the level of the synapse. This change may also predispose individuals to motor complications as the disease progresses.[40] This compensatory change was also exhibited in grafted neurons that consistently had decreases in DAT expression.

Another characteristic in grafted neurons was an increase in α-synuclein. A decrease in DAT was accompanied by an increase in cytoplasmic α-synuclein in 4-year-old grafted neurons. We hypothesize that decreases in DAT in grafted neurons may be compensated for with increases in some other synaptic proteins, in particular an augmentation of cytoplasmic α-synuclein. α-synuclein is normally seen mainly in presynaptic terminals. Thus we observed intense α-synuclein immunoreactivity within the perikarya of 4-year-old grafts. The increase in cytoplasmic α-synuclein appears to be associated with a decrease in DAT. The function of α-synuclein is still unknown, although several studies suggest that it plays an important role in synapse maturation and maintenance.[41–43] From co-immunoprecipitation studies, wild-type α-synuclein and its A30P mutant form were found to interact directly with the DAT, forming a protein:protein heteromeric complex in transfected cells, primary cultures of mesencephalic neurons and rat.[44] In cotransfected Ltk2 cells, α-synuclein negatively modulated

human dopamine transporter activity by attenuating the reuptake of dopamine and decreasing DAT levels.[45,46] This negative modulation was further verified by an inverse correlation between DAT expression in the striatum and the burden of pathological α-synuclein aggregates in the substantia nigra.[46] Increase in α-synuclein following a decrease in DAT in grafted neurons may initiate synucleinopathy.

Whether an increase in α-synuclein is beneficial or toxic to a cell is debated.[47,48] α-synuclein-knockout mice are grossly normal and display no neurodegenerative phenotype. However these mice display decreased numbers of synaptic vesicles and show subtle changes in dopamine homeostasis.[49,50] Dopaminergic mouse neurons and human neuroblastoma cells lacking α-synuclein have been shown to be resistant to the toxin 1-methyl-4-phenyl-1,2,3,6-tetrahydropyridine (MPTP) and its active metabolite 1-methyl-4-phenylpyridine (MPP+).[51,52] These data indicate that α-synuclein is a protein susceptible to neurotoxicity. Overexpression of wild-type or mutant α-synuclein in transgenic (tg) mice,[53] Drosophila,[54] and neurons[55] can cause alterations in nigrostriatal function and in some instances dopamine neuronal degeneration with inclusion bodies. Similarly targeted overexpression of α-synuclein in the nigrostriatal system of rats and nonhuman primates[56,57] induces α-synuclein inclusions and neuronal degeneration and mimics several of the pathological and behavioral features of PD. Age-related increase of cytoplasmic α-synuclein without aggregation[58] and decrease of DAT[59] in nigral neurons indicate that there may be an imbalance of presynaptic proteins in PD that does not occur in controls; effects mediated impaired lysosomal and proteasomal systems.

It is interesting that α-synuclein was robustly increased in 4-year-old grafted neurons and aggregated in 14-year-old grafted neurons. This accumulating α-synuclein could not be cleared by lysosomal and proteasomal systems. We hypothesized that the continued accumulation of α-synuclein in grafted neurons may be caused by active protein-modifying processes such as phosphorylation and oxidative stress since pathological modification of α-synuclein is a characteristic in familial and sporadic Lewy body disease.[60,61] Therefore we analyzed the specific forms of α-synuclein in grafted neurons using immunohistochemistry. We found heavy phosphorylated Ser-129 α-synuclein immunoreactive inclusions in 14-year-old grafts but not in 18-month-old grafts. Small amounts of phosphory-lated Ser129 α-synuclein were observed in 4-year-old grafted neurons. This cytosolic form of phos-phorylated α-synuclein may thus be the precursor to the predominant pathogenic form of α-synuclein in Lewy bodies. In order to understand whether accumulated α-synuclein in grafted neurons was ubiquitinated, ubiquitination was examined using immunohistochemistry. We found a pattern of la-beling for ubiquitin inclusions and neurites that was similar to that of α-synuclein labeling in 14-year-old grafted neuron but not in 18-month- and 4-year-old grafts. The absence of ubiquitin labeling in 4-year-old grafted neurons containing heavy cytoplas-mic α-synuclein immunostaining strongly suggests that ubiquitination occurs after α-synuclein aggre-gation. Immunoblots of two-dimensional polyacry-lamide gel electrophoresis (PAGE) gels stained with antibodies to synuclein and ubiquitin show that the major ubiquitinated species correspond in molec-ular mass to α-synuclein with ubiquitins attached in isolated Lewy bodies.[62,63] Ubiquitination was not detected in the soluble fraction of α-synuclein in de-mentia Lewy body brain.[63] It is possible that ubiq-uitinated α-synuclein with phosphorylated modi-fication may not go through the proteasome to be degraded and instead may accumulate to form Lewy bodies.

In summary, patients grafted with dopaminergic neurons experience improvements in their PD syn-drome for a decade and then show a progressive worsening of PD features. The neurochemical and morphological alterations of grafted dopaminergic neurons appeared to cause a decrease in dopamin-ergic phenotypes, especially in DAT, which caused an unbalance of proteins in grafted neurons. The decrease in DAT is accompanied by an increase in cytoplasmic α-synuclein. The increased cyto-plasmic α-synuclein was modified by oxidation or phosphorylation. In particular, the modified synuclein species Ser-129, which cannot be cleared through lysosomal and proteasomal systems, pref-erentially and consistently accumulates in the intra-cellular space and therefore may drive Lewy body formation.

Conflicts of interest

The authors declare no conflicts of interest.

References

1. Lindvall, O. *et al.* 1990. Fetal brain grafts and Parkinson's disease. *Science* **250:** 1435.

2. Lindvall, O. 1994. Clinical application of neuronal grafts in Parkinson's disease. *J. Neurol.* **242**(1 Suppl 1): S54–S56.

3. Peschanski, M. *et al.* 1994. Bilateral motor improvement and alteration of L-dopa effect in two patients with Parkinson's disease following intrastriatal transplanta-tion of foetal ventral mesencephalon. *Brain* **117:** 487–499.

4. Wenning, G.K. *et al.* 1997. Short- and long-term sur-vival and function of unilateral intrastriatal dopamin-ergic grafts in Parkinson's disease. *Ann. Neurol.* **42:** 95–107.

5. Kordower, J.H. *et al.* 1995. Neuropathological evidence of graft survival and striatal reinnervation after the trans-plantation of fetal mesencephalic tissue in a patient with Parkinson's disease. *N. Engl. J. Med.* **332:** 1118–1124.

6. Piccini, P. *et al.* 1999. Dopamine release from nigral transplants visualized in vivo in a Parkinson's patient. *Nat. Neurosci.* **2:** 1137–1140.

7. Mendez, I. *et al.* 2005. Cell type analysis of functional fe-tal dopamine cell suspension transplants in the striatum and substantia nigra of patients with Parkinson's disease. *Brain* **128:** 1498–1510.

8. Kordower, J.H. *et al.* 1998. Fetal nigral grafts survive and mediate clinical benefit in a patient with Parkinson's disease. *Mov. Disord.* **13:** 3833–3893.

9. Kordower, J.H. *et al.* 2008. Lewy body-like pathology in long-term embryonic nigral transplants in Parkinson's disease. *Nat. Med.* **14:** 504–506.

10. Kordower, J.H. *et al.* 2008. Transplanted dopaminergic neurons develop PD pathologic changes: a second case report. *Mov. Disord.* **23:** 2303–2306.

11. Li, J.Y. *et al.* 2008. Lewy bodies in grafted neurons in subjects with Parkinson's disease suggest host-to-graft disease propagation. *Nat. Med.* **14:** 501–503.

12. Olanow, C.W. *et al.* 2003. A double-blind controlled trial of bilateral fetal nigral transplantation in Parkinson's disease. *Ann Neurol.* **54:** 403–414.

13. Freed, C.R. *et al.* 2003. Do patients with Parkinson's dis-ease benefit from embryonic dopamine cell transplanta-tion? *J. Neurol.* **250**(Suppl 3): III44–III46.

14. Freed, C.R. *et al.* 2001. Transplantation of embryonic dopamine neurons for severe Parkinson's disease. *N. Engl. J. Med.* **344:** 710–719.

15. Anderson, J.P. *et al.* 2007. Phosphorylation of Ser-129 is the dominant pathological modification of α-synuclein

in familial and sporadic Lewy body disease. *J. Biol. Chem.* **281:** 29739–29752.

16. Chen, L. & M.B. Feany. 2005. α-synuclein phosphorylation controls neurotoxicity and inclusion formation in a Drosophila model of Parkinson disease. *Nat. Neurosci.* **8:** 657–663.

17. Engelender, S. 2008. Ubiquitination of α-synuclein and autophagy in Parkinson's disease. *Autophagy* **4:** 372–374.

18. Lee, J.T. *et al.* 2008. Ubiquitination of α-synuclein by Siah-1 promotes α-synuclein aggregation and apoptotic cell death. *Hum. Mol. Genet.* **17:** 906–917.

19. Imamura, K. *et al.* 2003. Distribution of major histocompatibility complex class II-positive microglia and cytokine profile of Parkinson's disease brains. *Acta Neuropathol.* **106:** 518–526.

20. Banati, R.B. *et al.* 1998. Glial pathology but absence of apoptotic nigral neurons in long-standing Parkinson's disease. *Mov. Disord.* **13:** 221–227.

21. Mirza, B. *et al.* 2000. The absence of reactive astrocytosis is indicative of a unique inflammatory process in Parkinson's disease. *Neuroscience* **95:** 425–432.

22. Fiszer, U. *et al.* 1994. Parkinson's disease and immunological abnormalities: increase of HLA-DR expression on monocytes in cerebrospinal fluid and of CD45RO+ T cells in peripheral blood. *Acta Neurol. Scand.* **90:** 160–166.

23. Bas, J. *et al.* 2001. Lymphocyte populations in Parkinson's disease and in rat models of parkinsonism. *J. Neuroimmunol.* **113:** 146–152.

24. McGeer, P.L. & E.G. McGeer. 2004. Inflammation and neurodegeneration in Parkinson's disease. *Parkinsonism Relat. Disord.* **10**(Suppl 1): S3–S7.

25. Bogerts, B. 1981. A brainstem atlas of catecholaminergic neurons in man, using melanin as a natural marker. *J. Comp. Neurol.* **197:** 63–80.

26. Mann, D.M. & P.O. Yates. 1974. Lipoprotein pigments–their relationship to ageing in the human nervous system. II. The melanin content of pigmented nerve cells. *Brain* **97:** 489–498.

27. Kordower, J.H. *et al.* 1996. Functional fetal nigral grafts in a patient with Parkinson's disease: chemoanatomic, ultrastructural, and metabolic studies. *J. Comp. Neurol.* **370:** 203–230.

28. Chu, Y. *et al.* 2006. Nurr1 in Parkinson's disease and related disorders. *J. Comp. Neurol.* **494:** 495–514.

29. Ichise, M. *et al.* 1999. SPECT imaging of pre and post-synaptic dopaminergic alterations in L-dopa-untreated PD. *Neurology* **52:** 1206–1214.

30. Seibyl, J.P. *et al.* 1995. Decreased single-photon emission computed tomographic [123-I] beta-CIT striatal uptake correlates with symptom severity in Parkinson's disease. *Ann. Neurol.* **38:** 589–598.

31. Bressan, R.A. *et al.* 2007. Can molecular imaging techniques identify biomarkers for neuropsychiatric disorders? *Rev. Bras. Psiquiatr.* **29:** 102–104.

32. Brundin, P. *et al.* 2008. Research in motion: the enigma of Parkinson's disease pathology spread. *Nat. Rev. Neurosci.* **9:** 741–745. Review.

33. Hasegawa, M. *et al.* 2002. Phosphorylated α-synuclein is ubiquitinated in α-synucleinopathy lesions. *J. Biol. Chem.* **277:** 49071–49076.

34. Aarms, J.R. *et al.* 2005. PET in LRRK2 mutations: comparison to sporadic Parkinson's disease and evidence for presymptomatic compensation. *Brain* **128:** 2760–2762.

35. Au, W.L. *et al.* 2005. Parkinson's disease: in vivo assessment of disease progression using positron emission tomography. *Brain Res. Mol. Brain Res.* **134:** 24–33.

36. Torres, G.E. *et al.* 2003. Oligomerization and trafficking of the human dopamine transporter. Mutational analysis identifies critical domains important for the functional expression of the transporter. *J. Biol. Chem.* **278:** 2731–2739.

37. Zhang, H. *et al.* 2009. Regulation of dopamine transporter activity by carboxypeptidase E. *Mol. Brain.* **2:** 1–13.

38. Kahlig, K.M. *et al.* 2005. Amphetamine induces dopamine efflux through a dopamine transporter channel. *Proc Natl. Acad. Sci. USA* 3495–3500.

39. Furman, C.A. *et al.* 2009. Opamine and amphetamine rapidly increase dopamine transporter trafficking to the surface: live-cell imaging using total internal reflection fluorescence microscopy. *J. Neurosci.* **29:** 3328–3336.

40. Sossi, V. *et al.* 2007. Dopamine transporter relation to dopamine turnover in Parkinson's disease: a positron emission tomography study. *Ann. Neurol.* **62:** 468–474.

41. George, J.M. 2002. The synucleins. *Genome Biol.* 3002.1–3002.6.

42. Perez, R.G. *et al.* 2002. A role for α-synuclein in the regulation of dopamine biosynthesis. *J. Neurosci.* 3090–3099.

43. Lotharius, J. & P. Brundin. 2002. Pathogenesis of Parkinson's disease: dopamine, vesicles and α-synuclein. *Nat. Rev. Neurosci.* **3:** 932–942.

44. Wersinger, C. & A. Sidhu. 2003. Attenuation of dopamine transporter activity by α-synuclein. *Neurosci. Lett.* **340:** 189–192.

45. Sidhu, A. *et al.* 2004. α-Synuclein regulation of the dopaminergic transporter: a possible role in the pathogenesis of Parkinson's disease. *FEBS Lett.* **565:** 1–5. Review.

46. Kovacs, G.G. *et al.* 2008. Nigral burden of α-synuclein correlates with striatal dopamine deficit. *Mov. Disord.* **23:** 1608–1612.

47. Sidhu, A. *et al.* 2004. The role of α-synuclein in both neuroprotection and neurodegeneration. *Ann. N. Y. Acad. Sci.* **1035:** 250–270. Review.

48. Cookson, M.R. 2009. α-Synuclein and neuronal death. *Mol. Neurodegener.* **4:** 1–14.

49. Abeliovich, A. *et al.* 2000. Mice lacking α-synuclein display functional deficits in the nigrostriatal dopamine system. *Neuron* **25:** 239–252.

50. Fountaine, T.M. & R. Wade-Martins. 2007. RNA interference-mediated knockdown of α-synuclein protects human dopaminergic neuroblastoma cells from MPP(+) toxicity and reduces dopamine transport. *J. Neurosci. Res.* **85:** 351–363.

51. Dauer, W. *et al.* 2002. Resistance of α-synuclein null mice to the parkinsonian neurotoxin MPTP. *Proc. Natl. Acad. Sci. USA* **99:** 14524–14529.

52. Fountaine, T.M. *et al.* 2008. The effect of α-synuclein knockdown on MPP+ toxicity in models of human neurons. *Eur. J. Neurosci.* **28:** 2459–2473.

53. Masliah, E. *et al.* 2000. Dopaminergic loss and inclusion body formation in α-synuclein mice: implications for neurodegenerative disorders. *Science* **287:** 1265–1269.

54. Feany, M.B. & W.W. Bender. 2000. A Drosophila model of Parkinson's disease. *Nature* **404:** 394–398.

55. Vekrellis, K. *et al.* 2009. Inducible over-expression of wild type α-synuclein in human neuronal cells leads to caspase-dependent non-apoptotic death. *J. Neurochem.* **109:** 1348–1362.

56. Kirik, D. *et al.* 2003. Nigrostriatal α-synucleinopathy induced by viral vector-mediated overexpression of human α-synuclein: a new primate model of Parkinson's disease. *Proc. Natl. Acad. Sci. USA* **100:** 2884–2889.

57. Chu, Y. *et al.* 2009. Alterations in lysosomal and proteasomal markers in parkinson's disease: relationship to α-synuclein inclusions. *Neurobiol. Dis.* **35:** 385–398.

58. Chu, Y. & H.J. Kordower. 2007. Age-associated increases of α-synuclein in monkeys and humans are associated with nigrostriatal dopamine depletion: Is this the target for Parkinson's disease? *Neurobiol. Dis.* **25:** 134–149.

59. Ma, S.Y. *et al.* 1999. Dopamine transporter-immunoreactive neurons decrease with age in the human substantia nigra. *J. Comp. Neurol.* **409:** 25–37.

60. Anderson, J.P. *et al.* 2006. Phosphorylation of Ser-129 is the dominant pathological modification of α-synuclein in familial and sporadic Lewy body disease. *J. Biol. Chem.* **281:** 29739–28752.

61. Gao, H.M. *et al.* 2008. Neuroinflammation and oxidation/nitration of α-synuclein linked to dopaminergic neurodegeneration. *J. Neurosci.* **28:** 7687–7698.

62. Nonaka, T. *et al.* 2005. Ubiquitination of α-synuclein. *Biochemistry* **44:** 361–368.

63. Engelender, S. 2008. Ubiquitination of α-synuclein and autophagy in Parkinson's disease. *Autophagy* **4:** 372–374.

Ann. N.Y. Acad. Sci. ISSN 0077-8923

ANNALS OF THE NEW YORK ACADEMY OF SCIENCES

Congenital heart disease and brain development

Patrick S. McQuillen[1] and Steven P. Miller[2,3]

[1]Departments of Pediatrics and [2]Neurology, University of California, San Francisco, California, USA. [3]Department of Pediatrics (Neurology), University of British Columbia, Vancouver, British Columbia, Canada

Address for correspondence: Steven P. Miller, MDCM, MAS, FRCPC, Associate Professor of Pediatrics (Neurology), University of British Columbia, BC Children's Hospital, Division of Neurology, K3–180, 4480 Oak St., Vancouver BC V6H 3V4 Canada. Voice: 604-875-2345 ext 5948; fax: 604-875-2285. smiller6@cw.bc.ca

Brain and heart development occur simultaneously in the human fetus. Given the depth and complexity of these shared morphogenetic programs, it is perhaps not surprising that disruption of organogenesis in one organ will impact the development of the other. Newborns with congenital heart disease show a high frequency of acquired focal brain injury on sensitive magnetic resonance imaging studies in the perioperative period. The surprisingly high incidence of white matter injury in these term newborns suggests a unique vulnerability and may be related to a delay in brain development. These abnormalities in brain development identified with MRI in newborns with congenital heart disease might reflect abnormalities in cerebral blood flow while *in utero*. A complete understanding of the mechanisms of white matter injury in the term newborn with congenital heart disease will require further investigation of the timing, extent, and causes of delayed fetal brain development in the presence of congenital heart disease.

Keywords: stroke; white matter injury; cardiopulmonary bypass; magnetic resonance imaging; hypoxia; ischemia; diffusion tensor imaging; spectroscopy

Introduction

Brain and heart development occur simultaneously in the human fetus through the orchestration of complex genetic programs followed by periods of morphologic refinement in response to physiologic function. Many genes and signaling pathways (e.g., FGF, Wnt, Bmp, Sonic hedgehog) and even cell lineages (derivatives of the embryonic neural crest) are shared by these developing organs. The developing brain is highly metabolic and dependent upon the heart for delivery of oxygen and nutrients. The heart in turn receives innervation and control from the autonomic nervous system. Given the depth and complexity of these shared morphogenetic programs, it is perhaps not surprising that disruption of organogenesis in one organ will have significant effects for the other. In this review, we will focus on disrupted brain development in congenital heart disease (CHD) by considering the problem from divergent perspectives including epidemiologic/societal, as well as developmental cardiovascular and neurobiology. We will review lessons learned from early

attempts to improve neurodevelopmental outcome by altering neonatal surgical and life support techniques. Finally, we will summarize results from recent investigations using advanced magnetic resonance imaging (MRI) of the brain in the perioperative period.

Widespread neurodevelopmental abnormalities are common following neonatal surgery for congenital heart disease

In North America, severe CHD is a common cause of childhood morbidity, occurring in 6–8 per 1,000 live births.[1,2] Up to 50% of newborns affected by CHD will require open-heart surgery to correct their cardiac defect.[1,2] Over the last three decades, most forms of CHD have become amenable to excellent anatomic surgical repair that results in good cardiac function.[3] Over this period, with the increased survival of newborns with CHD, it is increasingly recognized that neurological deficits occur frequently in these children. As will be described below, the

Ann. N.Y. Acad. Sci. 1184 (2010) 68–86 © 2009 New York Academy of Sciences.

neurodevelopmental deficits observed in term newborns with CHD share many features with those observed in premature newborns followed through childhood (reviewed in Ref. 4).

d-Transposition of the great arteries is one of the most commonly studied forms of CHD in regards to neurodevelopmental outcome. Newborns with d-transposition of the great arteries are an important subgroup of those affected by CHD to study because newborns with this lesion typically present in the neonatal period and typically receive corrective surgery that restores normal circulation in the first 2 weeks of life. Therefore, neurodevelopmental deficits in children surviving with d-transposition of the great arteries can be more clearly linked to perioperative events relating to a single corrective surgery with less concern that ongoing cyanosis, intracardiac shunt, or heart failure might contribute to the outcomes. Furthermore, genetic syndromes commonly associated with CHD (such as trisomy 21 and DiGeorge, Turner, and Noonan syndromes) are rarely found with d-transposition of the great arteries. The impact of disease-modifying alleles or other genetic factors, however, remains relevant. A recent study of two forms of cardiopulmonary bypass for the correction of d-transposition of the great arteries noted a neurological abnormality in more than one third of those enrolled.[5,6] The deficits identified in these newborns with d-transposition of the great arteries persisted throughout childhood with significant detriment to school performance. By 8 years of age, children with d-transposition of the great arteries corrected surgically as newborns had significantly lower scores than population means for fine motor skills, visual-spatial skills, and cognition, including memory, attention, and higher-order language skills.[7]

Long-term neurodevelopmental deficits seen in newborns with d-transposition of the great arteries cannot be attributed solely to abnormalities in cerebral blood flow associated with cardiopulmonary bypass, as these deficits are observed even when attempts are made to normalize cerebral blood flow during surgical correction of the heart lesion. In a cohort of 74 children with d-transposition of the great arteries repaired with full-flow cardiopulmonary bypass during the neonatal period, survivors at a median of 9 years were more likely than best-friend controls to have lower full-scale IQ scores, higher motor impairment scores, and lower

social-behavioral competence scores.[8] As reviewed by Bellinger, recent observations suggest that deficits in social cognition are often underrecognized yet prevalent neurodevelopmental morbidities in children with CHD.[9] Children with a variety of heart defects, including d-transposition of the great arteries, appear to have difficulties being able to infer the internal states of other people, and even their own internal states, and to interpret their action appropriately. The narratives of children with CHD often failed to include critical information required by a listener, and infrequently referred to internal states.[9] Studies are now addressing the burden of these deficits on social function and disability during adolescence.[9]

Neurodevelopmental disability is not limited to newborns with d-transposition of the great arteries. In a cohort of 131 infants with multiple types of CHD requiring surgery followed through early childhood, motor delays were documented in 42% and global developmental delay was seen in 23%.[10] A similar sized cohort of patients who underwent the Fontan operation between 1973 and 1991 for hypoplastic left heart syndrome, a common and severe form of CHD that requires three-staged palliative procedures during the first 3–5 years of life, had full-scale IQ testing at a median age of 11 years, with a mean full-scale IQ of 95.7 ± 17.4, ($P < 0.006$ versus normal), with 10 patients (7.8%) having a full scale IQ < 70 ($P = 0.001$).[11] In hypoplastic left heart syndrome, the incidence of major disabilities in survivors exceeds 60%.[12,13] Both the incidence and severity of deficits increases with increasing severity of CHD diagnosis and with palliative surgical procedure versus. complete repair (reviewed in Ref. 14).

Recently, the developmental and functional outcomes of children with CHD requiring open heart surgery have been reported at school entry. In a cohort of 94 children with CHD repaired in infancy and assessed at 5 years of age, mean IQ scores were in the low average range.[15] Often the magnitude of decrease in full-scale IQ scores seems to be modest. However, even modest decreases in overall IQ can translate into substantial burden to society. Studies of the impact of environmental lead exposure estimate that for each IQ point lost, lifetime productivity decreases by 1.8–2.4%.[16] Based upon estimates of lifetime earning potential and the prevalence of CHD survivors, even modest 5-point decreases in

IQ translate into losses to society of tens of billions of dollars. More striking were the behavioral difficulties seen in more than one fourth of the group. Furthermore, more than 10% of the cohort had limitations in at least one of the following areas: socialization, daily living skills, communication, or adaptive behavior. As with differences in IQ, limitations in these domains would be expected to have substantial effects on long-term school and work function. Particularly relevant to the clinician is that very few children had restricted mobility (<5%), the most easily recognizable functional limitation. Yet more than 20% of these children were more dependent than their peers in self-care and social cognition.[15]

Consistent with these findings is the burden of behavioral disorders observed during childhood in infants with CHD.[17] As part of the developmental assessment of 155 children observed in a randomized clinical trial of surgically corrected d-transposition of the great arteries were assessed with the Child Behavior Checklist between 4 and 8 years of age, completed by the parents and the Connors' Parent Rating Scale at 8 years of age.[17] Importantly, at 8 years of age, the child's teacher completed the Teacher's Report Form and the Connors' Teacher Rating Scale. All the children had undergone neonatal repair of their heart defect with the arterial switch operation, involving deep hypothermia with predominantly total circulatory arrest or predominantly low-flow continuous cardiopulmonary bypass. Approximately 20% of children had scores for Total Problem Behavior in the range of clinical concern on both the Child Behavior Checklist and the Teacher's Report Form.[17] Yet the methods of cardiopulmonary bypass (deep hypothermia with predominantly total circulatory arrest or predominantly low-flow continuous cardiopulmonary bypass) did not distinguish the children with behavioral problems.[17] Children with academic challenges at 8 years of age did however have a greater burden of behavioral limitations.[17] The impairments faced by these cohorts far exceed those measured with standard IQ tests and are a striking reminder that screening for disabilities in this population must consider domains other than motor skills.

These results underscore the wide range of developmental difficulties faced by childhood survivors of CHD repaired in infancy. Developmental and functional limitations in children with CHD undergoing surgery early in life were often preceded by recognizable clinical characteristics in the preoperative period (acyanotic heart lesion, maternal education), surgical factors (age at surgery, palliative surgery, duration of deep hypothermic circulatory arrest) and postoperative factors (abnormal postoperative neurologic examination, microcephaly).[15] It is now recognized that patient-specific factors, such as the presence of a genetic syndrome, low birth weight, and presence of the APOE epsilon2 allele, are important predictors of adverse neurodevelopmental outcome at 1 year of age.[18] While some of these predictors are not modifiable (e.g., type of heart defect, maternal education), several are amenable to postnatal intervention or modification of clinical care strategies (e.g., avoidance of prolonged deep hypothermic circulatory arrest). The broad global delays observed in these children also suggest the presence of brain abnormalities that are more diffuse than the focal brain injuries (e.g., stroke, WMI, intraventricular hemorrhage) observed most readily on conventional MRI. These observations have some parallel in the follow-up profiles of premature newborns in whom focal brain injuries observed with conventional MRI reflect only one component of a more diffuse brain abnormality.

Prenatal diagnosis and management of fetal cardiac anomalies

As described above, most neurodevelopmental outcome studies have addressed newborns with CHD recognized and diagnosed in the newborn period (i.e., after birth). Advances in echocardiography and the application of these technologies to the fetus have made the diagnosis of major congenital heart defects feasible from early gestation. Between 20–50% of all congenital cardiac defects may be identified prenatally, depending upon the population screened and screening strategy; serious cardiac malformations can be detected with accuracy as high as 96% when performed at experienced centers.[19] Some studies have shown that prenatal diagnosis has improved the postnatal outcome,[20,21] although this finding remains controversial.[22] Following prenatal diagnosis of d-transposition of the great arteries, 1-year neurodevelopmental testing was no different among newborns with a prenatal diagnosis and those infants diagnosed postnatally.[23] However prenatal diagnosis was associated with an increased rate of adverse outcomes for both newborn and mother, including lower rate of maternal spontaneous labor, lower infant birth weight and Apgar scores, and higher need for preoperative mechanical ventilation of the newborn. Overall, the effect of prenatal diagnosis of CHD on acute brain injury and long-term neurodevelopmental outcome remains unclear. The remainder of this review will address the occurrence of brain injury and abnormal brain development in newborns with CHD and will address potential mechanisms of abnormal *in utero* brain development.

The timing of brain injury in newborns with CHD

Over the last decade the etiology of neurological injury in children with CHD is being increasingly understood. It is apparent that the etiology of brain injury in this vulnerable population is multifactorial with regard to both when the injury occurs and the ultimate mechanism of injury. Earlier studies have focused on intraoperative factors as the primary "at-risk" period for newborns undergoing cardiac surgery, with intensive focus on mechanisms of injury related to cardiopulmonary bypass. Other major risks for brain injury in newborns are thought to be from pre- and postoperative hemodynamic instability and to postoperative complications including cardiac arrest.

Prolonged circulatory arrest time required for operative correction of the heart defect is identified as a major risk factor for subsequent neurodevelopmental impairments.[5,12,24,25] The seminal Boston Circulatory Arrest Trial examined two forms of cardiopulmonary bypass for the correction of d-transposition of the great arteries with the arterial-switch operation.[5] In this randomized trial, infants with d-transposition of the great arteries were randomized to corrective surgery with deep hypothermia and either total circulatory arrest or low-flow cardiopulmonary bypass.[5] Both of these techniques are intended to prevent energy failure of vital organs during heart surgery in infants. When examining the 1-year outcomes of the 155 infants who were evaluated, the infants assigned to circulatory arrest had lower Psychomotor Development Index scores of the Bayley Scales of Infant Development than those assigned low-flow bypass. Even after considering variations in the cardiac anatomy (presence or absence of a ventricular septal defect), a greater proportion of infants in the circulatory arrest group had scores two standard deviations below the normal population-based mean. Strengthening the causal inference of circulatory arrest with adverse neurodevelopmental outcome was the observation of a "dose-response": with longer duration of circulatory arrest, the Psychomotor Development Index declined and the risk of neurologic abnormalities increased.[5] These data drew critical attention to the potential impact of the cardiopulmonary bypass technique on the risk for adverse neurodevelopmental outcomes. Several other trials confirmed the importance of surgical technique and bypass strategy on the risk for neurological injury and neurodevelopmental outcome abnormalities.[12,24,25]

Cardiopulmonary bypass itself may result in brain injury due to embolism, cytokine release, and ischemia, resulting in impaired delivery of energy substrates (oxygen and glucose).[26] Near-infrared spectroscopy has been used extensively in newborns undergoing cardiopulmonary bypass to demonstrate a pronounced decrease of cytochrome oxidase during circulatory arrest[27] and consequently to limit the duration of circulatory arrest or to guide regional cerebral perfusion.[28] As will be discussed below, these changes often portend the identification of brain injury on postoperative brain MRI scans.

More recently has it been recognized that more than half of newborns with CHD have evidence of neurobehavioral and neurological abnormalities prior to surgery and that these abnormalities are a significant risk factor for later neurodevelopmental impairment.[10,29] In order to investigate the occurrence of abnormalities in neurobehavioral status before surgery in newborns with CHD, a standardized neonatal neurobehavioral assessment and a neurologic examination were performed in a series of 56 neonates prior to open heart surgery.[29] Neurobehavioral and neurological abnormalities were seen in more than half of the newborns.[29] These abnormalities included absent suck, changes in tone (hypo- or hypertonia), and motor asymmetries. Feeding difficulties were seen in more than one third of the newborns. Abnormal head size was seen in almost

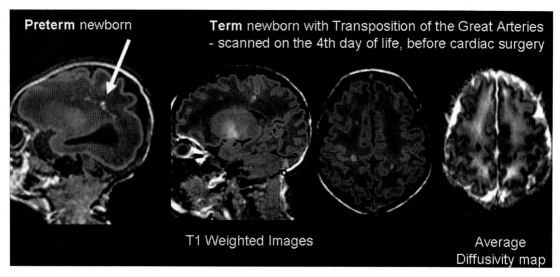

Figure 1. White matter injury on MRI. White matter injury in a premature newborn born at 28 weeks gestational age and scanned at 2 weeks of age, and in a term newborn with congenital heart disease scanned on the fourth day of life. The sagittal images from the T1-weighted volumetric scans show several foci of T1 hyperintensity in the periventricular white matter of the preterm newborn (*arrow*). Similar foci of abnormal T1 hyperintensity are evident on the sagittal and axial images from the T1-weighted volumetric scans and of the term newborn with heart disease. Additionally, several of the lesions in the newborn with heart disease demonstrate restricted diffusion on the average diffusivity map, suggesting that these lesions are acute.

half of the newborns, with microcephaly in more than one third.[29] These investigators then followed a larger cohort of newborns with CHD examined with similar preoperative assessments. When evaluated at 12–18 months of age, preoperative neurological and neurobehavioral abnormalities and the presence of microcephaly were associated with ongoing neurologic, motor, and developmental deficits.[10] Preoperative acidosis is also recognized as a risk for abnormal neurodevelopmental outcome.[25] In a study of 24 newborns with CHD studied with pre- and postoperative MRI, while more than half of the cohort had ischemic lesions postoperatively, 24% had preoperative ischemic lesions.[30] Taken together, these findings suggest that the neurological condition of the newborn with CHD prior to surgery is an important determinant of neurodevelopmental outcome later in infancy. These findings also highlight the potential of careful clinical and neuroimaging assessment of newborns with CHD to unravel the complex timing of brain abnormalities in this high-risk population. What is not clear from these investigations

is whether preoperative neurobehavioral abnormalities represent abnormal brain development or acute postnatally acquired injuries.

Pre- and postoperative brain injuries in newborns with CHD

Focal brain abnormalities (or "injuries") in the term newborn can be clearly and reliably detected with conventional MRI, and with greater resolution than with ultrasound or computed tomography.[31] Further, the extent of MRI abnormalities corresponds closely to histopathological changes found on postmortem examination.[32,33] In the newborn, acquired brain abnormalities, such as stroke and WMI, are often indicated by discrete (focal) areas of magnetic resonance (MR) signal abnormality (see Fig. 1). A number of cohort studies examining newborns with CHD before and after cardiac surgery, often with specialized transport equipment such as MR-compatible incubators and ventilators and trained personnel, demonstrate that brain abnormalities in critically ill newborns with CHD are safely and reliably detected using serial MRI.[30,34–37] In these studies, more than one third of newborns with CHD have brain injuries noted on MRI prior to cardiac surgery, with an additional one third of newborns acquiring brain injuries during or shortly after cardiac surgery. The spectra of brain injuries and their associated risk factors differ in the pre- and post-operative periods. Additionally, recent data suggest that separate potentially modifiable risk factors exist for each of the major patterns of brain injury: stroke and WMI.

Stroke and white matter injury are common in newborns with CHD prior to cardiac surgery

In some cohorts, stroke is the most common pattern of injury identified preoperatively (in more than half of those with injury), particularly in newborns with d-transposition of the great arteries.[35] Preoperative WMI is also observed with some frequency and may be particularly prevalent in newborns with single ventricle physiology.[30,35] In other series, WMI is the exclusive pattern of injury recognized prior to surgery.[38] It is important to recognize that the strokes and WMIs identified in these research studies are largely clinically silent and overlooked with routine clinical screening cranial ultrasounds. Some studies have identified that preoperative brain injury is strongly associated with balloon atrial septostomy, a therapeutic catheterization procedure required by many newborns with d-transposition of the great arteries. In fact, in one cohort, for newborns with d-transposition of the great arteries, all injuries followed balloon atrial septostomy and the majority of lesions appeared embolic.[35,36,39] However, in other studies, preoperative stroke has not been observed at all in newborns requiring balloon atrial septostomy.[38] Other risk factors for the preoperative brain injuries include lower Apgar scores and lower arterial oxygen saturations.[35,36] Elevated brain lactate on proton MR spectroscopy, indicating impaired cerebral metabolism, is detected in more than half of newborns preoperatively and is associated with brain injury on MRI.[30,39] In one cohort study in which WMI was the exclusive pattern of injury observed prior to surgery, the degree of hypoxemia (lower arterial oxygen saturations) and the time to surgical correction were the critical risk fac-

tors identified for preoperative brain injury.[38] These studies underscore the potential that differences in clinical care practices might result in different patterns of injury, each with different etiologic risk factors.

White matter injury is common in newborns with CHD following cardiac surgery

While brain injuries such as stroke and WMI are frequently recognized prior to surgery in newborns with CHD, injuries that were not evident before surgery are recognized postoperatively in an additional one third to one half of newborns with CHD.[30,35] In contrast with preoperative findings, the most common pattern of brain injury on postoperative MRI is WMI, particularly in neonates with single ventricle physiology and aortic arch obstruction.[30,35] The risk of detecting acquired brain injury postoperatively is associated with cardiopulmonary bypass with regional cerebral perfusion and with lower cerebral hemoglobin oxygen saturation during the myocardial ischemic period of bypass.[35] The findings detected with near-infrared spectroscopy (NIRS) are seen regardless of bypass method.[35] Just as with preoperative injuries, the risk factors for postoperative stroke need to be distinguished from those for WMI. In a recent study, all five postoperative strokes occurred following regional cerebral perfusion in single ventricle patients undergoing the Norwood procedure.[35] The strokes detected postoperatively were largely focal lesions involving < 1/3 of the arterial territory and had imaging characteristics suggesting embolism as a possible mechanism.[35] In contrast, new postoperative WMI is specifically associated with low blood pressure during the first postoperative day, and to relative cerebral desaturation detected by NIRS.[35,40,41] Relative cerebral desaturation refers to a failure of cerebral saturation to recover or normalize following the bypass period, measured by NIRS, at a time when systemic saturations, also measured by NIRS, normalize.[35,40,41] Thus, relative cerebral desaturation is apparent only when concurrent NIRS measures are obtained from the brain (head) and systemic organs (flank). Following cardiopulmonary bypass, this pattern of selective cerebral desaturation is frequently noted, especially with the bypass method of regional cerebral perfusion.[42,43] Additionally, during the first postoperative day in newborns with hypoplastic left heart syndrome, cerebral oxygen saturation below 45% for longer than 3 hours[41] and low diastolic blood pressure[40] are associated with brain injury, particularly WMI. In a recent series of newborns with hypoplastic left heart syndrome, those with adverse neurodevelopmental outcome had decreased systemic oxygen delivery postoperatively.[44] Postoperative seizures, a marker of brain injury, are also variably associated with adverse neurodevelopmental outcome, highlighting that the risk for cerebral energy failure and injury extend well beyond the period of cardiopulmonary bypass.[45–47] Together, these observations also suggest that intraoperative factors interact with postoperative risk factors such that events during cardiopulmonary bypass may predispose the brain to injury from postoperative low cardiac output.

It remains largely unknown how these focal brain injuries result in diffuse abnormalities of neurodevelopmental outcome, as seen in newborns with CHD. Recent observations related to WMI in the premature newborn (discussed below) suggest that the focal brain injuries observed with conventional MRI reflect only one component of a more diffuse brain abnormality. Recent observation in term newborns with CHD indicate that brain injury in the immature brain impairs subsequent white matter development. Using serial diffusion tensor imaging (DTI), an advanced quantitative MR technique, acquired brain injuries such as stroke and WMI in newborns with CHD are associated with impaired development of the corticospinal tracts, the primary white matter pathway subserving voluntary motor movements.[37] The corticospinal tract abnormalities were not evident on conventional MRI and were most apparent using the diffusion tensor tractography technique in those with the earliest brain injuries (i.e., preoperative injury). Newborns with injuries identified postoperatively had diffusion values in the corticospinal tract intermediate between those with normal scans and those with preoperative injuries. These findings are consistent with others in the premature newborn, highlighting the need to look beyond the focal abnormalities most readily appreciated with conventional MRI. These findings also highlight the important interplay between brain injury and abnormal brain development. This relationship is being most explicitly defined in regard to WMI in the developing brain.

White matter injury is the characteristic pattern of injury in premature newborns and is associated with adverse neurodevelopmental outcomes

WMI, including periventricular leukomalacia (PVL), is the characteristic pattern of brain injury in premature newborns without CHD.[48–50] The early descriptions of PVL referred to extensive cystic necrotic lesions that were frequently accompanied by white matter atrophy reflected in enlargement of the lateral ventricles. The cystic lesions of PVL were characteristically symmetric and located adjacent to the anterior and posterior horns of the lateral ventricles. The most commonly affected brain regions appeared to be the frontal and parietal-occipital periventricular white matter, including the optic radiations of the visual system. In the intensive care nursery, the cystic lesions of PVL and the accompanying enlargement of the ventricles are well detected by bedside brain ultrasound in premature newborns.[51] However, most children delivered preterm who eventually exhibit deficits in motor and cognitive outcomes do not have PVL identified sonographically in the neonatal period.[52] Furthermore, over the last decade a dramatic decline in the incidence of cystic PVL has been identified.[52] The decline in cystic PVL is related, at least in part, to changes in neonatal intensive care, such as a decrease in days of mechanical ventilation,[52] with the avoidance of hypocarbic alkalosis, a previously recognized risk factor for PVL.[53] However, with the increasing use of MRI tools, focal or diffuse noncystic WMIs are emerging as the predominant lesions with cystic PVL accounting for less than 5% of injuries in some series.[48,49,54]

Focal noncystic WMI is now recognized as one of the most common patterns of brain injury identified using MRI in the premature newborn.[48] On T1-weighted MRI, focal noncystic WMI appears as areas of hyperintensity. In some cohorts studied with MRI, focal noncystic WMI is identified in more than half of premature newborns.[48] As brain ultrasound, the traditional brain imaging technique for detecting PVL, has limited sensitivity for diagnosing focal noncystic WMI, these noncystic injuries were likely underrecognized in premature newborns in the past. WMI can now be considered a spectrum of brain injury ranging from the multifocal cystic lesions of PVL, to noncystic focal WMI, and diffuse myelination disturbances.[55] While neurodevelopmental deficits in premature newborns[4] might be attributed to PVL in some cases, most children who exhibit deficits in motor and cognitive outcomes do not have sonographically identified PVL.[52] In premature infants, the presence of WMI at term-equivalent age is also strongly associated with abnormal brain volumes, including smaller cerebral cortex volumes and smaller volumes of the basal ganglia.[56,57] This is consistent with the observation using serial DTI that focal noncystic WMI prior to term age is followed by diffuse abnormalities of white matter development and connectivity as the newborns develop to term-equivalent age.[58] These more widespread brain changes associated with the focal lesions of WMI might account for the observation that noncystic WMI on MRI is associated with diffuse abnormalities of early motor and cognitive function.[48]

Cellular and molecular mechanisms of white matter vulnerability in the premature newborn

The pathogenesis of WMI in premature newborns was previously considered to arise due to an ischemic vulnerability secondary to the immature brain's vascular anatomy. More recently, it has become recognized that the specific predilection for injury to the brain's white matter is strongly related to the vulnerability of specific developmentally regulated cell populations: specifically, late oligodendrocyte progenitor cells and subplate neurons. The late oligodendrocyte progenitor is the cell type predominating in the white matter during the high-risk period for WMI in premature newborns.[59] Neurons in the subplate zone (subplate neurons) are another developmentally regulated cell population that plays a critical role in normal visual thalamocortical development.[60,61] Subplate newborns are also exquisitely vulnerable to neonatal hypoxia-ischemia.[60,61] Similar to the developmental trajectory of the oligodendrocyte progenitors in human brain development, subplate neuron numbers peak at the onset of vulnerability for WMI.[62] Interestingly, subplate neurons are the first neurons of the cerebral cortex to express glutamatergic NMDA and AMPA receptors.[63,64] This is relevant, as oxidative stress and excitotoxicity are two mechanisms proposed for the selective vulnerability of these cell types.[60,65,66] Importantly, late oligodendrocyte progenitor cells also express N-methyl D-aspartate (NMDA) and α-amino-3-hydroxyl-5-methyl-4-isoxazole-propionate (AMPA) receptors and are blocking these receptors protects these cells from hypoxia-ischemia.[65,67] In a series of elegant experiments, Back and colleagues have demonstrated the selective vulnerability of the late oligodendrocyte progenitor cell to hypoxic ischemic injury.[66] In a sheep model of "preterm" hypoxic-ischemic brain injury, the distribution of these susceptible oligodendrocyte progenitor cells, rather than limitations in cerebral blood flow, underlies the spatial anatomy of WMI.[68] This observation suggests that the cell types populating the developing brain determine the pattern of brain injury following hypoxia-ischemia and that the immature brain's vascular anatomy is not sufficient to account for the preterm newborn's predilection to WMI. While earlier observations suggested that the late oligodendrocyte progenitor cells died following exposure to hypoxic-ischemic stress, more recent observations suggest that the myelination failure observed with WMI is the result of both delayed degeneration of the oligodendrocyte progenitor and an arrest in the maturation of the oligodendrocyte precursor pool.[69] These data imply that the persistence of oligodendrocyte precursors maintains a "susceptible" cell population leading to an ongoing white matter vulnerability to recurrent insults, such as that due to hypoxia-ischemia.[69] As will be discussed below, these issues are of direct relevance to the term newborn with CHD, in whom WMI is also observed with some frequency.

White matter injury in term newborns with CHD

While WMI is the characteristic pattern of brain injury in premature newborns, it is increasingly recognized in populations of term newborns such as those with CHD. As described above, full-term infants with CHD also have a strikingly high incidence of WMI on MRI and at autopsy.[30,35,40,70–72] For example, Galli and colleagues identified WMI in more that 54% of newborns with CHD early in the postoperative period,[40] and Miller and colleagues found WMI in 43% of infants with CHD 2 years after cardiac surgery.[72] The WMI lesions detected on MRI in term newborns with CHD have remarkably similar imaging characteristics to those observed in premature newborns.[35,48] This is consistent with autopsy data where WMI was noted in 25 of 33 children with CHD.[70] In order to address the impact of low-flow cardiopulmonary bypass, deep hypothermic circulatory arrest, and the age of the infants at the time of surgery on the severity of severity brain injury on neuropathology, Kinney and coworkers examined the brains of 38 infants dying after cardiac surgery.[71] WMI was the most prevalent pattern of brain injury in this series, with cerebral white matter gliosis seen in 79% and acute, organizing, or chronic PVL in 61%.[71] It should also be noted that acute neuronal injury in the cerebral cortex and hippocampal injuries were seen in more than 60% of cases.[71] Importantly infants with longer cardiopulmonary bypass time did not have more severe overall brain injury. Newborns undergoing surgery were at greater risk for WMI than older infants.[71] Acute PVL was seen in 34% of infants in the study, and this specific lesion occurred most frequently in infants who died at younger ages.[71] Together, these neuroimaging and neuropathology data suggest that WMI is common in the brain of term newborns with CHD and that it may result from a vulnerability of developmentally regulated cell populations in these newborns, analogous to the white matter vulnerability of the premature newborn.

Abnormal brain development in term newborns with CHD

As described above, the pattern of WMI in the premature newborn is attributed to developmentally regulated cell populations vulnerable to ischemia and oxidative stress.[51,60,68] Though predominant injury to neurons would be the expected response to these insults in term newborns with CHD,[31] WMI nonetheless occurs frequently. Similar to premature newborns, those with CHD are certainly at risk for impaired delivery of energy substrates due to ischemia, inflammation, and oxidative stress, particularly with cardiopulmonary bypass. Recent experimental and clinical research evidence suggests that term newborns with CHD retain a vulnerability to WMI because of impaired *in utero* brain development, possibly as a result of abnormal cerebral blood flow during early brain development. To address this issue *in vivo*, it is necessary to look beyond qualitative "diagnostic" MRI to more advanced quantitative MRI techniques. Insights into brain develop-

ment in term newborns with CHD from newborn brain imaging studies will be reviewed followed by experimental evidence relating to abnormal *in utero* cerebral blood flow in the fetus with CHD.

Advanced magnetic resonance imaging of brain development in newborns

Advanced MRI techniques, such as MR spectroscopic imaging (MRSI) and DTI, now provide an unprecedented dynamic window into neonatal brain development *in vivo* (Fig. 2).

Proton MRSI provides an *in vivo* measure of brain metabolism, measuring resonance from N-acetyl groups (predominantly N-acetylaspartate [NAA]), lactate, creatine, and tetramethylamines (predominantly choline-containing compounds).[73] NAA is found predominantly in neurons (cell body and axon), so that decreases and increases in NAA reflect neuronal metabolic integrity.[73] Particularly relevant to studies of brain development in the observation that NAA increases consistently with advancing cerebral maturity.[74] Elevations of lactate reflect ongoing metabolic disturbances as lactate provides an index of anaerobic glycolysis. However, lactate is detected in the brains of otherwise normal premature newborns in the absence of overt brain injury.[74] Because creatine increases with gestational age heterogeneously across brain regions, it does not provide an ideal internal reference for studies of newborn brain development.[73,74] In contrast, the choline peak is a useful internal reference in the newborn for pathological conditions that do not significantly change because it is relatively stable across the newborn period of brain development as measured by proton magnetic resonance spectroscopy (^{1}H-MRS).[74] Concentrations of these metabolites can now be quantified in the developing brain using sophisticated analysis of ^{1}H-MRS acquired at short echo times.[74] In the absence of such protocols for absolute quantitation of metabolites, levels of NAA and lactate may be expressed relative to the choline peak. In studies of neonatal brain injury, it is apparent that these metabolite ratios provide a dynamic measure of brain metabolism following hypoxia-ischemia. In the term newborn, in the first 24 hours following hypoxic-ischemic injury, lactate/choline increases, followed over the subsequent 72 hours by a decrease in NAA/choline.[75] In term newborns with

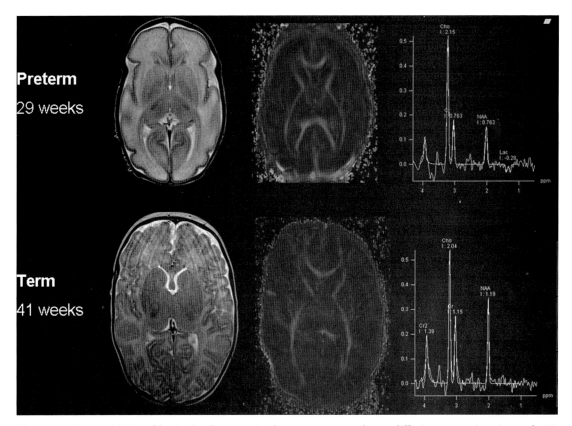

Figure 2. Advanced MRI of brain development in the premature newborn: diffusion tensor imaging and MR spectroscopic imaging. Axial T2-weighted, color-coded fractional anisotropy maps, and representative MR spectra from the thalamus in a premature neonate delivered at 28 weeks gestation and scanned at 29 weeks postmenstrual age and again at 41 weeks postmenstrual age. On the T2-weighted images note the dramatic increase in gyration of the cerebral cortex and early myelination in the posterior limb of the internal capsule. The color-coded fractional anisotropy maps represent the "directionality" of water diffusion, with brighter areas indicating more directionality (higher fractional anisotrophy [FA]). Water diffusion in the right–left plane is colored red, superior–inferior in blue, and anterior–posterior in green. The corticospinal tracts (blue region in the posterior limb of the internal capsule) and the optic radiations (green tract running from the thalamus to occipital cortex) are more clearly delineated with higher FA at term-equivalent age. In contrast, the cerebral cortex has high FA on the early scan, which is no longer detectable at term-equivalent age. The MR spectra from the thalamus demonstrate marked metabolic brain development, with a dramatic increase in N-acetylaspartate/choline ratio, and a loss of the lactate resonance, as the newborn develops to term-equivalent age.

encephalopathy presumed secondary to hypoxia-ischemia, lower NAA/choline and higher lactate/choline are associated with a greater risk for neurodevelopmental impairments.[76] A recent study showed that the ratios of lactate/NAA were even a better predictor of outcome than the abnormalities found with T_2 quantitative measure.[77] Together these studies demonstrate that changes in these metabolite ratios are an important reflector of brain development in the premature and term newborn,

and are predictive of neurodevelopmental outcomes following hypoxia-ischemia in the term newborn.

DTI can now be applied in the newborn to provide a sensitive measure of regional brain microstructural development. DTI characterizes the three-dimensional spatial distribution of water diffusion in each voxel of the MR image.[78] With increasing brain maturation, brain water content diminishes and developing neuronal and glial cell membranes increasingly restrict proton diffusion, resulting in a consistent decrease in average diffusivity (D_{av}) over time in gray and white matter regions[58,78] Fractional anisotropy (FA) is a measure of the directionality of proton diffusion. With increasing brain maturation, white matter FA increases coincident with the maturation of the oligodendrocyte lineage and early events of myelination.[58,79] Thus, changes in white matter FA provide a sensitive measure of white matter microstructural development. In the cerebral cortex, FA is high early in the third trimester and becomes undetectable by term. This loss of cortical diffusion anisotropy is thought to reflect a loss of the radial organization of the cerebral cortex in early brain development.[80,81] In addition to providing measures of microstructural brain development, these water diffusion parameters are also important reflectors of acute acquired brain injury. With acute brain injury, when a diffusion gradient is applied, intracellular water increases and water diffusion is "restricted" by the cell membrane. Areas of restricted diffusion can be visualized on the average diffusivity or the apparent diffusion coefficient (ADC) maps as areas of diminished signal intensity. In recent studies using serial diffusion MRI in term newborns with encephalopathy presumed secondary to hypoxia-ischemia, a characteristic evolution of D_{av} is observed over the first weeks of life.[75,82] Water diffusion abnormalities may be detected on D_{av} maps even when conventional MR images are largely normal, as expected on the first day following an insult.[75,82] More specifically, the diffusion abnormalities in a given region of the brain may be detectable in the first days of life but then normalize over the following 7–10 days. Additionally, the water diffusion abnormalities may progress to involve new brain areas over the first 2 weeks of life, as areas originally involved begin to normalize.[75] Even before the diffusion abnormalities begin to resolve, abnormalities become clearly evident on conventional MRI images.[31,75,82] Following hypoxic-ischemic encephalopathy in the term newborn, D_{av} values in the posterior limb of the internal capsule are a good indicator of the severity of brain injury and can be used as a predictor of neurodevelopmental outcome.[83] Thus, as with the MRSI metabolite parameters, the characteristics of water diffusion in the brain provide an important reflector of brain development in the premature and term newborn and a dynamic measure of the severity and extent of brain injury following hypoxia-ischemia in the term newborn.

Does abnormal brain development predispose newborns with CHD to white matter injury?

As described above, WMI is the characteristic pattern of brain injury observed after cardiac surgery, but may also be seen preoperatively in term newborns with CHD, suggesting that the white matter in these newborns shares vulnerability with that in premature newborns. Furthermore, CHD in newborns is associated with global developmental impairments identified as these infants develop through childhood. These observations suggest that term newborns with CHD may have more widespread abnormalities in brain development, as seen in premature newborns, in addition to the focal and multifocal brain injuries identified on MRI. Perhaps abnormal brain development predisposes newborns with CHD to WMI. Recently, using MRSI and DTI, brain metabolism and microstructure were characterized as measures of brain maturation in term newborns with CHD prior to heart surgery relative to normal controls.[34] In this study, 29 term newborns with d-transposition of the great arteries and 12 with single ventricle physiology, including hypoplastic left heart syndrome, were studied with MRI, 3-dimensional MRSI, and DTI before cardiac surgery. Sixteen normal term controls were studied at a similar postmenstrual age. N-acetylaspartate/choline ratios, lactate/choline ratios, average diffusivity, and white matter FA were calculated from several anatomically defined regions of interest. Relative to the normal control newborns, newborns with CHD had 10% lower NAA/choline ratios ($P = 0.003$). Newborns with CHD had higher lactate/choline, but the difference was not statistically significant (+28%, $P = 0.08$). Relative to controls, newborns with CHD had 4.5% higher D_{av} ($P < 0.001$), and 12% lower white matter FA ($P < 0.001$). These effects were similar in newborns with d-transposition of the great arteries and in those with single ventricle physiology relative to controls. WMI was observed in 13 (32%) newborns with CHD and in no controls. Among newborns with CHD, preoperative brain injury on MRI was not significantly associated with the MRSI or DTI measures. These data indicate that term newborns with CHD have widespread brain abnormalities prior to cardiac surgery. Impaired brain metabolism and microstructure were seen in this cohort, even in the absence of visible injury on MRI, and in uninvolved regions in those with injury. These impairments were widespread and did not conform to the patterns of brain injury typical of hypoxia-ischemia in the term newborn.[31] The pattern of lower NAA/choline, higher average diffusivity, and lower white matter FA observed in newborns with CHD is congruous with findings in premature newborns at an earlier age and may reflect delayed *in utero* brain development. Specifically, MRSI metabolite ratios in newborns with CHD are similar in value to those from premature newborns approximately 1 month prior to full term.[58,84] Thus data from this study suggest that abnormal brain development precedes surgery and even some acquired injuries in newborns with CHD, although further studies with fetal MRI are necessary to confirm this suggestion.

These *in vivo* observations using quantitative MR methods are consistent with neuropathology data that newborns with CHD are more likely to be microcephalic and have an immature cortical mantel.[85,86] In a study comparing fetal growth differences among 276 control infants with 69 infants with d-transposition of the great arteries, 66 with tetralogy of Fallot, 51 with hypoplastic left heart syndrome, and 65 with coarctation of the aorta, striking differences in head growth were found between groups.[85] Despite normal birth weight, infants with d-transposition of the great arteries had smaller head volume relative to birth weight. Those with tetralogy of Fallot were smaller overall but proportional in regard to head growth. Infants with hypoplastic left heart syndrome were smaller overall, but, even more striking, head volume was disproportionately lower relative to the already lower birth weight. In contrast, infants with coarctation of the aorta had, despite lower birth weight, larger head volume relative to birth weight. As will be discussed below, these findings indicate that abnormalities in *in utero* cerebral blood flow are associated with different patterns of abnormal fetal growth, including that of the brain.[85] These data are also consistent with neuropathology observation in 41 infants with the hypoplastic left heart syndrome.[86] In these newborns, brain weight was more than two standard deviations below the mean in 21%. While 29% of these infants had some abnormality of the central nervous system, major brain malformations were only seen in four (agenesis of the corpus callosum in three and

holoprosencephaly in one). Almost one fourth of these patients were described as having an immature cortical mantle.[86] Importantly for clinicians, brain malformations were not accurately predicted by the presence of dysmorphic features. Yet developmental abnormalities of the brain on neuropathology were more common in those infants who were small for gestational age, microcephalic, or had ocular abnormalities.[86] These data are consistent with those observed in imaging series, where overt brain malformations are uncommon on MRI, yet subtle abnormalities in brain development may be observed with more sophisticated imaging modalities.

In a recent study examining the hypothesis that newborns with CHD have delayed structural brain development *in utero*, 29 term newborns with d-transposition of the great arteries and 13 with hypoplastic left heart syndrome were scanned preoperatively with MRI.[87] The MR images were reviewed to assign a "total maturation score" describing myelination, cortical folding, involution of glial cell migration bands, and the presence of germinal matrix tissue. Consistent with previous observations, mean head circumference was one standard deviation below normal. The total maturation score for newborns with CHD was significantly lower than that reported previously in newborns without CHD. Consistent with the MRSI data described above, normative data in infants without congenital heart defects, corresponding to a delay of 1 month in structural brain development.[34,87] The mechanisms by which these heart lesions impact brain development are largely unknown but may relate to impairments in cerebral blood flow. In a group of 25 term newborns with CHD studied with pulsed arterial spin-label perfusion MRI prior to heart surgery, blood flow was low in the cohort as a whole and dramatically reduced in some newborns.[88] The occurrence of WMI was associated with lower cerebral blood flow values.[88] Experimental evidence for disrupted *in utero* cerebral blood flow as a result of CHD will be addressed below.

In addition to impairments in brain development evident prior to cardiac surgery in newborns with CHD, these newborns are also at risk of acquiring abnormalities in brain development postnatally. As noted above, the impact of preoperative brain injury on corticospinal tract development was examined in 25 newborns with CHD, imaged before and after surgery with diffusion tensor tractography of the corticospinal tracts.[37] Significant maturational increases of FA and decreases of average diffusivity in the pyramidal tract were measured in infants without brain injury. FA maturation rates were highest in newborns with normal scans, intermediate in those with postoperative injury, and lowest in those with preoperative injury, indicating a significant trend across brain injury groups.[37] Parallel to findings in the premature newborn, where WMI is associated with more widespread impairments in gray and white matter development, brain injury in newborns with CHD prior to surgery also impairs the subsequent development of the corticospinal tracts.[37] Together these data highlight the important connection of focal brain injuries with widespread abnormalities in subsequent brain development.

Taken together, these results point to a complex interplay between brain injury and abnormal brain development in newborns with CHD. In fact, focal brain injury may itself disturb subsequent brain development. Furthermore, there is now considerable evidence that newborns with CHD, particularly in those with d-transposition of the great arteries and single ventricle physiology, including hypoplastic left heart syndrome, have impaired *in utero* brain growth, possibly related to impaired fetal cerebral oxygen delivery.[89–91]

Review of fetal circulation

Blood flow in the fetus differs from the postnatal circulation in a number of respects that have significance for cerebral blood flow (reviewed in Ref. 91). In the following sections, we will review normal fetal circulation and then consider the effects of CHD, specifically d-transposition of the great arteries and forms of hypoplastic left heart syndrome. After birth, venous blood flows serially through the right ventricle to the lungs where it is oxygenated prior to returning to the left atrium. The left ventricle in turn pumps oxygenated blood to the body. Gas exchange in the fetus occurs through the placenta with blood supplied through the umbilical artery from the aorta, returning through the umbilical vein and ductus venosus to the portal vein, inferior vena cava and right atrium (Fig. 3A). Prior to birth, blood flow to the lungs is limited by elevated pulmonary vascular resistance. Two connections exist between the systemic and pulmonary cir-

culations: the foramen ovale connecting the right and left atria and the ductus arteriosus between the pulmonary trunk and descending aorta. Umbilical venous blood is preferentially directed through the ductus venosus. The left lobe of the liver receives predominantly umbilical venous blood, while the right lobe of the liver receives most of the portal venous blood and a substantial amount from the umbilical vein. As a consequence the oxygen saturation is higher in the left hepatic veins compared with the right as they join the inferior vena cava (IVC) resulting in streams of blood with different saturations. The more saturated stream containing blood from the ductus venosus is preferentially directed across the foramen ovale to the left atrium (Fig. 3A). This blood mixes with the limited amount of pulmonary venous blood returning from the lungs, resulting in a saturation in the fetal left ventricle of approximately 65%. Blood ejected by the right ventricle consists of venous blood from the superior vena cava as well as the relatively desaturated streams from the IVC and coronary sinus. The resulting saturation in the fetal right ventricle is about 55%.

Brain growth and changes in cerebral blood flow during gestation

Blood flow to the brain is estimated to be almost one fourth of the combined ventricular output in the third trimester.[91] Autoregulation of cerebral blood flow is thought to redistribute blood flow to the brain in the setting of placental insufficiency,[92] a phenomenon referred to as "brain sparing," resulting in a pattern of overall somatic growth restriction with relative preservation of head growth. In the setting of CHD, similar mechanisms give rise to lower cerebral to placental resistance ratios that would tend to preserve cerebral blood flow,[93] although very low cerebral blood flow has been measured in newborns with hypoplastic left heart syndrome and d-transposition of the great arteries using MRI.[88] Despite these regulatory mechanisms, newborns with certain forms of CHD have smaller head circumferences, possibly indicating impaired brain growth. However, growth patterns are specific to each form of CHD.[85] Newborns with d-transposition of the great arteries have small head circumference with normal birth weight. Newborns with hypoplastic left heart syndrome are smaller in

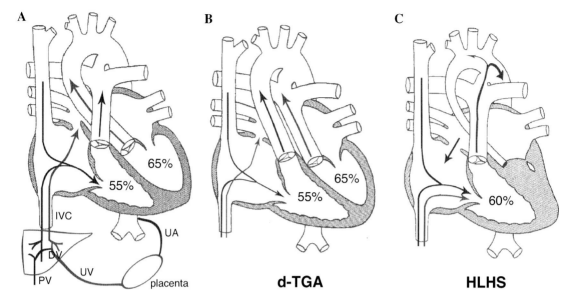

Figure 3. Normal fetal circulation and changes with congenital heart disease. Course of blood flow in a late gestation fetus with normal heart anatomy (**A**), d-transposition of the great arteries (**B**), and hypoplastic left heart syndrome due to aortic atresia (**C**). Blood flows to and from the placenta are shown only for the normal circulation (**A**). The course of relatively oxygenated (*red*) and deoxygenated blood (*blue*) is shown by arrows. Estimated hemoglobin oxygen saturation in percent is shown for each ventricle.

all dimensions, but head volume is disproportionately decreased. Surprisingly, infants with isolated aortic coarctation have a greater head volume relative to birth weight. Decline in head growth begins after midgestation in the majority of fetuses with hypoplastic left heart syndrome, as 78% of fetuses with hypoplastic left heart syndrome had normal head size on fetal ultrasound.[94] Midgestation through birth in human brain development coincides with periods of axonal pathfinding, synapse formation, and refinement (reviewed in Ref. 95). Neurogenesis of neocortex is complete, but generation of glia (oligodendrocytes and astrocytes) is ongoing.

d-Transposition of the great arteries

In d-transposition of the great arteries the aorta arises from the right ventricle and thus receives the relatively desaturated blood (∼55%) from the superior vena cava and lower saturation stream of blood in the IVC (Fig. 3B). The higher saturated stream from the left hepatic veins resulting from delivery of the oxygenated umbilical venous blood is directed normally across the foramen ovale to the

morphologic left ventricle. The left ventricle however is connected to the pulmonary trunk, and this higher saturated blood (∼65%) is delivered to the lungs and lower body (Fig. 3B). Some have proposed that delivery of this more saturated blood to the gastrointestinal tract and pancreas results in relative macrosomia in newborns with d-transposition of the great arteries.[96]

Hypoplastic left heart syndrome

Hypoplastic left heart syndrome includes a spectrum of conditions with obstruction to blood flow in the left ventricle. The condition is best represented by aortic atresia, but also includes critical aortic stenosis, mitral atresia, and Shone's complex (multiple left sided obstructive lesions). The fetal circulation is characterized by increased left atrial pressure, resulting in reversal of flow (left to right) across the foramen ovale (Fig. 3C). The left ventricle may be rudimentary in the cases of mitral or aortic atresia, or with preserved size but severely abnormal function in some cases of aortic stenosis. In both situations, left ventricular filling is impaired and there is no ventricular output or stroke volume is diminished. This results in diminished or absent flow into the ascending aorta. In the absence of preferential streaming of the well-saturated IVC blood into the left ventricle, all venous return mixes in the right ventricle and is ejected into the pulmonary trunk and ductus arteriosus (Fig. 3C). Although the resulting saturation is not as low as with d-transposition of the great arteries, a number of factors may restrict flow to the cerebral circulation, including presence of aortic atresia, severity of aortic and mitral stenosis, and coarctation of the aorta. In the setting of aortic atresia, flow to the head and neck vessels occurs only by retrograde flow into the transverse and ascending aorta (Fig. 3C). However, in a recent study ascending aortic diameter and not presence of aortic atresia or size of transverse aortic arch predicted the degree of microcephaly in newborns with hypoplastic left heart syndrome.[97]

Summary and conclusions

In summary, newborns with CHD show a high frequency of acquired focal brain injury on sensitive MRI studies in the peri-operative period. These injuries are clinically silent and include small focal strokes and WMI. The surprisingly high incidence of WMI in these term newborns suggests a unique vulnerability and may be related to findings suggesting a delay in brain development. A complete understanding of the mechanisms of WMI in the term newborn with CHD will require further investigation of the timing, extent, and causes of delayed fetal brain development in the presence of CHD. Lessons learned from these studies will have relevance for current clinical practice (e.g., timing and nature of surgical intervention) as well as for newly proposed fetal therapies for CHD. It will also be critical to determine the specific contribution of peri-operative focal brain injuries and the more widespread disturbances in brain development to the neurodevelopmental abnormalities identified in childhood survivors of CHD.

Newborns with CHD are an important population in whom to evaluate emerging therapies to prevent brain injury, as there is a temporally planned and quantifiable exposure to ischemia with cardiopulmonary bypass. The feasibility of studying brain protective agents in this population has been demonstrated.[98] A better understanding of brain injury in newborns with CHD, and when the injury is acquired, will be critical to the optimal application of emerging brain-protection strategies. The imaging findings outlined in this review also suggest that a number of potentially modifiable risk factors for brain injury in this population exist. Therefore, the ability to quantify brain injury and identify modifiable risk factors should enable the design and testing of new strategies for preventing or treating brain injury. These interventions will ultimately improve outcomes and reduce the healthcare costs associated with caring for newborns with CHD. How patient-specific factors, such as genetic traits, interact with risk factors for brain injury and the neurodevelopmental sequelae of brain abnormalities will require larger "gene environment" studies. Ultimately, the development of accurate *in vivo* measures of brain injury in newborns with CHD should also help parents and physicians to better care for these newborns by providing important prognostic information so that rehabilitation strategies can be implemented as early as possible.

Acknowledgments

The authors thank Dr. Abraham M. Rudolph for critical review of the manuscript. SPM is supported by a Canadian Institutes of Health Clinician Scientist Phase 2 award (40747) and a Michael Smith Foundation for Health Research Scholar award (CI-SCH-065 (05–1)). PSM is supported by NIH K02 NS047098. Research reported here is funded by the March of Dimes Foundation (#5-FY05–1231), the American Heart Association (0365018Y), the Larry L. Hillblom Foundation (2002/3E), Dana Foundation (Brain & Immuno Imaging), Canadian Institutes for Health Research (CIHR; CHI 151135), and NIH grants RO1 NS40117, 5 M01 RR-01271, and P50 NS35902.

Conflicts of interest

The authors declare no conflicts of interest.

References

1. Hoffman, J.I. & S. Kaplan. 2002. The incidence of congenital heart disease. *J. Am. Coll. Cardiol.* **39:** 1890–1900.
2. Samanek, M. 2000. Congenital heart malformations: prevalence, severity, survival, and quality of life. *Cardiol. Young.* **10:** 179–185.

3. Castaneda, A.R., J.R., J.E. Mayer & F.L. Hanley. 1994. *Cardiac Surgery of the Neonate and Infant*. W.B. Saunders. Philadelphia.

4. Saigal, S. & L.W. Doyle. 2008. An overview of mortality and sequelae of preterm birth from infancy to adulthood. *Lancet* **371:** 261–269.

5. Bellinger, D.C., R.A. Jonas, L.A. Rappaport, *et al*. 1995. Developmental and neurologic status of children after heart surgery with hypothermic circulatory arrest or low-flow cardiopulmonary bypass. *N. Engl. J. Med.* **332:** 549–555.

6. Jonas, R., J.W. Newburger & J.J. Volpe. 1996. *Brain Injury and Pediatric Cardiac Surgery*. Butterworth-Heinimann. Boston.

7. Bellinger, D.C., D. Wypij, A.J. Duplessis, *et al*. 2003. Neurodevelopmental status at eight years in children with dextro-transposition of the great arteries: the Boston Circulatory Arrest Trial. *J. Thorac. Cardiovasc. Surg.* **126:** 1385–1396.

8. Karl, T.R., S. Hall, G. Ford, *et al*. 2004. Arterial switch with full-flow cardiopulmonary bypass and limited circulatory arrest: neurodevelopmental outcome. *J. Thorac. Cardiovasc. Surg.* **127:** 213–222.

9. Bellinger, D.C. 2008. Are children with congenital cardiac malformations at increased risk of deficits in social cognition? *Cardiol. Young.* **18:** 3–9.

10. Limperopoulos, C., A. Majnemer, M.I. Shevell, *et al*. 2002. Predictors of developmental disabilities after open heart surgery in young children with congenital heart defects. *J. Pediatr.* **141:** 51–58.

11. Wernovsky, G., K.M. Stiles, K. Gauvreau, *et al*. 2000. Cognitive development after the Fontan operation. *Circulation* **102:** 883–889.

12. Miller, G., J.R. Tesman, J.C. Ramer, *et al*. 1996. Outcome after open-heart surgery in infants and children. *J. Child Neurol.* **11:** 49–53.

13. Rogers, B.T., M.E. Msall, G.M. Buck, *et al*. 1995. Neurodevelopmental outcome of infants with hypoplastic left heart syndrome. *J. Pediatr.* **126:** 496–498.

14. Wernovsky, G. 2006. Current insights regarding neurological and developmental abnormalities in children and young adults with complex congenital cardiac disease. *Cardiol. Young.* **16**(Suppl 1): 92–104.

15. Majnemer, A., C. Limperopoulos, M. Shevell, *et al*. 2008. Developmental and functional outcomes at school entry in children with congenital heart defects. *J. Pediatr.* **153:** 55–60.

16. Grosse, S.D., T.D. Matte, J. Schwartz, *et al*. 2002. Economic gains resulting from the reduction in children's exposure to lead in the United States. *Environ. Health Perspect.* **110:** 563–569.

17. Bellinger, D.C., J.W. Newburger, D. Wypij, *et al*. 2009. Behaviour at eight years in children with surgically corrected transposition: The Boston Circulatory Arrest Trial. *Cardiol. Young.* **19:** 86–97.

18. Gaynor, J.W., G. Wernovsky, G.P. Jarvik, *et al*. 2007. Patient characteristics are important determinants of neurodevelopmental outcome at one year of age after neonatal and infant cardiac surgery. *J. Thorac. Cardiovasc. Surg.* **133:** 1344–1353, 1353 e1341–1343.

19. Gardiner, H.M. 2001. Fetal echocardiography: 20 years of progress. *Heart* **86**(Suppl 2): II12–II22.

20. Tworetzky, W., D.B. McElhinney, V.M. Reddy, *et al*. 2001. Improved surgical outcome after fetal diagnosis of hypoplastic left heart syndrome. *Circulation* **103:** 1269–1273.

21. Mahle, W.T., R.R. Clancy, S.P. McGaurn, *et al*. 2001. Impact of prenatal diagnosis on survival and early neurologic morbidity in neonates with the hypoplastic left heart syndrome. *Pediatrics* **107:** 1277–1282.

22. Kumar, R.K., J.W. Newburger, K. Gauvreau, *et al*. 1999. Comparison of outcome when hypoplastic left heart syndrome and transposition of the great arteries are diagnosed prenatally versus when diagnosis of these two conditions is made only postnatally. *Am. J. Cardiol.* **83:** 1649–1653.

23. Bartlett, J.M., D. Wypij, D.C. Bellinger, *et al*. 2004. Effect of prenatal diagnosis on outcomes in D-transposition of the great arteries. *Pediatrics* **113:** e335–e340.

24. Oates, R.K., J.M. Simpson, T.B. Cartmill, *et al*. 1995. Intellectual function and age of repair in cyanotic congenital heart disease. *Arch. Dis. Child.* **72:** 298–301.

25. Hovels-Gurich, H.H., M.C. Seghaye, R. Schnitker, *et al*. 2002. Long-term neurodevelopmental outcomes in school-aged children after neonatal arterial switch operation. *J. Thorac. Cardiovasc. Surg.* **124:** 448–458.

26. Newman, M.F., J.L. Kirchner, B. Phillips-Bute, *et al*. 2001. Longitudinal assessment of neurocognitive function after coronary- artery bypass surgery. *N. Engl. J. Med.* **344:** 395–402.

27. Nollert, G., R.A. Jonas & B. Reichart. 2000. Optimizing cerebral oxygenation during cardiac surgery: a review of experimental and clinical investigations with near infrared spectrophotometry. *Thorac. Cardiovasc. Surg.* **48:** 247–253.

28. Andropoulos, D.B., S.A. Stayer, E.D. McKenzie, *et al*. 2003. Novel cerebral physiologic monitoring to guide low-flow cerebral perfusion during neonatal aortic arch

reconstruction. *J. Thorac. Cardiovasc. Surg.* **125:** 491–499.

29. Limperopoulos, C., A. Majnemer, M.I. Shevell, *et al.* 1999. Neurologic status of newborns with congenital heart defects before open heart surgery. *Pediatrics* **103:** 402–408.

30. Mahle, W.T., F. Tavani, R.A. Zimmerman, *et al.* 2002. An MRI study of neurological injury before and after congenital heart surgery. *Circulation* **106:** I109–I114.

31. Chau, V., K.J. Poskitt, M.A. Sargent, *et al.* 2009. Comparison of computer tomography and magnetic resonance imaging scans on the third day of life in term newborns with neonatal encephalopathy. *Pediatrics* **123:** 319–326.

32. Schouman-Claeys, E., M.C. Henry-Feugeas, F. Roset, *et al.* 1993. Periventricular leukomalacia: correlation between MR imaging and autopsy findings during the first 2 months of life. *Radiology* **189:** 59–64.

33. Felderhoff-Mueser, U., M.A. Rutherford, W.V. Squier, *et al.* 1999. Relationship between MR imaging and histopathologic findings of the brain in extremely sick preterm infants. *AJNR Am. J. Neuroradiol.* **20:** 1349–1357.

34. Miller, S.P., P.S. McQuillen, S. Hamrick, *et al.* 2007. Abnormal brain development in newborns with congenital heart disease. *N. Engl. J. Med.* **357:** 1928–1938.

35. McQuillen, P.S., A.J. Barkovich, S.E. Hamrick, *et al.* 2007. Temporal and anatomic risk profile of brain injury with neonatal repair of congenital heart defects. *Stroke* **38:** 736–741.

36. McQuillen, P.S., S.E. Hamrick, M.J. Perez, *et al.* 2006. Balloon atrial septostomy is associated with preoperative stroke in neonates with transposition of the great arteries. *Circulation* **113:** 280–285.

37. Partridge, S.C., D.B. Vigneron, N.N. Charlton, *et al.* 2006. Pyramidal tract maturation after brain injury in newborns with heart disease. *Ann. Neurol.* **59:** 640–651.

38. Petit, C.J., J.J. Rome, G. Wernovsky, *et al.* 2009. Preoperative brain injury in transposition of the great arteries is associated with oxygenation and time to surgery, not balloon atrial septostomy. *Circulation* **119:** 709–716.

39. Miller, S.P., P.S. McQuillen, D.B. Vigneron, *et al.* 2004. Preoperative brain injury in newborns with transposition of the great arteries. *Ann. Thorac. Surg.* **77:** 1698–1706.

40. Galli, K.K., R.A. Zimmerman, G.P. Jarvik, *et al.* 2004. Periventricular leukomalacia is common after neonatal cardiac surgery. *J. Thorac. Cardiovasc. Surg.* **127:** 692–704.

41. Dent, C.L., J.P. Spaeth, B.V. Jones, *et al.* 2006. Brain magnetic resonance imaging abnormalities after the Norwood procedure using regional cerebral perfusion. *J. Thorac. Cardiovasc. Surg.* **131:** 190–197.

42. Hoffman, G.M., E.A. Stuth, R.D. Jaquiss, *et al.* 2004. Changes in cerebral and somatic oxygenation during stage 1 palliation of hypoplastic left heart syndrome using continuous regional cerebral perfusion. *J. Thorac. Cardiovasc. Surg.* **127:** 223–233.

43. McQuillen, P.S., M.S. Nishimoto, C.L. Bottrell, *et al.* 2007. Regional and central venous oxygen saturation monitoring following pediatric cardiac surgery: Concordance and association with clinical variables*. *Pediatr. Crit. Care Med.* **8:** 154–160.

44. Hoffman, G.M., K.A. Mussatto, C.L. Brosig, *et al.* 2005. Systemic venous oxygen saturation after the Norwood procedure and childhood neurodevelopmental outcome. *J. Thorac. Cardiovasc. Surg.* **130:** 1094–1100.

45. Rappaport, L.A., D. Wypij, D.C. Bellinger, *et al.* 1998. Relation of seizures after cardiac surgery in early infancy to neurodevelopmental outcome. Boston Circulatory Arrest Study Group. *Circulation* **97:** 773–779.

46. Gaynor, J.W., G.P. Jarvik, J. Bernbaum, *et al.* 2006. The relationship of postoperative electrographic seizures to neurodevelopmental outcome at 1 year of age after neonatal and infant cardiac surgery. *J. Thorac. Cardiovasc. Surg.* **131:** 181–189.

47. Clancy, R.R., S.A. McGaurn, G. Wernovsky, *et al.* 2003. Risk of seizures in survivors of newborn heart surgery using deep hypothermic circulatory arrest. *Pediatrics* **111:** 592–601.

48. Miller, S.P., D.M. Ferriero, C. Leonard, *et al.* 2005. Early brain injury in premature newborns detected with MRI: relationship with early neurodevelopmental outcome. *J. Pediatr.* **147:** 609–616.

49. Woodward, L.J., P.J. Anderson, N.C. Austin, *et al.* 2006. Neonatal MRI to predict neurodevelopmental outcomes in preterm infants. *N. Engl. J. Med.* **355:** 685–694.

50. Banker, B.Q. & J.C. Larroche. 1962. Periventricular leukomalacia of infancy. A form of neonatal anoxic encephalopathy. *Arch Neurol.* **7:** 386–410.

51. Volpe, J. 2001. *Neurology of the Newborn*, 4th edn. W.B. Saunders Company. Philadelphia.

52. Hamrick, S.E., S.P. Miller, C. Leonard, *et al.* 2004. Trends in severe brain injury and neurodevelopmental outcome in premature newborn infants: the role of cystic periventricular leukomalacia. *J. Pediatr.* **145:** 593–599.

53. Fujimoto, S., H. Togari, N. Yamaguchi, *et al.* 1994. Hypocarbia and cystic periventricular leukomalacia in premature infants. *Arch. Dis. Child.* **71:** F107–F110.

54. Counsell, S.J., J.M. Allsop, M.C. Harrison, *et al.* 2003. Diffusion-weighted imaging of the brain in preterm infants with focal and diffuse white matter abnormality. *Pediatrics* **112:** 1–7.

55. Volpe, J.J. 2001. Neurobiology of periventricular leukomalacia in the premature infant. *Pediatr. Res.* **50:** 553–562.

56. Inder, T.E., S.K. Warfield, H. Wang, *et al.* 2005. Abnormal cerebral structure is present at term in premature infants. *Pediatrics* **115:** 286–294.

57. Boardman, J.P., S.J. Counsell, D. Rueckert, *et al.* 2006. Abnormal deep grey matter development following preterm birth detected using deformation-based morphometry. *Neuroimage* **32:** 70–78.

58. Miller, S.P., D.B. Vigneron, R.G. Henry, *et al.* 2002. Serial quantitative diffusion tensor MRI of the premature brain: Development in newborns with and without injury. *J. Magn. Reson. Imaging* **16:** 621–632.

59. Back, S.A., N.L. Luo, N.S. Borenstein, *et al.* 2001. Late oligodendrocyte progenitors coincide with the developmental window of vulnerability for human perinatal white matter injury. *J. Neurosci.* **21:** 1302–1312.

60. McQuillen, P.S., R.A. Sheldon, C.J. Shatz, *et al.* 2003. Selective vulnerability of subplate neurons after early neonatal hypoxia-ischemia. *J. Neurosci.* **23:** 3308–3315.

61. McQuillen, P.S. & D.M. Ferriero. 2004. Selective vulnerability in the developing central nervous system. *Pediatr. Neurol.* **30:** 227–235.

62. Kostovic, I., V. Judas, M. Rados, *et al.* 2002. Laminar organization of the human fetal cerebrum revealed by histochemical markers and magnetic resonance imaging. *Cereb. Cortex* **12:** 536–544.

63. Catalano, S.M., C.K. Chang & C.J. Shatz. 1997. Activity-dependent regulation of NMDAR1 immunoreactivity in the developing visual cortex. *J. Neurosci.* **17:** 8376–8390.

64. Talos, D.M., P.L. Follett, R.D. Folkerth, *et al.* 2006. Developmental regulation of alpha-amino-3-hydroxy-5-methyl-4-isoxazole-propionic acid receptor subunit expression in forebrain and relationship to regional susceptibility to hypoxic/ischemic injury. II. Human cerebral white matter and cortex. *J. Comp. Neurol.* **497:** 61–77.

65. Follett, P.L., P.A. Rosenberg, J.J. Volpe, *et al.* 2000. NBQX attenuates excitotoxic injury in developing white matter. *J. Neurosci.* **20:** 9235–9241.

66. Back, S.A., B.H. Han, N.L. Luo, *et al.* 2002. Selective vulnerability of late oligodendrocyte progenitors to hypoxia- ischemia. *J. Neurosci.* **22:** 455–463.

67. Manning, S.M., D.M. Talos, C. Zhou, *et al.* 2008. NMDA receptor blockade with memantine attenuates white matter injury in a rat model of periventricular leukomalacia. *J. Neurosci.* **28:** 6670–6678.

68. Riddle, A., N.L. Luo, M. Manese, *et al.* 2006. Spatial heterogeneity in oligodendrocyte lineage maturation and not cerebral blood flow predicts fetal ovine periventricular white matter injury. *J. Neurosci.* **26:** 3045–3055.

69. Segovia, K.N., M. McClure, M. Moravec, *et al.* 2008. Arrested oligodendrocyte lineage maturation in chronic perinatal white matter injury. *Ann. Neurol.* **63:** 520–530.

70. Gilles, F.H., A. Leviton & J. Jammes. 1973. Age-dependent changes in white matter in congenital heart disease. *J. Neuropathol. Exp. Neurol.* **32:** 179.

71. Kinney, H.C., A. Panigrahy, J.W. Newburger, *et al.* 2005. Hypoxic-ischemic brain injury in infants with congenital heart disease dying after cardiac surgery. *Acta Neuropathol. (Berl.)* **110:** 563–578.

72. Miller, G., A.C. Mamourian, J.R. Tesman, *et al.* 1994. Long-term MRI changes in brain after pediatric open heart surgery. *J. Child. Neurol.* **9:** 390–397.

73. Novotny, E., S. Ashwal & M. Shevell. 1998. Proton magnetic resonance spectroscopy: an emerging technology in pediatric neurology research. *Pediatr. Res.* **44:** 1–10.

74. Kreis, R., L. Hofmann, B. Kuhlmann, *et al.* 2002. Brain metabolite composition during early human brain development as measured by quantitative in vivo 1H magnetic resonance spectroscopy. *Magn. Reson. Med.* **48:** 949–958.

75. Barkovich, A.J., S.P. Miller, A. Bartha, *et al.* 2006. MR imaging, MR spectroscopy, and diffusion tensor imaging of sequential studies in neonates with encephalopathy. *AJNR Am. J. Neuroradiol.* **27:** 533–547.

76. Miller, S.P., N. Newton, D.M. Ferriero, *et al.* 2002. Predictors of 30-month outcome after perinatal depression: role of proton MRS and socioeconomic factors. *Pediatr. Res.* **52:** 71–77.

77. Shanmugalingam, S., J.S. Thornton, O Iwata, *et al.* 2006. Comparative prognostic utilities of early quantitative magnetic resonance imaging spin-spin relaxometry and proton magnetic resonance spectroscopy in neonatal encephalopathy. *Pediatrics* **118:** 1467–1477.

78. Beaulieu, C. 2002. The basis of anisotropic water diffusion in the nervous system–a technical review. *NMR Biomed.* **15:** 435–455.

79. Drobyshevsky, A., S.K. Song, G. Gamkrelidze, *et al.* 2005. Developmental changes in diffusion anisotropy coincide with immature oligodendrocyte progression and maturation of compound action potential. *J. Neurosci.* **25:** 5988–5997.

80. Deipolyi, A.R., P. Mukherjee, K. Gill, *et al.* 2005. Comparing microstructural and macrostructural development

of the cerebral cortex in premature newborns: Diffusion tensor imaging versus cortical gyration. *Neuroimage* **27:** 579–586.

81. McKinstry, R.C., A. Mathur, J.H. Miller, *et al.* 2002. Radial organization of developing preterm human cerebral cortex revealed by non-invasive water diffusion anisotropy MRI. *Cereb. Cortex* **12:** 1237–1243.

82. McKinstry, R.C., J.H. Miller, A.Z. Snyder, *et al.* 2002. A prospective, longitudinal diffusion tensor imaging study of brain injury in newborns. *Neurology* **59:** 824–833.

83. Hunt, R.W., J.J. Neil, L.T. Coleman, *et al.* 2004. Apparent diffusion coefficient in the posterior limb of the internal capsule predicts outcome after perinatal asphyxia. *Pediatrics* **114:** 999–1003.

84. Vigneron, D.B. 2006. Magnetic resonance spectroscopic imaging of human brain development. *Neuroimaging Clin. N. Am.* **16:** 75–85, viii.

85. Rosenthal, G.L. 1996. Patterns of prenatal growth among infants with cardiovascular malformations: possible fetal hemodynamic effects. *Am. J. Epidemiol.* **143:** 505–513.

86. Glauser, T.A., L.B. Rorke, P.M. Weinberg, *et al.* 1990. Congenital brain anomalies associated with the hypoplastic left heart syndrome. *Pediatrics* **85:** 984–990.

87. Licht, D.J., D.M. Shera, R.R. Clancy, *et al.* 2009. Brain maturation is delayed in infants with complex congenital heart defects. *J. Thorac. Cardiovasc. Surg.* **137:** 529–536; discussion 536–527.

88. Licht, D.J., J. Wang, D.W. Silvestre, *et al.* 2004. Preoperative cerebral blood flow is diminished in neonates with severe congenital heart defects. *J. Thorac. Cardiovasc. Surg.* **128:** 841–849.

89. Donofrio, M.T., Y.A. Bremer, R.M. Schieken, *et al.* 2003. Autoregulation of cerebral blood flow in fetuses with congenital heart disease: the brain sparing effect. *Pediatr. Cardiol.* **24:** 436–443.

90. Jouannic, J.M., A. Benachi, D. Bonnet, *et al.* 2002. Middle cerebral artery Doppler in fetuses with transposition of the great arteries. *Ultrasound Obstet. Gynecol.* **20:** 122–124.

91. Rudolph, A. 2001. *Congenital Diseases of the Heart: Clinical-Physiological Considerations*, 2nd edn. Futura Publishing Company. Armonk.

92. Groenenberg, I.A., J.W. Wladimiroff & W.C. Hop. 1989. Fetal cardiac and peripheral arterial flow velocity waveforms in intrauterine growth retardation. *Circulation* **80:** 1711–1717.

93. Donofrio, M.T., Y.A. Bremer, R.M. Schieken, *et al.* 2003. Autoregulation of cerebral blood flow in fetuses with congenital heart disease: the brain sparing effect. *Pediatr. Cardiol.* **24:** 436–443.

94. Hinton, R.B., G. Andelfinger, P. Sekar, *et al.* 2008. Prenatal head growth and white matter injury in hypoplastic left heart syndrome. *Pediatr. Res.* **64:** 364–369.

95. McQuillen, P.S. & D.M. Ferriero. 2005. Perinatal subplate neuron injury: implications for cortical development and plasticity. *Brain Pathol.* **15:** 250–260.

96. Naeye, R.L. 1966. Transposition of the great arteries and prenatal growth. *Arch. Pathol.* **82:** 412–418.

97. Shillingford, A.J., R.F. Ittenbach, B.S. Marino, *et al.* 2007. Aortic morphometry and microcephaly in hypoplastic left heart syndrome. *Cardiol. Young.* **17:** 189–195.

98. Clancy, R.R., S.A. McGaurn, J.E. Goin, *et al.* 2001. Allopurinol neurocardiac protection trial in infants undergoing heart surgery using deep hypothermic circulatory arrest. *Pediatrics* **108:** 61–70.

Ann. N.Y. Acad. Sci. ISSN 0077-8923

ANNALS OF THE NEW YORK ACADEMY OF SCIENCES

The tuberous sclerosis complex

Ksenia A. Orlova and Peter B. Crino

Departments of Neurology and Neuroscience, University of Pennsylvania School of Medicine, Philadelphia, Pennsylvania, USA

Address for correspondence: Peter B. Crino, M.D., Ph.D., Department of Neurology, 3 West Gates Bldg., 3400 Spruce St., University of Pennsylvania Medical Center, Philadelphia, PA 19104. Voice: 215-349-5312. peter.crino@uphs.upenn.edu

Tuberous sclerosis complex (TSC) is an autosomal dominant disorder that results from mutations in the *TSC1* or *TSC2* genes and is associated with hamartoma formation in multiple organ systems. The neurological manifestations of TSC are particularly challenging and include infantile spasms, intractable epilepsy, cognitive disabilities, and autism. Progress over the past 15 years has demonstrated that the TSC1 or TSC2 encoded proteins modulate cell function via the mTOR signaling cascade and serve as keystones in regulating cell growth and proliferation. The mTOR pathway provides an intersection for an intricate network of protein cascades that respond to cellular nutrition, energy levels, and growth-factor stimulation. In the brain, TSC1 and TSC2 have been implicated in cell body size, dendritic arborization, axonal outgrowth and targeting, neuronal migration, cortical lamination, and spine formation. Antagonism of the mTOR pathway with rapamycin and related compounds may provide new therapeutic options for TSC patients.

Keywords: tuberous sclerosis complex (TSC); focal cortical malformations (FCMs); *TSC1* genes; *TSC2* genes; rapamycin

Focal malformations of cortical development

Focal cortical malformations (FCMs) are the most common cause of medically intractable epilepsy (resistant to antiepileptic drug polytherapy) in the pediatric patient population.[1] FCMs, including tubers in the tuberous sclerosis complex (TSC), focal cortical dysplasia (FCD) with balloon cells (BCs), and hemimegalencephaly (HMEG), are of particular interest because these developmental malformations affect restricted regions of the cerebral cortex, share certain histopathological features[2–4] and are linked to abnormalities in the mammalian target of rapamycin (mTOR) cell signaling. Tubers, FCD, and HMEG often require neurosurgical resection to achieve adequate seizure control. Unfortunately, Class I outcomes following resection of FCMs are less often attained than for standard temporal lobectomy surgery. FCDs have been classified into subtypes I and II based on distinguishing histopathological features, such as the presence of dysmorphic neurons (DNs) and BCs in type II FCDs but not in type I.[5] FCDs are often visualized by pre- operative brain MRI although some milder type I FCDs are not detected by routine neuroimaging. HMEG is highly associated with severe intractable neonatal seizures and infantile spasms, a devastating epilepsy syndrome in infants; a classification scheme for HMEG has not yet been formulated. Perhaps most compelling is a recent study demonstrating that of 89 neocortical resections (mean patient age ∼25 years), 58 exhibited some type of FCM by neuropathological examination despite a normal preoperative brain MRI.[6] Thus, FCMs may be responsible for the development and manifestation of seizures in patients with presumed nonlesional neocortical epilepsy. Clearly, FCMs are associated with significant healthcare impact for patients including cost, morbidity, and even mortality.

TSC is an autosomal dominant disorder resulting from mutations in one or two genes (*TSC1* and *TSC2*), whereas FCD and HMEG are sporadic disorders that form by unknown mechanisms (for review, see Ref. 4). TSC serves as an important disease model for FCMs because of the similarities in histopathology and cell signaling abnormalities. As we advance our understanding of the neurobiology of TSC, it is likely that new insights into other FCMs associated with epilepsy, cognitive, disability, and autism will follow.

Tuberous sclerosis complex: clinical presentation and pathophysiology

TSC is characterized by formation of hamartomas in multiple organ systems.[7] The birth incidence of TSC is estimated to be approximately 1 in 6000.[8] Although the majority of organs are susceptible, most patients exhibit dermatological, renal, and/or neurological manifestations.[9] Dermatological abnormalities are evident in the pediatric population and include hypomelanotic macules, which are found in over 90% of TSC patients, and facial angiofibromas, present in 75% of patients.[10] Renal lesions, collectively occurring in 50–80% of patients with TSC,[11–13] include angiomyolipomas (AMLs), renal cysts, renal cell carcinoma, and oncocytomas.[14] Multiple bilateral AMLs, comprising abnormally organized blood vessels, smooth muscle cells, and adipose tissue, occur in approximately 80% of individuals with TSC[12] and represent the leading cause of mortality in the TSC patient population secondary to spontaneous hemorrhage.[7,15] Although the overall incidence of renal cell carcinoma approximates that of the general population, it occurs, on average, 25 years earlier in TSC patients.[14]

Neurological abnormalities including epilepsy,[16] neurocognitive dysfunction,[17] and pervasive developmental disorders such as autism[18] are perhaps the most devastating and therapeutically challenging manifestations of TSC. The neurological features of TSC are believed to reflect structural brain abnormalities. Histopathological examination of TSC brain specimens reveals cortical tubers, subependymal nodules, and subependymal giant cell astrocytomas (SEGAs). Cortical tubers are focal developmental malformations of the cerebral cortex exhibiting loss of normal hexalaminar structure and containing several abnormal cellular elements including DNs, excessive numbers of astrocytes, and giant cells (GCs).[7,19] Radiological studies demonstrated the presence of tubers *in utero* by 20 weeks gestation, suggesting that tubers form during embryonic cortical development.[20] In contrast, subependymal nodules are benign proliferative lesions protruding from the ventricular surface into the ventricular lumen and are believed to

be asymptomatic. Subependymal nodules may undergo transformation into SEGAs, which are found in 10% of patients, and may lead to progressive hydrocephalus and death.[21]

Analysis of surgically resected and postmortem TSC-associated lesions provides pivotal clues into the neuropathogenesis of TSC. GCs found in cortical tubers are highly immunoreactive for immature neuroglial markers[19,22] and show aberrant hyperactivation of the mTOR signaling cascade.[23,24] For example, GCs and DNs within tubers are highly immunoreactive for the phosphorylated isoforms of S6K, S6, 4E-BP1, and express abundant vascular endothelial growth factor (VEGF) (Fig. 1). This phosphorylation profile indicates abnormal signaling through the mTOR cascade (see below), which may be responsible for many of the neurological abnormalities found in TSC and implicates rapamycin (an inhibitor of mTOR) as a potential therapeutic agent. Single-cell microdissection of GCs and DNs from tubers coupled with *in situ* reverse transcription to generate cDNA revealed expression of immature marker proteins such as nestin and vimentin as well as proliferation markers PCNA and Ki-67,[25] suggesting that these cells may be capable of cell division. Recent expression studies of glutamate receptor subtypes revealed an abnormal distribution of GluR subunits in GCs and DNs, implicating aberrant glutamate signaling in TSC-associated epilepsy.[26,27]

Epilepsy, which usually manifests during the first year of life in TSC patients, is the most common neurological disorder in TSC, occurring in 60–90% of individuals.[28] A variety of seizure types have been documented, including infantile spasms, simple partial, complex partial, and generalized tonic-clonic seizures.[28] Although it is widely believed that tubers are the epileptogenic foci, recent data have raised some controversy.[28] While seizures clearly originate from radiographically identified tubers and surgical resection of tubers can alleviate seizures in patients with medically intractable epilepsy,[29,30] some patients continue to seize following tuberectomy.[30] Furthermore, epilepsy has been shown to occur in TSC patients in the absence of cortical tubers. A recent study of three TSC patients who underwent detailed intracranial electrocorticography revealed the tubers were electrically silent while the surrounding perituberal cortex demonstrated epileptiform activity.[31]

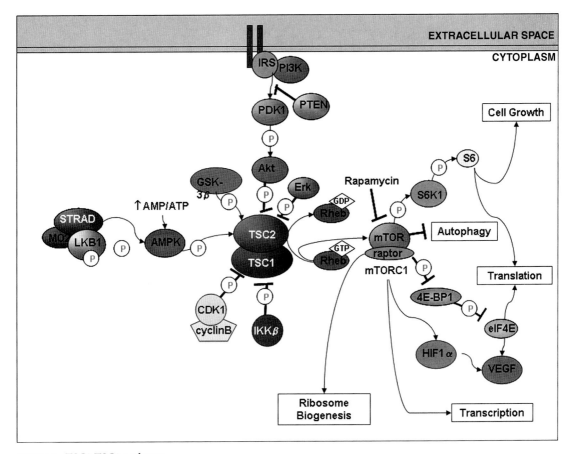

Figure 1. TSC2:TSC1 pathway.

Neurocognitive and behavioral disturbances are also prevalent in the TSC patient population, but exhibit highly variable expression and severity. Patients with TSC exhibit a bimodally distributed intelligence quotient (IQ), with 55% of patients falling within the normal range, 14% exhibiting mild to severe impairment, and 30.5% exhibiting profound mental retardation.[32]

Other clinical manifestations of TSC include lymphangioleiomyamatosis (LAM), which exclusively affects the female patient population and is distinguished by abnormal proliferation of smooth muscle cells and cystic changes within the lung parenchyma.[33] Cardiac rhabdomyomas are common, affecting 50–70% of infants but are rarely symptomatic.[34] Retinal astrocytic hamartomas are present in approximately 50% of TSC patients[35] and may arise from undifferentiated glial precursors during retinal embryogenesis.[36] Despite the recent advent of neurogenetic testing for TSC gene muta-

tions, diagnosis remains based on clinical criteria (Table 1). For example, definitive diagnosis of TSC can be made in a patient who exhibits two major or one major and two minor features of the diagnostic criteria.

Tuberous sclerosis complex: genetics

TSC results from inactivating mutations in either *TSC1*, located on chromosome 9q34,[37] or *TSC2*, located on chromosome 16p13.3.[38] *TSC1* encodes a 130-kDa protein TSC1/hamartin[37] and *TSC2* encodes a 200-kDa protein TSC2/tuberin, which contains a C-terminal GTPase activating protein domain (GAP).[39] The *TSC1*-encoded protein hamartin and *TSC2*-encoded protein tuberin bind to each other via their respective coiled-coil domains to form a functional heterodimer (TSC2:TSC1).[40] TSC exhibits an autosomal dominant pattern of inheritance, but the majority of cases result from

Table 1. Diagnostic criteria for tuberous sclerosis complex

Major	Minor
Cardiac rhabdomyoma	Multiple pits in dental enamel
Cortical tuber	Hamartomatous rectal polyps
Facial angiofibroma	Bone cysts
Hypomelanotic macule	Radial migration lines in
Lymphangiomyomatosis	cerebral white matter
Renal angiomyolipoma	Gingival fibromas
Retinal hamartomas	Retinal achromatic patches
Shagreen patch	"Confetti" skin lesions
Subependymal	Multiple renal cysts
giant-cell tumor	
Subependymal nodule	
Ungual fibromas	

Definite TSC: Two major or one major plus two minor criteria.
Probable TSC: One major plus one minor criteria.
Possible TSC: One major or two minor features.

sporadic germline mutations. Although *TSC1* and *TSC2* mutations are equally represented in familial TSC, mutations in the *TSC2* gene are more common in sporadic cases.[41] While large deletions and missense mutations have been identified in *TSC2*, the majority of mutations in *TSC1* are small and result in expression of a truncated protein.[41]

The TSC2:TSC1 complex functions in a common signaling pathway (Fig. 1), thus inactivating mutations in either gene give rise to the same clinical disorder. Binding of TSC1 to TSC2 appears to stabilize intracellular TSC2 levels since uncomplexed TSC2 is subject to ubiquitin-mediated degradation.[42,43] Missense mutations in the *TSC2* gene that disrupt its ability to bind to TSC1 have been documented in TSC patients.[44,45] Furthermore, studies in *Drosophila* revealed that inactivating mutations in the *Drosophila* orthologs of *TSC1* and *TSC2* (*dTSC1* and *dTSC2*) give rise to indistinguishable phenotypes and suggested that the protein products of these genes regulate a myriad of cellular processes, including cell size, cell cycle, and cellular proliferation.[46–49] dTSC2 and dTSC1 form a protein complex, and concomitant overexpression of both TSC2 and TSC1—but not individually—results in attenuation of cell size and number.[48] Cells lacking dTSC1 or dTSC2 are cytomegalic, retain normal ploidy,

and continue to inappropriately enter S phase in normally quiescent cell types, suggesting that these proteins play an essential role in facilitating exit from the cell cycle.[47] TSC1 and TSC2 are known to bind to at least 40 additional proteins,[50] and thus there are numerous potential and yet undefined effects of *TSC* gene mutations.

Upstream regulation of TSC2:TSC1

The TSC2:TSC1 heterodimer serves as a nexus for integrating the energy status of the cell with nutritional availability and extracellular growth factor signaling (Fig. 2). Both TSC2 and TSC1 are regulated by phosphorylation. TSC1 is phosphorylated at multiple sites (Thr[417], Ser[584], and Thr[1047]) by cyclin-dependent kinase 1 (CDK1)/cyclin B during the G_2/M phase of the cell cycle.[51] TSC1 has been shown to localize to the centrosome and interact with the mitotic polo-like kinase (Plk1), the levels of which are negatively regulated by TSC1.[52] TSC1 has also been shown to interact with actin-binding proteins belonging to the ezrin-radixin-moesin (ERM) family and regulate focal adhesion formation through a Rho-mediated mechanism.[53] Additionally, TSC1 is negatively regulated through IKKβ-mediated phosphorylation on Ser487 and Ser511 and is possibly linked to cellular inflammatory responses.[54] Many upstream kinases regulate the activity of TSC2 by phosphorylation, including extracellular signaling-regulated kinase (Erk),[55,56] Akt,[57–60] AMP-activated kinase (AMPK),[61–63] and glycogen synthase kinase 3 (GSK3).[64] Growth factors generally serve to inhibit TSC2 by activating the MAP kinase (Ras-Raf-MEK1/2-Erk1/2) and PI3K (PI3K-PDK1-Akt) signaling pathways.

Phosphorylation of TSC2 by Erk on Ser664 results in dissociation of the TSC2:TSC1 complex, leading to diminished inhibition of mTOR and hindering the ability of TSC2 to inhibit cell proliferation and oncogenic transformation.[55,56] This Erk-mediated phosphorylation and inactivation of TSC2 offers an intriguing alternative to loss-of-heterozygosity (LOH) as a pathogenic mechanism underlying tumorigenesis of $TSC2^{+/-}$ CNS lesions. Specifically, the protein product of the wild-type allele may be posttranslationally inactivated by Erk-mediated phosphorylation to produce a functionally null phenotype.[55] Interestingly, tubers and SEGAs have been shown to be highly immunoreactive for the

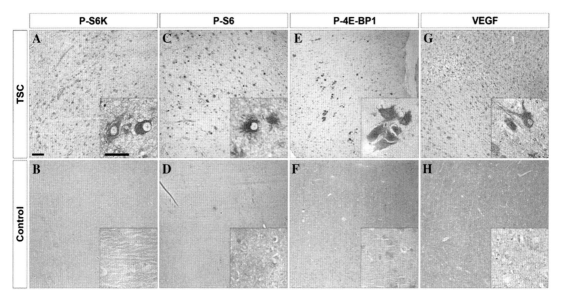

Figure 2. IHC of tubers for PS6K, PS6, P4EBP1, VEGF. Tubers from TSC patients exhibit hyperactive mTOR signaling. Tuber (*top panel*) and epilepsy-control (*bottom panel*) cortical tissue was probed with antibodies recognizing the phosphorylated isoforms of S6K (**A,B**), S6 (**C,D**), 4E-BP1 (**E,F**), and VEGF (**G,H**). Large panels were taken at 5× (scale bar: 200 μm), and insets were taken at 40× (scale bar: 50 μm).

phosphorylated isoforms of Mek1/2 and Erk1/2, suggesting abnormally hyperactive MAP kinase signaling.[65,66] Thus, hyperactive MAP signaling in TSC may result in Erk-mediated inactivation of the wild-type allele resulting in functional LOH, producing TSC-associated lesion formation. The exact biological mechanism by which TSC2:TSC1 regulates MAP kinase activation has not been fully elucidated.

Insulin or insulin-like growth factors (IGFs) inhibit the TSC2:TSC1 complex primarily through Akt-mediated phosphorylation and inactivation of TSC2. In brief, binding of IGFs to their receptors results in recruitment and phosphorylation of the insulin receptor substrate (IRS) and subsequent activation of phosphoinositide 3-kinase (PI3K).[67,68] Activated PI3K converts phosphatidylinositol (4,5) bi-phosphate (PIP2) into phosphatidylinositol (3,4,5) tri-phosphate (PIP3), and leads to recruitment of Akt to the plasma membrane where it is phosphorylated and activated by PDK1.[67] The PI3K-mediated conversion of PIP2 into PIP3 is inhibited by the lipid phosphatase phosphatase and tensin homolog deleted on chromosome 10 (PTEN), which removes the D3 phosphate from PIP3 to regenerate PIP2.[69,70] The role of the TSC2:TSC1 heterodimer in the insulin-signaling

pathway was first revealed by genetic epistasis experiments in *Drosophila*. Overexpression of dTSC1 and dTSC2 suppressed the lethal phenotype of overexpressed *Drosophila* insulin receptor (dinr) and overexpression of dS6K, which lies downstream from dTSC2:dTSC1 (see below) on a *dTSC1*-mutant background reversed the *dTSC1*-null phenotype.[48] Additionally, although loss of Akt, which is downstream from the insulin receptor, led to a decrease in cell size, cells lacking both Akt and dTSC1 were similar in size to those lacking dTSC1 alone, confirming that dTSC2:dTSC1 lies downstream of and antagonizes insulin-mediated Akt signaling.[49] This signaling pathway is well conserved across species.

Addition of growth factors or serum supplementation of mammalian cell lines results in phosphorylation of TSC2 in a PI3K-dependent manner. Addition of PI3K inhibitors LY294002 and wortmannin yields accelerated gel mobility of TSC2, suggesting decreased phosphorylation of TSC2 in response to PI3K inhibition.[60] This is directly mediated by Akt, which binds to and phosphorylates TSC2.[58,60] *In vitro* kinase assays revealed that Akt is capable of phosphorylating TSC2 on seven distinct residues.[60] Mutations of two of these residues, Ser939 and Thr1462, to alanine (TSC2^S939A/T1462A), which renders them nonphosphorylatable, as well as expression of a dominant negative form of Akt, inhibits insulin-induced phosphorylation of S6K.[58] Exogenous expression of Akt enhances phosphorylation of TSC2 while expression of kinase-inactive Akt (Akt-KM) or treatment with a PI3K inhibitor LY294002 decreases phosphorylation of TSC2.[59] TSC1 or TSC2-depleted cells fail to attenuate downstream mTOR signaling in response to amino acid depletion, serum starvation or growth factor withdrawal.[71–73] Additionally, exogenous expression of PTEN, an inhibitor of the PI3K-Akt signaling results in decreased phosphorylation of TSC2 and cell lines derived from PTEN-null (PTEN$^{-/-}$) mouse embryos exhibit constitutively phosphorylated TSC2 on Thr1462.[58,59] Phosphorylation of TSC2 by Akt may inhibit the function of the TSC2:TSC1 complex either by decreasing the interaction between TSC2 and TSC1 or enhancing the degradation of the heterodimeric complex by the ubiquitin-proteasome pathway.[59,60]

PTEN inhibits insulin signaling by removing the 3′ phosphate of phosphatidylinositol (3,4,5) triphosphate (PIP3) to generate phosphatidylinositol (4,5) bi-phosphate (PIP2), thus reversing the PI3K-mediated phosphorylation of PIP2.[74] *Drosophila* mutants harboring inactivating mutations in the *Drosophila* ortholog of PTEN (dPTEN) exhibit cellular and organ hypertrophy.[75,76] Overexpression of dPTEN results in attenuated cell size but does not rescue the cytomegalic phenotype of dTSC1-null cell,[48] while overexpression of dPTEN along with dTSC2 and dTSC1 is additive in the reduction of cell size,[47] indicating that dPTEN acts upstream of dTSC2:dTSC1. Mice harboring homozygous deletions in *PTEN* (PTEN$^{-/-}$) die during embryogenesis, while heterozygous mutants (PTEN$^{+/-}$) contain dysplastic changes in the gastrointestinal tract, prostate gland, and skin and develop cancer in multiple organ systems.[77] Human mutations in *PTEN* cause several distinct disorders, including Cowden syndrome (CS), an autosomal dominant disorder characterized by hamartomatous lesions in the skin, thyroid, and breast tissue, macrocephaly, and increased incidence of cancer.[78] Germline mutations in *PTEN* have also been reported in autistic individuals with concomitant macrocephaly.[79] Mice harboring a conditional deletion of *PTEN* in differentiated cortical and hippocampal neurons (Nse-cre; Pten$^{loxP/loxP}$) display abnormal social interactions as evidenced by impairments in learning to recognize a previously encountered mouse, diminished nesting, attenuated interaction with a social target, and deficits in maternal behavior.[80] Macrocephaly in Nse-cre; Pten$^{loxP/loxP}$ mice was found to be secondary to neuronal soma hypertrophy, and cells lacking PTEN exhibited enhanced immunoreactivity for the phosphorylated isoforms of Akt, S6 (Ser235/Ser236) and TSC2 (Ser939), suggesting aberrant hyperactivation of the PI3K-Akt-mTOR pathway.[80] PTEN-deficient neurons displayed markedly abnormal characteristics, including hypertrophy of the dendritic arborizations, increased dendritic spine density, and abnormal axonal projections in the dentate gyrus of the hippocampus.[80]

In addition to Akt-mediated inhibition, the TSC2:TSC1 complex is negatively regulated by other signaling pathways. For example, TSC2 has recently been shown to bind to the death-associated protein kinase (DAPK), which subsequently phosphorylates TSC2 and leads to dissociation of the TSC2:TSC1 complex.[81] DAPK is a serine-threonine kinase with a diverse repertoire of functions, including regulation of apoptosis in response to a variety of death signals and promotion of autophagy.[82] Exogenous expression of DAPK in HEK293 cells results in enhanced phosphorylation of S6K and S6 following serum starvation while siRNA-mediated knockout of DAPK attenuates phosphorylation of S6K and S6 primarily secondary to epidermal growth factor (EGF)-mediated activation of the Erk signaling.[82] Interestingly, DAPK has also been shown to directly phosphorylate S6 on Ser235.[83] Additionally, the TSC2:TSC1 complex is inhibited by binding of the forkhead transcription factor FoxO1 to TSC2, leading to subsequent activation of the mTOR-signaling cascade.[84] FoxO1 belongs to a family of FOXO transcription factors that are degraded in the presence of insulin or growth factors by Akt- and GSK-mediated phosphorylation and translocate into the nucleus upon growth factor withdrawal to regulate cell cycle arrest and DNA repair.[85]

The TSC2:TSC1 complex is activated by AMPK and GSK3. Fluxes in cellular energy stores signal to TSC2:TSC1 through AMPK, which activates TSC2 by phosphorylation on Thr1227 and Ser1345.[61] Depletion of ATP by the glucose analog 2-deoxyglucose (2DG) results in enhanced phosphorylation of TSC2 and decreased phosphorylation of mTOR effectors, including S6K and 4E-BP1.[61] TSC2 is required for inhibition of S6K in response to energy stress since energy depletion fails to decrease S6K phosphorylation in TSC2-null fibroblasts or following siRNA-mediated TSC2 knockdown.[61] AMPK is activated by two conditions: elevation of AMP/ATP and subsequent phosphorylation on its activation loop (Thr173) by upstream kinases. Elevated AMP/ATP levels result in a conformational change of AMPK, rendering it a suitable substrate for upstream kinases, such as LKB1 and CaMKK.[63,86] Interestingly, in addition to inactivating TSC2, Akt has been shown to inhibit AMPK by decreasing the cellular AMP/ATP ratio.[62] LKB1-deficient mouse embryonic fibroblasts (LKB1[−/−] MEFs) fail to phosphorylate and activate AMPK, resulting in aberrant downstream signaling.[63] Moreover, LKB1[−/−] MEFs are similar to TSC2-deficient MEFs in their inability to attenuate downstream mTOR signaling and inhibit apoptosis during periods of energy depletion.[87] Exogenous expression of LKB1 attenuates signaling downstream from mTOR in an AMPK-dependent manner, since the addition of compound C (an inhibitor of AMPK) or a dominant negative AMPK construct ameliorates the ability of LKB1 to decrease phosphorylation of S6K (Thr389).[88] Thus, energy depletion induces LKB1-dependent activation of AMPK, which in turn serves to activate the TSC2:TSC1 complex.

Mutations in the LKB1 gene cause the autosomal dominant disorder Peutz-Jeghers syndrome (PJS), characterized by intestinal polyposis and increased incidence of cancer.[89] Like TSC-associated lesions, PJS polyps exhibit enhanced activation of the mTOR signaling pathway, as evidenced by hyperphosphorylated S6K and S6.[87] The activity and subcellular localization of LKB1 is regulated by the pseudokinase STRADα, which relocalizes LKB1 from the nuclear to the cytoplasmic compartment and significantly augments the catalytic activity of LKB1.[90,91] Homozygous deletions in the STRADα gene have recently been shown to cause Pretzel syndrome (PS), an autosomal recessive disorder characterized by macrocephaly, intractable epilepsy, and severe psychomotor retardation.[92] PS brain tissue, like TSC- and PJS-associated lesions, is highly immunoreactive for the phosphorylated isoform of S6.[92] Thus, hyperactive mTOR signaling, secondary to attenuated TSC2:TSC1-mediated inhibition, may serve as the foundation for the pathogenesis of TSC, PJS, and PS.

Like energy and serum deprivation, hypoxia also inhibits mTOR signaling by a TSC2:TSC1-dependent mechanism. In response to hypoxia, TSC2[−/−] MEFs and TSC2-depleted HEK293 and HeLa cells fail to decrease phosphorylation of S6K and S6.[93] Hypoxia modulates mTOR signaling by upregulating regulated in development and DNA damage responses (Redd1) mRNA, which appears to signal to mTOR through the TSC2:TSC1 complex. Exogenous or inducible expression of Redd1 is sufficient to attenuate phosphorylation of S6K and S6 in wild-type but not TSC2-depleted HEK293 cells.[93] Genetic experiments in *Drosophila* indicate that Redd1-homologs inhibit dTOR upstream of the dTSC2:dTSC1 complex.[94] In fact, overexpression of the mTOR-activator Rheb, which is inactivated by TSC2:TSC1 complex, prevents Redd1 from inhibiting mTOR signaling.[95] Interestingly, Redd1-deficient cells also fail to attenuate mTOR activity secondary to energy (2DG) or glucose depletion, suggesting a broader role for Redd1 in transferring information about the overall energy status of the cell to mTOR through the TSC2:TSC1 complex.[95]

Phosphorylation of TSC2 by AMPK primes the former kinase for subsequent phosphorylation and activation by GSK3, thus demonstrating a link between Wnt signaling and TSC2:TSC1.[64] Wnt signaling regulates multiple aspects of cellular physiology including proliferation, differentiation, cell growth, and development.[96] Wnts are secreted glycoproteins that bind to members of the Frizzled (FZ) family of receptors, leading to activation of disheveled (DSH) and subsequent phosphorylation and inactivation of GSK3.[96] Exogenous expression of Wnt-1 or application of purified recombinant Wnt-3a to several cell lines yields enhanced phosphorylation of S6K and 4E-BP1 in a rapamycin-dependent manner.[64] Wnt-mediated activation of mTOR was demonstrated to be dependent on GSK3-mediated phosphorylation of TSC2 on Ser1337 and Ser1341 after a priming phosphorylation of TSC2 on Ser1345 by AMPK.[64] Moreover, the effects of TSC2 activation by AMPK and GSK3 appear to be additive, since 5-aminoimidazole-4-carboxamide-1-β-riboside (AICAR)-mediated activation of AMPK results in enhanced Wnt-3 mediated phosphorylation of S6K while inhibition of AMPK results in attenuation of GSK3-mediated inhibition of mTOR signaling.[64] Thus, the TSC2:TSC1 complex integrates information provided by AMPK and GSK3 signaling.

Genomic stress also acts through the AMPK signaling pathway to enhance activation of the TSC2:TSC1 complex, thus leading to attenuation of mTOR signaling. Several factors, such as DNA damage, hypoxia, and ribonucleoside triphosphase depletion, lead to stabilization and activation of p53.[97] p53 activation results in phosphorylation of AMPK (Thr172) and leads to mTOR inhibition in a TSC2:TSC1-dependent manner.[98] The p53-mediated phosphorylation and activation of AMPK is orchestrated by two transcriptional targets of p53, Sestrin1 and Sestrin2.[99] Overexpression of Sestrin1 and Sestrin2 along with S6K1 results in decreased phosphorylation of S6K1 on Thr389 and enhances the phosphorylation of AMPK, while inhibition of AMPK using compound C or shRNA-mediated knockdown of AMPK eliminates Sestrin1- and Sestrin2-dependent attenuation of S6K1 phosphorylation.[99] In fact, Sestrins form a complex with both AMPK and TSC2:TSC1, thus enhancing the ability of AMPK to phosphorylate and activate the TSC2:TSC1 complex.[99] Interestingly, p53 regulates expression of several inhibitors of the mTOR-signaling pathway, including AMPK, PTEN, and TSC2.[100] However, the ability of p53 to inhibit downstream mTOR signaling appears to be largely dependent on Sestrins since Sestrin2-null cells and Sestrin1 and Sestrin2 depleted cells fail to downregulate phosphorylation of mTOR effectors in response to genotoxic stress.[100]

Downstream from mTOR

The TSC2:TSC1 complex is the principal cellular inhibitor of the mammalian target of rapamycin. The TSC2 protein acts as a GTPase activating protein toward Ras homolog enriched in brain (Rheb), a Ras family GTPase.[101,102] GTP-bound Rheb activates mTOR[103] by preventing the association of mTOR with its endogenous inhibitor FKBP38.[104] TSC2:TSC1 inhibits mTOR activity by stimulating the conversion of active Rheb-GTP to the inactive form, Rheb-GDP.[101] Exogenous expression of Rheb enhanced phosphorylation of mTOR effectors S6K and 4E-BP1 in a rapamycin-dependent manner, while co-expression of Rheb with TSC2:TSC1 attentuates Rheb-mediated mTOR activation.[101,105]

mTOR is an evolutionarily conserved 280-kDa Ser/Thr protein kinase that regulates a myriad of energy-expansive biological processes including cell growth, translation, transcription, ribosome biogenesis, autophagy, and metabolism.[67] mTOR is a central component of two complexes: TORC1, which also contains raptor and is inhibited by rapamycin [106] and TORC2, which contains rictor and is not sensitive to rapamycin.[107] TORC2 is implicated in the regulation of actin organization in yeast[108] and mammalian systems[109] and has recently been shown to activate Akt.[110] Much more is known about the function of mTOR within the context of TORC1, which is simply referred to as "mTOR" within this manuscript.

The best-characterized effectors of mTOR are S6K1 and 4E-BP1. The catalytic activity of S6K1 is regulated by multiple phosphorylation events, including an mTOR-dependent phosphorylation on Thr371 and Thr389.[111] Phosphorylation of Thr389 correlates well with the catalytic activity of S6K1.[112] *Drosophila* deficient in the *Drosophila* ortholog of S6K (dS6K) display a small-body phenotype secondary to diminished cellular size.[113] Overexpression of dS6K along with dTSC2 and dTSC1 suppresses the aberrant small phenotype of cells overexpressing dTSC2 and dTSC1 in isolation, suggesting that the dTSC2:dTSC1 regulate cell size by decreasing dS6K activity.[48] Mice harboring homozygous deletions in S6K1 (S6K1$^{-/-}$) are viable but exhibit a significant reduction in overall body size.[114] The S6K1-dependent regulation of cellular size is mediated by ribosomal protein S6, which is phosphorylated by S6K1 and the closely related S6K2 on Ser235/Ser236.[115,116] Mice harboring serine-to-alanine substitutions in all five phosphorylation sites (rpS6$^{P-/-}$) are viable but MEFs derived from rpS6$^{P-/-}$ embryos were significantly smaller than controls (rpS6$^{P+/+}$).[115] In addition to serving as an activating kinase toward S6, S6K1 establishes a negative feedback loop on mTOR signaling by negative regulation of insulin receptor substrate-1(IRS1) function.[117] Thus, enhanced activation of the PI3K-AKT pathway leads to activation of the mTOR cascade, which results in enhanced phosphorylation of S6K1, which subsequently leads to attenuated PI3K-AKT signaling.

mTOR also regulates translation by inhibition of 4E-BP1, which in its nonphosphorylated state binds to and inhibits the eukaryotic initiation factor 4E (eIF4E).[118,119] eIF4E, as part of the eIF4F complex, recognizes and binds to the 7-methylguanosine cap present on the 5' end of mRNAs. 4E-BP1 undergoes consecutive phosphorylation events beginning on Thr37/Thr46 and proceeding to Ser65/Thr70, the phosphorylation of which is greatly enhanced following serum stimulation in a PI3K and rapamycin-sensitive manner.[119] Phosphorylation of 4E-BP1 by mTOR results in release of eIF4E from 4E-BP1 and permits the initiation of cap-dependent translation. 4E-BP1 knockout mice are viable and fertile but display several metabolic abnormalities, including hypoglycemia, enhanced metabolic rate and a significant reduction in white adipose tissue, implicating this mTOR effector in regulation of metabolism and adipogenesis.[120]

mTOR signaling plays a pivotal role in promoting angiogenesis. One of the principal players in mTOR-mediated angiogenesis is VEGF. mTOR regulates VEGF expression at both the transcriptional and translational level. Inactivation of TSC2:TSC1 results in enhanced mTOR signaling, which triggers increased intracellular levels of the transcription factor HIF1α, which in turn turns on expression of VEGF.[121] HIF1α levels are tightly regulated by oxygen tension, so that during periods of oxygen abundance, oxygen results in hydroxylation of HIF1α, subsequently leading to its degradation via pVHL-mediated ubiquitination.[122,123] TSC2-deficient MEFs exhibit increased levels of HIF1α and VEGF, which normalize following treatment with rapamycin.[121] Reconstitution of TSC2 expression in TSC2$^{-/-}$ MEFs is sufficient to rescue HIF1α levels.[121] Interestingly, mice heterozygous for the TSC1 gene (TSC1$^{+/-}$) or the TSC2 gene (TSC2$^{+/-}$) display a range of vascular abnormalities, including hepatic hemangiomas and angiosarcomas.[73,124–126] Hepatic hemangiomas from TSC1$^{+/-}$ and TSC2$^{+/-}$ mice are strongly immunoreactive for VEGF and TSC2, and TSC1-null fibroblasts have been shown to secrete excess VEGF *in vitro*.[127] Additionally, serum obtained from TSC1$^{+/-}$ animals contains high levels of circulating VEGF, suggesting a potential utilization of VEGF as a biomarker for abnormal TSC2:TSC1 function.[127] Treatment of TSC1$^{+/-}$ animals with repeated doses of rapamycin attenuates serum VEGF levels, and more importantly, results in readily apparent histological changes in tumor appearance.[127] In addition to transcriptional regulation, mTOR activation modulates translation

of VEGF by inactivating 4E-BP1, which in turn leads to initiation of VEGF mRNA translation.[128,129] mTOR-mediated initiation of angiogenesis is also regulated by inflammatory pathways that converge on TSC1.[54] TSC1 is phosphorylated on Ser487 and Ser511 by IKKβ, which is one of the principal downstream effectors in the TNFα inflammatory signaling cascade.[130] Phosphorylation of TSC1 by IKKβ results in dissociation of the TSC2:TSC1 complex, enhanced levels of GTP-bound Rheb, and subsequently increased activation of mTOR, ultimately resulting in increased VEGF production and accelerated angiogenesis.[54]

The neurobiology of TSC2:TSC1

The function of TSC2:TSC1 in the brain is currently an active area of investigation. Clearly, both TSC1 and TSC2 play pivotal roles in several processes that are crucial for normal brain development, including regulation of somatic size, dendritogenesis, formation of dendritic spines, axon outgrowth, astrocyte proliferation, and cortical lamination. In addition, because TSC1 and TSC2 are widely expressed throughout the mature brain, these proteins likely serve important homeostatic regulatory functions in neurons during adult life.

Cre-mediated deletion of exons 17 and 18 in the mouse *TSC1* gene (Tsc1$^{C/C}$) in cultured mouse hippocampal neurons results in enhanced phosphorylation of S6 and increased neuronal soma size.[131] Additionally, Tsc1$^{C/C}$ neurons as well as TSC2-depleted neurons display enhanced dendritic spine length and head width and diminished dendritic spine density.[131] These morphological changes appear to be regulated by phosphorylation of the actin-binding protein cofilin on Ser3, as this phosphorylated isoform is increased in TSC2-deficient neurons and, more importantly, expression of a Ser-to-Ala mutant cofilin (S3A) rescues soma size, dendritic spine length and head width. Most interestingly, neurons harboring a single deleted copy of the *TSC1* gene (Tsc1$^{C/+}$) exhibit morphological changes characteristic of TSC1- and TSC2-depleted neurons, suggesting that haploinsufficiency rather than LOH may contribute to the neuropathogenesis of TSC.[131] Tsc1$^{C/C}$ neurons also exhibit increased amplitude of spontaneous miniature excitatory postsynaptic currents (mEPSC), suggesting enhanced neurotransmitter sensitivity that may contribute to the epileptogenic phenotype of patients with TSC.

The TSC2:TSC1 complex has been recently implicated in the regulation of axonogenesis.[132] Exogenous expression of TSC2 and TSC1 in rodent hippocampal neurons inhibits axon formation, whereas shRNA-mediated knockdown of TSC2 and TSC1 results in supernumerary axons in a rapamycin-dependent manner.[132] Moreover, mice lacking TSC1 in postmitotic neurons (Syn-Cre; Tsc1$^{flox/flox}$) display ectopic axonal localization throughout the developing brain.[132] Interestingly, knockdown of TSC2:TSC1 results in increased expression of synapses of amphids defective-A (SAD-A), which has been demonstrated to be required for axonogenesis *in vivo*.[133] shRNA-mediated knockdown of SAD-A and SAD-B (SAD-A/B) kinases prevents the formation of supernumerous axons in TSC2-deficient hippocampal neurons.[132] SAD-A and SAD-B kinases belong to the AMPK-related kinase family and are activated by LKB1-mediated phosphorylation.[134] Conditional knockout of LKB1 in dorsal telencephalic progenitors (Emx1$^{Cre/+}$;LKB1$^{F/F}$) results in a global suppression of axon formation *in vivo* in a SAD-A/B-dependent manner.[135] Thus, LKB1 seems to regulate axonogenesis by multiple pathways, promoting axonal differentiation by phosphorylation of SAD-A/B kinases and inhibiting axonogenesis during periods of cellular energy deficiency by way of AMPK-TSC2:TSC1 activation.

Several animal models of TSC have been generated by knockout of either *TSC1* or *TSC2* genes. The original reported TSC1-knockout mouse (Tsc1$^{-/-}$) was constructed by gene targeting in embryonic stem cells (ESCs), replacing exons 6 through 8 with an IRES-EGFP-pA sequence and a neo-expression cassette.[136] These homozygous Tsc1$^{-/-}$ mice exhibit embryonic lethality, with the majority of embryos dying between embryonic day 10.5 and 11.5, although several Tsc1$^{-/-}$ animals lived until E13.5. Tsc1$^{-/-}$ embryos are all smaller compared to age-matched controls, and histological analysis reveals abnormal closure of the neural tube in approximately one-third of the Tsc1$^{-/-}$ embryos. Additional developmental defects include aberrant appearance of the cardiac myocytes and liver hypoplasia. All mice heterozygous for the deletion in the *TSC1* allele (Tsc1$^{+/-}$) developed renal cysts by 15–18 months of age. Renal tumor formation

was noted in several animals, the genetic analysis of which revealed LOH in two out of six samples. Tumor development in several other organs was also reported, including liver, tail, and uterus. There was no increase in mortality at 18 months of Tsc1$^{+/-}$ animals when compared with controls, although sudden death of several animals older than 18 months was noted.[136]

Another TSC1 knockout mouse was subsequently engineered by deletion of exons 17 and 18, which is virtually identical in phenotype to the original Tsc1$^{-/-}$ knockout mouse with several notable exceptions.[73] Namely, neural tube defects were not detected and impressive vascular dilation was evident in several internal organs. Unlike the original Tsc1$^{+/-}$ mice, these heterozygotes (Tsc1$^{+/-}$), exhibited enhanced incidence of mortality with a clear female predominance (45% of female Tsc1$^{+/-}$ compared to 10% of male Tsc1$^{+/-}$ and 10% of wild types) probably secondary to rupture of liver hemangiomas with subsequent hemorrhage. Similar to the original Tsc1$^{+/-}$ animals, all Tsc1$^{+/-}$ mice exhibited renal cystadenomas, the histological examination of which revealed high expression of gelsolin. MEFs developed from E10.5 Tsc1$^{-/-}$ embryos fail to attenuate phosphorylation of S6K and S6 following serum starvation and do not enhance phosphorylation of AKT following serum stimulation in a rapamycin-dependent manner.[73]

A third TSC1-knockout was recently developed by deletion of exons 6 through 8 in ES cells by substitution with a β-galactoside reporter/neomycin selection cassette, which unexpectedly produced an aberrantly spliced construct with fusion of exons 5 and 9, resulting in creation of a premature stop codon within exon 9.[125] Homozygous Tsc1$^{-/-}$ mice exhibited a lethal phenotype that was similar to the original Tsc1$^{-/-}$ mice, including exencephaly and myocyte anomalies, although liver hypoplasia was not noted. Interestingly, several abnormalities of the heterozygous animals proved to be background specific. For example, the authors report a 27% increase in postnatal mortality of Tsc1$^{+/-}$ mice that were backcrossed onto a C57BL/6 background when compared to Tsc1$^{+/-}$ mice backcrossed onto Balb/c and C3H backgrounds. Additionally, Tsc1$^{+/-}$ on a C3H background developed significantly more renal lesions, both microscopic and macroscopic, when compared with those on a C57BL/6 and Balb/c backgrounds by 15–18 months. Genetic analysis revealed loss of heterozygosity in 42% of renal regions and western blot analysis showed enhanced phosphorylation of mTOR and S6 in all lesions examined when compared to adjacent normal kidney tissue, consistent with hyperactivation of mTOR. Thus, disparate genetic modifiers may contribute to the phenotypic expression of TSC.

Several conditional knockout animals have also been generated. An astrocyte-specific TSC1 conditional knockout mouse was designed by interbreeding mice harboring two LoxP sites flanking exons 17 and 18 (Tsc1$^{c/c}$) with transgenic mice that express glial fibrillary acidic protein (GFAP)-driven Cre recombinase (GFP-Cre) to produce Tsc1$^{c/c}$; GFP-Cre mice.[137] By 2 months of age, these mice exhibit spontaneous EEG-confirmed seizures and 50% of Tsc1$^{c/c}$; GFP-Cre mice die by 3 months of age. Histological analysis of cortical and hippocampal tissue revealed enhanced astrocyte proliferation, as evidenced by increased immunostaining for GFAP and PCNA, and aberrant organization of the hippocampus, owing primarily to abnormal positioning of pyramidal neurons in the dentate hilar region. Tubers, however, were not identified in this mouse model. Further analysis demonstrated reduced expression of astrocytic glutamate transporters, GLT-1 and GLAST, and decreased density of glutamate transport currents.[138] This may disturb glutamate homeostasis and contribute to the epileptogenic phenotype characteristic of this mouse models and patients with TSC.

Recently, a neuronal-specific TSC1 knockout mouse was engineered by crossing Tsc1$^{c/c}$ with mice expressing Cre recombinase under the Synapsin1 promoter (Tsc1$^{c/c}$; Syn1-Cre).[139] Histological analysis of Tsc1$^{c/c}$; Syn1-Cre brains revealed normal hexalaminar cortical architecture absence of tubers. However, electrophysiological recordings from nontuberous cortical tissue slices revealed bicuculline-induced α-amino-3-hydroxyl-5-methyl-4-isoxazole-proprionate (AMPA)-mediated long-duration polyspike responses and periodical epileptiform discharge. A recently reported conditional knockout mouse in which *TSC1* was deleted from a subset of postnatal forebrain neurons was constructed by crossing Tsc1$^{c/c}$ with a transgenic mouse expressing Cre recombinase under a αCAMPKII promoter.[140] A small percentage of the Tsc1$^{c/c}$; αCAMPKII–Cre mice that survived past the first postnatal week exhibited macrocephaly

secondary to neuronal hypertrophy and astrogliosis. Seizures were not reported in this strain.

Mutations in the *TSC2* gene have also been utilized to model TSC. The Eker rat has a naturally occurring inactivating germline mutation in the TSC2 gene (Tsc2$^{+/-}$)[124,141] resulting from retrotransposition of a rat intracisternal-A particle.[142] The functionally heterozygous Eker rats spontaneously develop myriad tumors, most notably renal cell carcinomas[143] and uterine and pituitary tumors.[144] The majority of nonbrain lesions found in the Eker rat model exhibit LOH.[145] Although no neurological abnormalities have been documented, including spontaneous seizures, several groups documented neurohistopathological findings that approximate those found in human brain samples from patients with TSC. One group reported the occurrence of subependymal hamartomas and subcortical hamartomas in Eker rats between the ages of 18 and 24 months that were mainly composed of GFAP immunoreactive glia, although no classical cortical tubers were noted.[146] Only one study to date of the Eker model reported the finding of a cortical tuber (in one rat only) that closely resembles human tubers in TSC patients.[147] Immunohistologial analysis of renal tumors in Eker rats revealed abnormally enhanced phosphorylation of S6 and 4E-BP1, lending credence to the notion that TSC-specific lesions exhibit hyperactivated mTOR signaling.[148] An interesting recent study of Eker rats suggests that tuber formation may not be necessary for manifestation of TSC-associated cognitive dysfunction and epilepsy since Eker rats were found to exhibit increased episodic-like memory and augmented responses to pharmacologically induced plasticity.[149]

Since most TSC-associated lesions are postulated to result from either LOH or a "second hit" event, some investigators have employed various methods to enhance the probability of rate-limiting mutagenesis to study the progression of TSC-associated neuropathology. For example, one group irradiated Eker rats at 3 days of age and analyzed their brain tissue at 3 months of age.[150] Irradiated Eker brains contained NeuN/NF immunoreactive large DNs within layers II-VI of the cortical plate, giant GFAP-positive astrocytes, and subependymal and subcortical hamartomas composed primarily of glial cells. Others have utilized *in utero* exposure to carcinogens, such as hydroquinone (HQ), as well as the natural aging process.[151] Although intraperitoneal injections of HQ did not result in tuber formation or any measurable histological anomalies, analysis of aged (18–24 months) Eker rats demonstrated the presence of NeuN positive cytomegalic neurons and GFAP/vimentin/nestin immunoreactive GCs.

The earliest reported *TSC2* knockout mouse was engineered by deletion of exons 2 through 5 by homologous recombination in ES cells, with subsequent chimeras bred onto a C57BL/6J background.[152] The Tsc2$^{-/-}$ phenotype was embryonic lethal around E10.5, with exencephaly noted in 50% of embryos. Some embryos exhibited abnormally thickened myocardia. All heterozygous animals developed renal cell carcinoma by 10 months of age, and 80% of Tsc2$^{+/-}$ had hepatic hemangiomas by 1.5 years of age. The second TSC2-null mouse was constructed by insertion of a neomycin resistance cassette into exon 2 of the *TSC2* gene.[126] Three different strains of transgenic mice were produced by backcrossing onto C57BL/6, BALB/c, and Black Swiss backgrounds. Homozygous Tsc2$^{-/-}$ exhibited an embryonic lethal phenotype—no viable embryos were observed after E12.5—and had pronounced developmental delay, including exencephaly, hepatic hypoplasia, absence of the diaphragm, and severe vasodilatation. Embryos exhibited pallor, and the cause of death was attributed to liver hypoplasia with secondary anemia. Heterozygous animals (Tsc2$^{+/-}$) developed normally but incurred a substantial burden of cyst and tumor development in several organs, including kidneys, liver, lungs, and extremities. Renal cysts and adenomas, occurring in all mice by 15 months of age, were confined to the renal cortex, and the intercalated cell was defined as the cell of origin by virtue of intense staining for gelsolin. Progression to overt carcinoma was noted in fewer than 10% of cases. Half of Tsc2$^{+/-}$ animals developed liver hemangiomas by 15 months of age. Some strain-specific differences were noted, most notably with respect to renal cystadenoma size and frequency of angiosarcomas. LOH was observed in 30% of the examined cysts and tumors. A population of nestin-positive neuroepithelial cells that were morphologically similar to GCs in human tubers was derived from the *Tsc2* null mice by growth factor stimualtion.[24] These cells exhibited high levels of S6 phosphorylation and expression profiles of a variety of candidate genes including neurotransmitter receptors approximated human GCs.

To mimic the genotype of TSC patients, a novel conditional knockout mouse was recently created that harbors a heterozygous deletion of *TSC2* in all cells and a homozygous deletion of *TSC2* in radial glia cells (RGCs) beginning at E12 in the hippocampus and E13.5–E14.0 in the cortex (Tsc2$^{flox/ko}$; hGFAP-Cre).[153] This mouse model phenocopies many aspects of the neurological pathology associated with TSC, including macrocephaly, cellular cytomegaly, lamination defects, astrogliosis, hypomyelination, and hyperphosphorylated S6.[153] Additionally, the mutant brains exhibit abnormal distribution of the layer II–IV marker Cux1 and a reduction in the layer VI-specific FoxP2-positive cells, which is accompanied by an increased population of Trb2-positive progenitors cells.[153] These results indicate that loss of TSC2 in RGCs results in expansion of progenitor cells that give rise to later-born neurons designated for superficial layers of the cortical plate at the expense of earlier-born neurons, which are specified for deeper layers. Additionally, this mouse model lends support to the LOH hypothesis that requires a second hit to occur prior to development of TSC-associated lesions.

Recently, Ehniger and colleagues described several hippocampal-dependent learning deficits in TSC2$^{+/-}$ mice.[140] Specifically, TSC2$^{+/-}$ animals exhibited spatial learning deficits in the Morris water maze, working memory deficits in the win-shift version of the eight-arm radial maze, and abnormal context discrimination in a context-conditioning paradigm. These behavioral changes correlated with extracellular field recordings in hippocampal slices that revealed decreased threshold for late-long term potentiation induction. Most notably, rapamycin treatment prior to induction of hippocampal-dependent learning resulted in substantial reversal of behavioral deficits. Furthermore, the threshold for L-LTP induction of TSC2$^{+/-}$ hippocampal slices perfused with rapamycin approximated those of wild-type controls. Thus, inactivation of TSC2 may result in abnormal learning and memory, contributing to the cognitive deficits associated with TSC, which may be ameliorated by rapamycin treatment.

TSC as a model disease

The histopathological similarities between tubers and several other types of nonsyndromic focal cortical malformations have provided new insights into the molecular pathogenesis of FCD and HMEG. Unifying features of these disorders are the presence of disorganized cortical lamination, cytomegalic cells, and intractable epilepsy. For example, both FCD type IIB and HMEG exhibit near complete loss of lamination and both contain BCs and cytomegalic neurons. Recent studies have demonstrated that BCs in FCD and HMEG exhibit robust phosphorylation of S6 protein in a pattern similar to GCs in cortical tubers.[23,154–156] In fact, these groups have suggested that phosphorylation of S6 in FCD and HMEG is consistent with the hypothesis that these focal malformations may form as a result of aberrant mTOR signaling. Indeed, we have described TSC, FCD, and HMEG as "TORopathies" to reflect the abnormal mTOR activation.

However, while mTOR signaling seems to be hyperactive in FCD and HMEG, several challenges remain. For example, while TSC results from identified gene mutations, no genetic association for either FCD or HMEG has been identified. In fact, screening the *TSC1* and *TSC2* genes in FCD and HMEG has not revealed mutations. Thus, if FCD and HMEG result from single gene defects, it is reasonable to propose that the causative gene, at least in some manner, affects mTOR signaling. Since virtually all identified genetic cortical malformation syndromes result from loss of function mutations, it seems logical that gene mutations in FCD and HMEG that lead to enhanced mTOR signaling must occur within negative modulators of mTOR function. Another distinction is that although S6 phosphorylation reflects hyperactive mTOR activity and potentially a unifying molecular event, the histopathology and transcriptional profiles of tubers versus FCD, BCs in FCD versus HMEG, or BCs versus GCs in TSC are not identical. There are well-characterized differences in mRNA and protein expression that distinguish these lesions and cell types. Thus, a comprehensive analysis of genetic, genomic (e.g., SNPs), and transcriptional similarities and differences between TSC, FCD, and HMEG will likely yield new insights.

Rapamycin and clinical trials

In light of the role that the TSC1 and TSC2 proteins play in regulation of mTOR kinase activity, a logical progression is to consider the widely available medication rapamycin in clinical trials for TSC. Rapamycin is a macrolide antibiotic that was identified in the 1970s as a product of the bacterium *Streptomyces hygroscopicus* in a soil sample from Easter Island. Rapamycin was initially developed as an antifungal agent but was subsequently shown to have important regulatory effects on cell growth, proliferation, and inflammation via its inhibitory action on mTOR. Rapamycin has been used as an immunomodulatory agent following organ transplantation and has a moderate-risk side effect profile.

The first use of rapamycin in a clinical setting was a case report of four TSC patients with SEGAs and one with pilocytic astrocytoma.[157] All were treated with oral rapamycin (serum levels 5–15 ng/mL) from 2.5 to 20 months and all showed some degree of tumor shrinkage by serial neuroimaging. One patient exhibited tumor recurrence when rapamycin was discontinued, but retreatment led again to tumor reduction. This report demonstrated that rapamycin could be used to treat SEGAs and possibly alleviate the need for resective surgery.

The first formal clinical trial of rapamycin examined a cohort of 25 patients with TSC or sporadic lymphangioleiomyomatosis (LAM) over a 24-month period.[158] Rapamycin was administered for 12 months with a 12-month follow-up period. Outcome measures included progression of LAM by pulmonary function testing (PFT) and chest computed tomography, change in volume of renal AML and neuroimaging to evaluate cortical tubers. The results were promising in the 18 patients who completed the trial and demonstrated a clear reduction in AML volume and modest improvement in PFT following 12 months of therapy that persisted in some patients at 24 months. There was no change in tuber volume. For some patients, however, renal AML size increased in the 12-month period without rapamycin treatment, echoing previous reports in both preclinical and clinical case series. An accompanying letter[159] reported interim findings at 12 months for 13 patients with TSC-associated LAM or sporadic LAM following rapamycin therapy in a UK-based initiative. All patients exhibited a reduction in AML volume (mean 26%), but none exhibited clear improvement in lung function by PFT. Assessment of memory and executive function in this cohort did not reveal a decrease in cognitive function following rapamycin therapy. In both trials, adverse effects were minimal and included aphthous oral ulcers, hyperlipidemia, peripheral edema, and increase rate of infection.

Both preclinical and clinical trial data suggest that rapamycin may provide a possible therapy for TSC. If so, this would represent a new frontier for therapeutics based on discoveries relating to functional cell cascades. However, several important questions remain to be answered before widespread rapamycin therapy is instituted. First, when should rapamycin therapy be initiated? Should all TSC patients be treated with rapamycin as a prophylaxis or should rapamycin be started for specific symptoms (e.g., dyspnea, seizures, or hematuria) or disease features (e.g., confirmed LAM, tubers, SEGAs, or AMLs)? A benefit of rapamycin in human epilepsy, cognitive disability, or autism has not been shown, yet many clinicians are eager to perform case–control trials. Should rapamycin be initiated if tubers are detected by MRI in the newborn period or even fetal life in a selected group of patients? A particularly devastating problem in TSC is the high incidence of infantile spasms (IS). There is clinical evidence that IS in TSC are linked to subsequent intractable seizures and cognitive disabilities and thus, early rapamycin treatment could be an effective prevention of both. Perhaps more problematic than therapy initiation is when, if ever, to stop rapamycin treatment? Current evidence suggests that the benefits of rapamycin in a preclinical or clinical setting may only be realized during active therapy and that any gains may be lost if the medication is discontinued. Furthermore, rapamycin has side effects that may prevent long-term treatment in some patients.

Summary/future directions

The identification of the *TSC1* and *TSC2* genes provides a unique example of how translational efforts spanning gene cloning in human patients, model generation in *Drosophila*, and extensive *in vitro* and *in vivo* investigation of mTOR signaling have culminated in a new and exciting potential therapy for TSC. Although much has been accomplished, a daunting amount of future work remains. Many fundamental questions regarding disease variability and heterogeneity, genotype–phenotype correlation, and organ-specific pathology are still unanswered.

Acknowledgments

This work was supported by the Tuberous Sclerosis Alliance, National Institutes of Health (R01NS04502), and Department of Defense.

Conflicts of Interest

The authors declare no conflicts of interest.

References

1. Krsek, P. *et al.* 2008. Different features of histopathological subtypes of pediatric focal cortical dysplasia. *Ann. Neurol.* **63:** 758–769.

2. Mischel, P.S. *et al.* 1995. Cerebral cortical dysplasia associated with pediatric epilepsy. Review of neuropathologic features and proposal for a grading system. *J. Neuropathol. Exp. Neurol.* **54:** 137–153.

3. Andermann, F. 2000. Cortical dysplasias and epilepsy: a review of the architectonic, clinical, and seizure patterns. *Adv. Neurol.* **84:** 479–496.

4. Sarnat, H.B. & L. Flores-Sarnat. 2001. A new classification of malformations of the nervous system: an integration of morphological and molecular genetic criteria as patterns of genetic expression. *Eur. J. Paediatr. Neurol.* **5:** 57–64.

5. Palmini, A. *et al.* 2004. Terminology and classification of the cortical dysplasias. *Neurology* **62:** S2–S8.

6. Lee, S.K. *et al.* 2005. Surgical outcome and prognostic factors of cryptogenic neocortical epilepsy. *Ann. Neurol.* **58:** 525–532.

7. Crino, P.B. *et al.* 2006. The tuberous sclerosis complex. *N. Engl. J. Med.* **355:** 1345–1356.

8. Osborne, J.P. *et al.* 1991. Epidemiology of tuberous sclerosis. *Ann. N.Y. Acad. Sci.* **615:** 125–127.

9. Curatolo, P. *et al.* 2008. Tuberous sclerosis. *Lancet* **372:** 657–668.

10. Jozwiak, S. *et al.* 2000. Usefulness of diagnostic criteria of tuberous sclerosis complex in pediatric patients. *J. Child Neurol.* **15:** 652–659.

11. Cook, J.A. *et al.* 1996. A cross sectional study of renal involvement in tuberous sclerosis. *J. Med. Genet.* **33:** 480–484.

12. Rakowski, S.K. *et al.* 2006. Renal manifestations of tuberous sclerosis complex: Incidence, prognosis, and predictive factors. *Kidney Int.* **70:** 1777–1782.

13. O'Callaghan, F.J. *et al.* 2004. An epidemiological study of renal pathology in tuberous sclerosis complex. *BJU Int.* **94:** 853–857.

14. Henske, E.P. 2005. Tuberous sclerosis and the kidney: from mesenchyme to epithelium, and beyond. *Pediatr. Nephrol.* **20:** 854–857.

15. Shepherd, C.W. *et al.* 1991. Causes of death in patients with tuberous sclerosis. *Mayo Clin. Proc.* **66:** 792–796.

16. Thiele, E.A. 2004. Managing epilepsy in tuberous sclerosis complex. *J. Child Neurol.* **19:** 680–686.

17. Prather, P. & P.J. de Vries. 2004. Behavioral and cognitive aspects of tuberous sclerosis complex. *J. Child Neurol.* **19:** 666–674.

18. Smalley, S.L. 1998. Autism and tuberous sclerosis. *J. Autism. Dev. Disord.* **28:** 407–414.

19. Crino, P.B. *et al.* 1996. Embryonic neuronal markers in tuberous sclerosis: single-cell molecular pathology. *Proc. Natl. Acad. Sci.* **93:** 14152–14157.

20. Park, S.H. *et al.* 1997. Tuberous sclerosis in a 20-week gestation fetus: immunohistochemical study. *Acta Neuropathol.* **94:** 180–186.

21. Goh, S. *et al.* 2004. Subependymal giant cell tumors in tuberous sclerosis complex. *Neurology* **63:** 1457–1461.

22. Mizuguchi, M. *et al.* 2002. Doublecortin immunoreactivity in giant cells of tuberous sclerosis and focal cortical dysplasia. *Acta Neuropathol.* **104:** 418–424.

23. Baybis, M. *et al.* 2004. mTOR cascade activation distinguishes tubers from focal cortical dysplasia. *Ann. Neurol.* **56:** 478–487.

24. Onda, H. *et al.* 2002. Tsc2 null murine neuroepithelial cells are a model for human tuber giant cells, and show activation of an mTOR pathway. *Mol. Cell. Neurosci.* **21:** 561–574.

25. Lee, A. *et al.* 2003. Markers of cellular proliferation are expressed in cortical tubers. *Ann. Neurol.* **53:** 668–673.

26. Talos, D.M. *et al.* 2008. Cell-specific alterations of glutamate receptor expression in tuberous sclerosis complex cortical tubers. *Ann. Neurol.* **63:** 454–465.

27. Boer, K. *et al.* 2008. Cellular localization of metabotropic glutamate receptors in cortical tubers and subependymal giant cell tumors of tuberous sclerosis complex. *Neuroscience* **156:** 203–215.

28. Holmes, G.L. & C.E. Stafstrom. 2007. Tuberous sclerosis complex and epilepsy: recent developments and future challenges. *Epilepsia* **48:** 617–630.

29. Koh, S. *et al.* 2000. Epilepsy surgery in children with tuberous sclerosis complex: presurgical evaluation and outcome. *Epilepsia* **41:** 1206–1213.

30. Jansen, F.E. *et al.* 2007. Epilepsy surgery in tuberous sclerosis: a systematic review. *Epilepsia* **48:** 1477–1484.

31. Philippe Major, S.R., M.V. Simon, M.L. Cheng, *et al.* 2009. Are cortical tubers epileptogenic? Evidence from electrocorticography. *Epilepsia* **50:** 147–154.

32. Joinson, C. *et al.* 2003. Learning disability and epilepsy in an epidemiological sample of individuals with tuberous sclerosis complex. *Psychol. Med.* **33:** 335–344.

33. Ryu, J.H. *et al.* 2006. The NHLBI lymphangioleiomyomatosis registry: characteristics of 230 patients at enrollment. *Am. J. Respir. Crit. Care Med.* **173:** 105–111.

34. Smythe, J.F. *et al.* 1990. Natural history of cardiac rhabdomyoma in infancy and childhood. *Am. J. Cardiol.* **66:** 1247–1249.

35. Mennel, S. *et al.* 2007. Current treatment modalities for exudative retinal hamartomas secondary to tuberous sclerosis: review of the literature. *Acta Ophthalmol. Scand.* **85:** 127–132.

36. Gunduz, K. *et al.* 1999. Invasive giant cell astrocytoma of the retina in a patient with tuberous sclerosis. *Ophthalmology* **106:** 639–642.

37. van Slegtenhorst, M. *et al.* 1997. Identification of the tuberous sclerosis gene TSC1 on chromosome 9q34. *Science* **277:** 805–808.

38. Kandt, R.S. *et al.* 1992. Linkage of an important gene locus for tuberous sclerosis to a chromosome 16 marker for polycystic kidney disease. *Nat. Genet.* **2:** 37–41.

39. Maheshwar, M.M. *et al.* 1997. The GAP-related domain of tuberin, the product of the TSC2 gene, is a target for missense mutations in tuberous sclerosis. *Hum. Mol. Genet.* **6:** 1991–1996.

40. van Slegtenhorst, M. *et al.* 1998. Interaction between hamartin and tuberin, the TSC1 and TSC2 gene products. *Hum. Mol. Genet.* **7:** 1053–1057.

41. Jones, A.C. *et al.* 1997. Molecular genetic and phenotypic analysis reveals differences between TSC1 and TSC2 associated familial and sporadic tuberous sclerosis. *Hum. Mol. Genet.* **6:** 2155–2161.

42. Benvenuto, G. *et al.* 2000. The tuberous sclerosis-1 (TSC1) gene product hamartin suppresses cell growth and augments the expression of the TSC2 product tuberin by inhibiting its ubiquitination. *Oncogene* **19:** 6306–6316.

43. Chong-Kopera, H. *et al.* 2006. TSC1 stabilizes TSC2 by inhibiting the interaction between TSC2 and the HERC1 ubiquitin ligase. *J. Biol. Chem.* **281:** 8313–8316.

44. Jones, A.C. *et al.* 1999. Comprehensive mutation analysis of TSC1 and TSC2-and phenotypic correlations in 150 families with tuberous sclerosis. *Am. J. Hum. Genet.* **64:** 1305–1315.

45. Nellist, M. *et al.* 2001. TSC2 missense mutations inhibit tuberin phosphorylation and prevent formation of the tuberin-hamartin complex. *Hum. Mol. Genet.* **10:** 2889–2898.

46. Ito, N. & G.M. Rubin. 1999. Gigas, a *Drosophila* homolog of tuberous sclerosis gene product-2, regulates the cell cycle. *Cell* **96**: 529–539.

47. Tapon, N. *et al.* 2001. The *Drosophila* tuberous sclerosis complex gene homologs restrict cell growth and cell proliferation. *Cell* **105**: 345–355.

48. Potter, C.J. *et al.* 2001. *Drosophila* Tsc1 functions with Tsc2 to antagonize insulin signaling in regulating cell growth, cell proliferation, and organ size. *Cell* **105**: 357–368.

49. Gao, X. & D. Pan. 2001. TSC1 and TSC2 tumor suppressors antagonize insulin signaling in cell growth. *Genes Dev.* **15**: 1383–1392.

50. Rosner, M. *et al.* 2008. The tuberous sclerosis gene products hamartin and tuberin are multifunctional proteins with a wide spectrum of interacting partners. *Mutat. Res.* **658**: 234–246.

51. Astrinidis, A. *et al.* 2003. Cell cycle-regulated phosphorylation of hamartin, the product of the tuberous sclerosis complex 1 gene, by cyclin-dependent kinase 1/cyclin B. *J. Biol. Chem.* **278**: 51372–51379.

52. Astrinidis, A. *et al.* 2006. Hamartin, the tuberous sclerosis complex 1 gene product, interacts with polo-like kinase 1 in a phosphorylation-dependent manner. *Hum. Mol. Genet.* **15**: 287–297.

53. Lamb, R.F. *et al.* 2000. The TSC1 tumour suppressor hamartin regulates cell adhesion through ERM proteins and the GTPase Rho. *Nat. Cell. Biol.* **2**: 281–287.

54. Lee, D.F. *et al.* 2007. IKK beta suppression of TSC1 links inflammation and tumor angiogenesis via the mTOR pathway. *Cell* **130**: 440–455.

55. Ma, L. *et al.* 2005. Phosphorylation and functional inactivation of TSC2 by Erk implications for tuberous sclerosis and cancer pathogenesis. *Cell* **121**: 179–193.

56. Ma, L. *et al.* 2007. Identification of S664 TSC2 phosphorylation as a marker for extracellular signal-regulated kinase mediated mTOR activation in tuberous sclerosis and human cancer. *Cancer Res.* **67**: 7106–7112.

57. Potter, C.J. *et al.* 2002. Akt regulates growth by directly phosphorylating Tsc2. *Nat. Cell. Biol.* **4**: 658–665.

58. Manning, B.D. *et al.* 2002. Identification of the tuberous sclerosis complex-2 tumor suppressor gene product tuberin as a target of the phosphoinositide 3-kinase/Akt pathway. *Mol. Cell* **10**: 151–162.

59. Inoki, K. *et al.* 2002. TSC2 is phosphorylated and inhibited by Akt and suppresses mTOR signalling. *Nat. Cell Biol.* **4**: 648–657.

60. Dan, H.C. *et al.* 2002. Phosphatidylinositol 3-kinase/Akt pathway regulates tuberous sclerosis tumor suppressor complex by phosphorylation of tuberin. *J. Biol. Chem.* **277**: 35364–35370.

61. Inoki, K. *et al.* 2003. TSC2 mediates cellular energy response to control cell growth and survival. *Cell* **115**: 577–590.

62. Hahn-Windgassen, A. *et al.* 2005. Akt activates the mammalian target of rapamycin by regulating cellular ATP level and AMPK activity. *J. Biol. Chem.* **280**: 32081–32089.

63. Shaw, R.J. *et al.* 2004. The tumor suppressor LKB1 kinase directly activates AMP-activated kinase and regulates apoptosis in response to energy stress. *Proc. Natl. Acad. Sci.* **101**: 3329–3335.

64. Inoki, K. *et al.* 2006. TSC2 integrates Wnt and energy signals via a coordinated phosphorylation by AMPK and GSK3 to regulate cell growth. *Cell* **126**: 955–968.

65. Maldonado, M. *et al.* 2003. Expression of ICAM-1, TNF-alpha, NF kappa B, and MAP kinase in tubers of the tuberous sclerosis complex. *Neurobiol. Dis.* **14**: 279–290.

66. Han, S. *et al.* 2004. Phosphorylation of tuberin as a novel mechanism for somatic inactivation of the tuberous sclerosis complex proteins in brain lesions. *Cancer Res.* **64**: 812–816.

67. Wullschleger, S. *et al.* 2006. TOR signaling in growth and metabolism. *Cell* **124**: 471–484.

68. Manning, B.D. & L.C. Cantley. 2007. AKT/PKB signaling: navigating downstream. *Cell* **129**: 1261–1274.

69. Myers, M.P. *et al.* 1998. The lipid phosphatase activity of PTEN is critical for its tumor supressor function. *Proc. Natl. Acad. Sci.* **95**: 13513–13518.

70. Keniry, M. & R. Parsons. 2008. The role of PTEN signaling perturbations in cancer and in targeted therapy. *Oncogene* **27**: 5477–5485.

71. Gao, X. *et al.* 2002. Tsc tumour suppressor proteins antagonize amino-acid-TOR signalling. *Nat. Cell Biol.* **4**: 699–704.

72. Jaeschke, A. *et al.* 2002. Tuberous sclerosis complex tumor suppressor-mediated S6 kinase inhibition by phosphatidylinositide-3-OH kinase is mTOR independent. *J. Cell Biol.* **159**: 217–224.

73. Kwiatkowski, D.J. *et al.* 2002. A mouse model of TSC1 reveals sex-dependent lethality from liver hemangiomas, and up-regulation of p70S6 kinase activity in Tsc1 null cells. *Hum. Mol. Genet.* **11**: 525–534.

74. Maehama, T. & J.E. Dixon. 1998. The tumor suppressor, PTEN/MMAC1, dephosphorylates the lipid second messenger, phosphatidylinositol 3,4,5-trisphosphate. *J. Biol. Chem.* **273**: 13375–13378.

75. Gao, X. *et al.* 2000. *Drosophila* PTEN regulates cell growth and proliferation through PI3K-dependent and -independent pathways. *Dev. Biol.* **221:** 404–418.

76. Goberdhan, D.C. *et al.* 1999. *Drosophila* tumor suppressor PTEN controls cell size and number by antagonizing the Chico/PI3-kinase signaling pathway. *Genes Dev.* **13:** 3244–3258.

77. Di Cristofano, A. *et al.* 1998. Pten is essential for embryonic development and tumour suppression. *Nat. Genet.* **19:** 348–355.

78. Waite, K.A. & C. Eng. 2002. Protean PTEN: form and function. *Am. J. Hum. Genet.* **70:** 829–844.

79. Butler, M.G. *et al.* 2005. Subset of individuals with autism spectrum disorders and extreme macrocephaly associated with germline PTEN tumour suppressor gene mutations. *J. Med. Genet.* **42:** 318–321.

80. Kwon, C.H. *et al.* 2006. Pten regulates neuronal arborization and social interaction in mice. *Neuron* **50:** 377–388.

81. Stevens, C. *et al.* 2009. Peptide combinatorial libraries identify TSC2 as a death-associated protein kinase (DAPK) death domain-binding protein and reveal a stimulatory role for DAPK in mTORC1 signaling. *J. Biol. Chem.* **284:** 334–344.

82. Bialik, S. & A. Kimchi. 2006. The death-associated protein kinases: structure, function, and beyond. *Annu. Rev. Biochem.* **75:** 189–210.

83. Schumacher, A.M. *et al.* 2006. Death-associated protein kinase phosphorylates mammalian ribosomal protein S6 and reduces protein synthesis. *Biochemistry (Mosc.)* **45:** 13614–13621.

84. Cao, Y. *et al.* 2006. Interaction of FoxO1 and TSC2 induces insulin resistance through activation of the mammalian target of rapamycin/p70 S6K pathway. *J. Biol. Chem.* **281:** 40242–40251.

85. Greer, E.L. & A. Brunet. 2005. FOXO transcription factors at the interface between longevity and tumor suppression. *Oncogene* **24:** 7410–7425.

86. Hardie, D.G. *et al.* 2003. Management of cellular energy by the AMP-activated protein kinase system. *FEBS Lett.* **546:** 113–120.

87. Shaw, R.J. *et al.* 2004. The LKB1 tumor suppressor negatively regulates mTOR signaling. *Cancer Cell* **6:** 91–99.

88. Corradetti, M.N. *et al.* 2004. Regulation of the TSC pathway by LKB1: evidence of a molecular link between tuberous sclerosis complex and Peutz-Jeghers syndrome. *Genes Dev.* **18:** 1533–1538.

89. Hemminki, A. *et al.* 1998. A serine/threonine kinase gene defective in Peutz-Jeghers syndrome. *Nature* **391:** 184–187.

90. Dorfman, J. & I.G. Macara. 2008. STRADalpha regulates LKB1 localization by blocking access to importin-alpha, and by association with Crm1 and exportin-7. *Mol. Biol. Cell.* **19:** 1614–1626.

91. Hawley, S.A. *et al.* 2003. Complexes between the LKB1 tumor suppressor, STRAD alpha/beta and MO25 alpha/beta are upstream kinases in the AMP-activated protein kinase cascade. *J. Biol.* **2:** 28.

92. Puffenberger, E.G. *et al.* 2007. Polyhydramnios, megalencephaly and symptomatic epilepsy caused by a homozygous 7-kilobase deletion in LYK5. *Brain* **130:** 1929–1941.

93. Brugarolas, J. *et al.* 2004. Regulation of mTOR function in response to hypoxia by REDD1 and the TSC1/TSC2 tumor suppressor complex. *Genes Dev.* **18:** 2893–2904.

94. Reiling, J.H. & E. Hafen. 2004. The hypoxia-induced paralogs Scylla and Charybdis inhibit growth by downregulating S6K activity upstream of TSC in *Drosophila*. *Genes Dev.* **18:** 2879–2892.

95. Sofer, A. *et al.* 2005. Regulation of mTOR and cell growth in response to energy stress by REDD1. *Mol. Cell. Biol.* **25:** 5834–5845.

96. Moon, R.T. *et al.* 2004. WNT and beta-catenin signalling: diseases and therapies. *Nat. Rev. Genet.* **5:** 691–701.

97. Levine, A.J. 1997. p53, the cellular gatekeeper for growth and division. *Cell* **88:** 323–331.

98. Feng, Z. *et al.* 2005. The coordinate regulation of the p53 and mTOR pathways in cells. *Proc. Natl. Acad. Sci.* **102:** 8204–8209.

99. Budanov, A.V. & M. Karin. 2008. p53 target genes sestrin1 and sestrin2 connect genotoxic stress and mTOR signaling. *Cell* **134:** 451–460.

100. Feng, Z. *et al.* 2007. The regulation of AMPK beta1, TSC2, and PTEN expression by p53: stress, cell and tissue specificity, and the role of these gene products in modulating the IGF-1-AKT-mTOR pathways. *Cancer Res.* **67:** 3043–3053.

101. Inoki, K. *et al.* 2003. Rheb GTPase is a direct target of TSC2 GAP activity and regulates mTOR signaling. *Genes Dev.* **17:** 1829–1834.

102. Garami, A. *et al.* 2003. Insulin activation of Rheb, a mediator of mTOR/S6K/4E-BP signaling, is inhibited by TSC1 and 2. *Mol. Cell.* **11:** 1457–1466.

103. Long, X. *et al.* 2005. Rheb binds and regulates the mTOR kinase. *Curr. Biol.* **15:** 702–713.

104. Bai, X. *et al.* 2007. Rheb activates mTOR by antagonizing its endogenous inhibitor, FKBP38. *Science* **318:** 977–980.

105. Castro, A.F. *et al.* 2003. Rheb binds tuberous sclerosis complex 2 (TSC2) and promotes S6 kinase activation in a rapamycin- and farnesylation-dependent manner. *J. Biol. Chem.* **278:** 32493–32496.

106. Kim, D.H. *et al.* 2002. mTOR interacts with raptor to form a nutrient-sensitive complex that signals to the cell growth machinery. *Cell* **110:** 163–175.

107. Sarbassov, D.D. *et al.* 2004. Rictor, a novel binding partner of mTOR, defines a rapamycin-insensitive and raptor-independent pathway that regulates the cytoskeleton. *Curr. Biol.* **14:** 1296–5131302.

108. Fadri, M. *et al.* 2005. The pleckstrin homology domain proteins Slm1 and Slm2 are required for actin cytoskeleton organization in yeast and bind phosphatidylinositol-4,5-bisphosphate and TORC2. *Mol. Biol. Cell.* **16:** 1883–1900.

109. Jacinto, E. *et al.* 2004. Mammalian TOR complex 2 controls the actin cytoskeleton and is rapamycin insensitive. *Nat. Cell Biol.* **6:** 1122–1128.

110. Sarbassov, D.D. *et al.* 2005. Phosphorylation and regulation of Akt/PKB by the rictor-mTOR complex. *Science* **307:** 1098–1101.

111. Dufner, A. & G. Thomas. 1999. Ribosomal S6 kinase signaling and the control of translation. *Exp. Cell Res.* **253:** 100–109.

112. Proud, C.G. 2007. Signalling to translation: how signal transduction pathways control the protein synthetic machinery. *Biochem. J.* **403:** 217–234.

113. Montagne, J. *et al.* 1999. *Drosophila* S6 kinase: a regulator of cell size. *Science* **285:** 2126–2129.

114. Shima, H. *et al.* 1998. Disruption of the p70(s6k)/p85(s6k) gene reveals a small mouse phenotype and a new functional S6 kinase. *EMBO J.* **17:** 6649–6659.

115. Ruvinsky, I. *et al.* 2005. Ribosomal protein S6 phosphorylation is a determinant of cell size and glucose homeostasis. *Genes Dev.* **19:** 2199–2211.

116. Ruvinsky, I. & O. Meyuhas. 2006. Ribosomal protein S6 phosphorylation: from protein synthesis to cell size. *Trends Biochem. Sci.* **31:** 342–348.

117. Um, S.H. *et al.* 2004. Absence of S6K1 protects against age- and diet-induced obesity while enhancing insulin sensitivity. *Nature* **431:** 200–205.

118. Gingras, A.C. *et al.* 1998. 4E-BP1, a repressor of mRNA translation, is phosphorylated and inactivated by the Akt(PKB) signaling pathway. *Genes Dev.* **12:** 502–513.

119. Gingras, A.C. *et al.* 2001. Hierarchical phosphorylation of the translation inhibitor 4E-BP1. *Genes Dev.* **15:** 2852–2864.

120. Tsukiyama-Kohara, K. *et al.* 2001. Adipose tissue reduction in mice lacking the translational inhibitor 4E-BP1. *Nat. Med.* **7:** 1128–1132.

121. Brugarolas, J.B. *et al.* 2003. TSC2 regulates VEGF through mTOR-dependent and -independent pathways. *Cancer Cell* **4:** 147–158.

122. Ivan, M. *et al.* 2001. HIFalpha targeted for VHL-mediated destruction by proline hydroxylation: implications for O2 sensing. *Science* **292:** 464–468.

123. Jaakkola, P. *et al.* 2001. Targeting of HIF-alpha to the von Hippel-Lindau ubiquitylation complex by O2-regulated prolyl hydroxylation. *Science* **292:** 468–472.

124. Kobayashi, T. *et al.* 1995. A germline insertion in the tuberous sclerosis (Tsc2) gene gives rise to the Eker rat model of dominantly inherited cancer. *Nat. Genet.* **9:** 70–74.

125. Wilson, C. *et al.* 2005. A mouse model of tuberous sclerosis 1 showing background specific early post-natal mortality and metastatic renal cell carcinoma. *Hum. Mol. Genet.* **14:** 1839–1850.

126. Onda, H. *et al.* 1999. Tsc2(+/−) mice develop tumors in multiple sites that express gelsolin and are influenced by genetic background. *J. Clin. Invest.* **104:** 687–695.

127. El-Hashemite, N. *et al.* 2003. Loss of Tsc1 or Tsc2 induces vascular endothelial growth factor production through mammalian target of rapamycin. *Cancer Res.* **63:** 5173–5177.

128. Chung, J. *et al.* 2002. Integrin (alpha 6 beta 4) regulation of eIF-4E activity and VEGF translation: a survival mechanism for carcinoma cells. *J. Cell Biol.* **158:** 165–174.

129. Klos, K.S. *et al.* 2006. ErbB2 increases vascular endothelial growth factor protein synthesis via activation of mammalian target of rapamycin/p70S6K leading to increased angiogenesis and spontaneous metastasis of human breast cancer cells. *Cancer Res.* **66:** 2028–2037.

130. Chen, G. & D.V. Goeddel. 2002. TNF-R1 signaling: a beautiful pathway. *Science* **296:** 1634–1635.

131. Tavazoie, S.F. *et al.* 2005. Regulation of neuronal morphology and function by the tumor suppressors Tsc1 and Tsc2. *Nat. Neurosci.* **8:** 1727–1734.

132. Choi, Y.J. *et al.* 2008. Tuberous sclerosis complex proteins control axon formation. *Genes Dev.* **22:** 2485–2495.

133. Kishi, M. *et al.* 2005. Mammalian SAD kinases are required for neuronal polarization. *Science* **307:** 929–932.

134. Lizcano, J.M. *et al.* 2004. LKB1 is a master kinase that activates 13 kinases of the AMPK subfamily, including MARK/PAR-1. *EMBO J.* **23:** 833–843.

135. Barnes, A.P. *et al.* 2007. LKB1 and SAD kinases define a pathway required for the polarization of cortical neurons. *Cell* **129:** 549–563.

136. Kobayashi, T. *et al.* 2001. A germ-line Tsc1 mutation causes tumor development and embryonic lethality that are similar, but not identical to, those caused by Tsc2 mutation in mice. *Proc. Natl. Acad. Sci.* **98:** 8762–8767.

137. Uhlmann, E.J. *et al.* 2002. Astrocyte-specific TSC1 conditional knockout mice exhibit abnormal neuronal organization and seizures. *Ann. Neurol.* **52:** 285–296.

138. Wong, M. *et al.* 2003. Impaired glial glutamate transport in a mouse tuberous sclerosis epilepsy model. *Ann. Neurol.* **54:** 251–256.

139. Wang, Y. *et al.* 2007. Neocortical hyperexcitability in a human case of tuberous sclerosis complex and mice lacking neuronal expression of TSC1. *Ann. Neurol.* **61:** 139–152.

140. Ehninger, D. *et al.* 2008. Reversal of learning deficits in a Tsc2+/- mouse model of tuberous sclerosis. *Nat. Med.* **14:** 843–848.

141. Yeung, R.S. *et al.* 1994. Predisposition to renal carcinoma in the Eker rat is determined by germ-line mutation of the tuberous sclerosis 2 (TSC2) gene. *Proc. Natl. Acad. Sci.* **91:** 11413–11416.

142. Xiao, G.H. *et al.* 1995. Germ-line Tsc2 mutation in a dominantly inherited cancer model defines a novel family of rat intracisternal-A particle elements. *Oncogene* **11:** 81–87.

143. Hino, O. *et al.* 1993. Spontaneous and radiation-induced renal tumors in the Eker rat model of dominantly inherited cancer. *Proc. Natl. Acad. Sci.* **90:** 327–331.

144. Yeung, R.S. 2004. Lessons from the Eker rat model: from cage to bedside. *Curr. Mol. Med.* **4:** 799–806.

145. Yeung, R.S. *et al.* 1995. Allelic loss at the tuberous sclerosis 2 locus in spontaneous tumors in the Eker rat. *Mol. Carcinog.* **14:** 28–36.

146. Yeung, R.S. *et al.* 1997. Subependymal astrocytic hamartomas in the Eker rat model of tuberous sclerosis. *Am. J. Pathol.* **151:** 1477–1486.

147. Mizuguchi, M. *et al.* 2000. Novel cerebral lesions in the Eker rat model of tuberous sclerosis: cortical tuber and anaplastic ganglioglioma. *J. Neuropathol. Exp. Neurol.* **59:** 188–196.

148. Kenerson, H.L. *et al.* 2002. Activated mammalian target of rapamycin pathway in the pathogenesis of tuberous sclerosis complex renal tumors. *Cancer Res.* **62:** 5645–5650.

149. Waltereit, R. *et al.* 2006. Enhanced episodic-like memory and kindling epilepsy in a rat model of tuberous sclerosis. *J. Neurochem.* **96:** 407–413.

150. Wenzel, H.J. *et al.* 2004. Morphology of cerebral lesions in the Eker rat model of tuberous sclerosis. *Acta Neuropathol.* **108:** 97–108.

151. Takahashi, D.K. *et al.* 2004. Abnormal cortical cells and astrocytomas in the Eker rat model of tuberous sclerosis complex. *Epilepsia* **45:** 1525–1530.

152. Kobayashi, T. *et al.* 1999. Renal carcinogenesis, hepatic hemangiomatosis, and embryonic lethality caused by a germ-line Tsc2 mutation in mice. *Cancer Res.* **59:** 1206–1211.

153. Way, S.W. *et al.* 2009. Loss of Tsc2 in radial glia models the brain pathology of tuberous sclerosis complex in the mouse. *Hum. Mol. Genet.* **18:** 1252–1265.

154. Miyata, H. *et al.* 2004. Insulin signaling pathways in cortical dysplasia and TSC-tubers: tissue microarray analysis. *Ann. Neurol.* **56:** 510–519.

155. Ljungberg, M.C. *et al.* 2006. Activation of mammalian target of rapamycin in cytomegalic neurons of human cortical dysplasia. *Ann. Neurol.* **60:** 420–429.

156. Aronica, E. *et al.* 2007. Co-expression of cyclin D1 and phosphorylated ribosomal S6 proteins in hemimegalencephaly. *Acta Neuropathol.* **114:** 287–293.

157. Franz, D.N. *et al.* 2006. Rapamycin causes regression of astrocytomas in tuberous sclerosis complex. *Ann. Neurol.* **59:** 490–498.

158. Bissler, J.J. *et al.* 2008. Sirolimus for angiomyolipoma in tuberous sclerosis complex or lymphangioleiomyomatosis. *N. Engl. J. Med.* **358:** 140–151.

159. Davies, D.M. *et al.* 2008. Sirolimus therapy in tuberous sclerosis or sporadic lymphangioleiomyomatosis. *N. Engl. J. Med.* **358:** 200–203.

Ann. N.Y. Acad. Sci. ISSN 0077-8923

ANNALS OF THE NEW YORK ACADEMY OF SCIENCES

Neurological complications of immune reconstitution in HIV-infected populations

Tory Johnson[1,2] and Avindra Nath[1,3]

Departments of [1]Neurology, [2]Pathology, and [3]Neuroscience, Johns Hopkins University, Baltimore, Maryland, USA

Address for correspondence: Avindra Nath, MD, 509 Pathology, 600 N. Wolfe St, Baltimore, MD 21287. Voice: 443-287-4656; fax: 410-502-8075. anath1@jhmi.edu

The introduction of highly active antiretroviral therapy (HAART) for human immunodeficiency virus (HIV) infection has transformed this disease from a fatal infection to a chronic yet manageable condition by restoring immune function. All the same, this restoration of immune response in some may be associated with deterioration in clinical status, which has been termed immune reconstitution inflammatory syndrome (IRIS). This syndrome often occurs in the context of an underlying opportunistic infection and develops after an interval of weeks to months after the initiation of HAART. Occasionally, IRIS may occur in the brain without any opportunistic infection, which presents as a T cell–mediated encephalitis. This paradoxical infiltration of previously immune suppressed patients with T cells represents a diagnostic challenge and a treatment dilemma. Nonetheless, CNS-IRIS with or without an opportunistic infection can range in severity. Severe cases can be fatal and hence require intervention with steroid treatment. This review discusses the diagnosis, clinical manifestations, risk factors, pathophysiology, and potential treatment strategies of the various forms of IRIS that involve the nervous system.

Keywords: HIV; brain; IRIS; HAART; immune reconstitution; encephalitis; meningitis; PML

Introduction

The term *immune reconstitution inflammatory syndrome* (IRIS) has been defined as "a paradoxical deterioration in clinical status attributable to the recovery of the immune system during HAART."[1] The disorder, in the context of human immunodeficiency virus (HIV) infection, was first described in 1992 when a patient developed an acute *Mycobacterium avium-intracellulare* infection after the initiation of antiretroviral therapy.[2] Subsequently, IRIS was recognized in patients with a wide variety of presentations and associated pathogens.[3–13] IRIS is also referred to as immune restoration disease (IRD) or immune reconstitution syndrome (IRS), however all names refer to a disease process due to the reemergence of a functional immune system as opposed to a disorder due to immune suppression. Neurological syndromes with immune restoration had been recognized prior to the HIV era, mainly in the context of bacterial infections such as tuberculous or bacterial meningitis, where after initiation of antimicrobial therapy clinical deterioration may oc-cur due to a heightened immune response, and have often been termed hypersensitivity reactions. The Jarisch-Herxheimer reaction which occurs following treatment for syphilis is another example. A similar "leprosy reaction" is known to occur in patients with lepromatous leprosy who develop neurological deterioration following treatment. For the purpose of this review, we have used the acronym IRIS for the umbrella of disorders arising from the reconstitution of the immune system after the advent of highly active antiretroviral therapy (HAART).[1]

Two distinct forms of IRIS are typically discussed in the literature. The first form is termed "unmasking" IRIS, in which an immune-suppressed individual is unable to respond to an opportunistic infection (OI), and once HAART is commenced a robust, inflammatory immune response occurs against the offending pathogen, but also a worsening of clinical condition in the patient.[15] The other form of IRIS is termed "paradoxical" because these patients have a deterioration of clinical status due to an inflammatory process against an antigen that was previously controlled or treated.[1,14] This form of IRIS

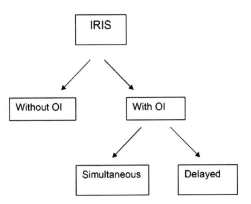

Figure 1. Types of IRIS: IRIS following initiation of HAART may occur in the presence or absence of an opportunistic infection (OI). In some, the OI may first become clinically apparent concurrently with the IRIS and hence termed "simultaneous IRIS." In others, the OI predates the initiation of HAART but subsequently results in IRIS. This has been termed "delayed IRIS."

may be due to an overesponsive immune system. Additionally, the antigens driving IRIS are often OIs, although cases have been documented in which no pathogen was identified, leading to the hypothesis that IRIS can be a result of HIV-specific immune responses or autoantigens.[15] IRIS itself is defined as a paradoxical worsening of clinical condition due to the restoration of the immune system, and therefore both "unmasking" and "paradoxical" IRIS are by definition contradictory in nature. Using the term *paradoxical IRIS* is therefore redundant and ultimately may obscure the difference between the multiple forms of IRIS. We suggest using terms to clarify the differences between the forms of IRIS associated with OIs: *simultaneous IRIS* for patients who develop IRIS and a newly diagnosed OI at the same time and *delayed IRIS* to describe patients with an OI in which the IRIS manifests sometime thereafter (Fig. 1).

Epidemiology

IRIS occurs in approximately 15–35% of HIV-infected adult patients initiating HAART, with similar percentages occurring in children.[16–18] A recent study, however, determined that CNS-IRIS occurs at much lower frequencies, with approximately 0.9% of adults developing some CNS-IRIS after initiating HAART.[19] This group also determined that within the subgroup of patients with a CD4$^+$ T cell nadir of <200 cells/mm^3 the incidence of CNS-IRIS rose

to 1.5%, confirming that lower CD4$^+$ T cell nadir is an important risk factor for development of IRIS.[19] The wide range of occurrence may also reflect the challenge of recognizing and diagnosing IRIS. In developing countries, where antiretroviral therapy is often initiated only when severe immunosuppression is present, there is a higher risk for developing IRIS,[20,21] but epidemiological data on CNS-IRIS from these regions are currently lacking.

Risk factors

The current standard of care for HIV infection is the initiation of HAART when CD4$^+$ T cell counts are less than 350 cells/mm^3 or if the individual has an AIDS-defining illness.[22] When HAART is initiated in individuals with severe immune suppression there is a greater risk for developing IRIS. There are several factors that increase this risk, including a low CD4$^+$ nadir, the presence of subclinical or fulminate OIs, which may be responsible for driving the immune response, and a rapid response to HAART therapy indicated by a prompt decline in viral load and increase in CD4$^+$ T cells.[18,23,24] There may also be genetic risk factors that are as yet unidentified, because some people develop IRIS and others, with similar clinical status and risk factors, do not. Several studies using a simian immunodeficiency virus (SIV) model indicate differential expression of viral peptides by distinct MHC alleles, which could influence the aggressiveness of the immune response directed toward SIV.[25] This may extend to the human condition in which some MHC genotypes could be more inflammatory in the context of HIV and therefore could contribute to the development of IRIS. Additional support for a genetic contribution to the development of IRIS comes from a study that examined cytokine polymorphisms within the context of certain HLA alleles.[26]

Clinical manifestations of CNS-immune reconstitution inflammatory syndrome

Diagnosis of CNS-IRIS is difficult since it remains a clinical syndrome with varying presentations and severities and the CNS is a region of limited access. The ideal criteria for diagnosing CNS-IRIS include a history of HIV infection, worsening of clinical neurological status, either new neuroradiological findings or deterioration of previous findings unexplainable by previous illness or therapy, a log-fold or greater decrease in viral load, and HAART often with increasing CD4$^+$ cell counts. If available, histopathologic findings demonstrating T cell infiltrates into the CNS would confirm a CNS-IRIS diagnosis.[27] Depending on the severity of CNS-IRIS it maybe classified as (1) asymptomatic, where only radiological changes such as increased enhancement may be present; (2) symptomatic, where clinical deterioration in neurological function occurs, most often accompanied by new changes on MRI scan of brain; or (3) catastrophic, where severe neurological deficits occur such as coma and imminent signs of cerebral herniation.

Biomarkers for IRIS

It is imperative that pre-HAART therapy risk-assessment screening for IRIS be developed and implemented. Useful biomarkers for diagnosing and monitoring CNS-IRIS progression are much needed. Some immune correlates have been demonstrated. Most consistent is the finding of elevated plasma IL-6 levels during IRIS.[28,29] Further cytokine profiles may indicate several dependable markers irrelevant of the type of IRIS that may be present. Recent work demonstrates potential in developing genetic markers and gene expression profiles for IRIS.[30] Definitive diagnosis for CNS-IRIS requires pathological confirmation and hence is difficult to ascertain without invasive procedures. However, if correlates to CNS-IRIS exist with peripheral markers a clearer picture of CNS-IRIS may emerge

Immunobiology of IRIS

Restoration of the immune system

An HIV-infected, immune-suppressed individual who commences antiretroviral therapy undergoes a biphasic pattern of immune reconstitution. Initial recovery of the immune system is seen as an increase in memory T cells followed by an increase in thymic production of naive T cells, both of which result in an overall increase in the number of CD4$^+$ T cells present in circulation[31–33] (Fig. 2A). In addition, there is recovery of reduced or damaged secondary lymphoid organs such as the gut and mesenteric-associated lymphoid tissue, which are often lost due to chronic HIV-mediated inflammation.[34] Immune recovery can continue for 3–5 years,[35] as CD4$^+$ T naive and memory cell production resumes. However, there is typically an initial and rapid rise of CD4$^+$ T cells, composed of memory cells being re-

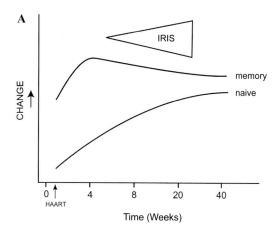

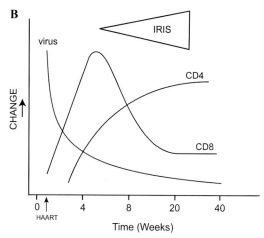

Figure 2. Immune restoration after HAART is biphasic. (**A**) Initial recovery of immune cells is dominated by a rapid increase in memory cells as these are released from compartments into circulation. This is followed by a gradual yet steady increase in naive cell production that can continue for several years. (**B**) A rapid decline in viral load is accompanied by a rapid rise in circulating numbers of CD8$^+$ T cells, although these return to slightly above baseline levels. CD4$^+$ T cells rise more slowly and continually.

leased from lymphoid tissues,[31] within 3–6 months of initiation of HAART therapy.[31–33] CD8$^+$ T cells also increase during the first 2 months of HAART, although these levels tend to return to baseline after 4 months of HAART[33] (Fig. 2B). Additionally, reconstitution of the immune system tends to take longer in patients with very low nadir CD4$^+$ counts and may also be incomplete in as much as one-third of patients, even after stably reducing viral loads.[35,36]

Onset of CNS-IRIS

The majority of patients who develop IRIS do so within the first 3 to 6 months of initiation of HAART,[15] although later cases may develop. During the early weeks of HAART the major immune component that is restored is the memory T cell subset.[31–33] Memory T cells are both phenotypically and functionally distinct from naive T cells. Memory T cells respond to their antigen more readily than naive cells and exhibit effector functions faster than naive cells. Indeed, these characteristics are important for the normal function of immunological memory; however, within the context of immune suppression and restoration, the release of memory cells from immune compartments may be detrimental. Since these cells are more easily stimulated, needing less costimulation and less antigen load,[37] a mild OI may appear as an overwhelming infection to memory cells, triggering a very robust immune response. The correlation between the timing of the onset of IRIS and the release of memory cells needs further study to address the extent that this subset of cells is involved in CNS-IRIS. Later in immune restoration, as naive T cells increase, they may also contribute to the development or continuation of IRIS. In a recent study, patients who developed CNS-IRIS after 6 weeks of HAART initiation had a CD4$^+$ T cell nadir of less than 25 cells/mm^3, indicating that restoration of the CD4$^+$ T cell component is important in the pathobiology of IRIS.[19]

Opportunistic infections and IRIS

The inflammatory response seen during this phase is often directed at OIs present prior to the advent of HAART. These immune responses may represent a normal pathogen-directed immune response that is in excess or may indicate a failure of the immune system to properly regulate the potency of the immune response. There are several OIs, including viral, parasitic, bacterial, and fungal, that are well recognized to contribute to CNS-IRIS development. While many pathogens are recognized to contribute to the development of IRIS, it remains unclear if the disease mechanisms associated with IRIS are the same for each OI or if there are microbial-driven specific immune responses that result it different pathologies for each pathogen.

Viral pathogens associated with CNS-IRIS

JC virus

JC virus is one of the most neurologically devastating of the OIs associated with IRIS, resulting in upwards of 42% mortality.[38] Survivors of PML often demonstrate severe neurological impairment and require long-term care. Of the approximate 5% of HIV+ patients who develop PML,[39] up to an estimated 19% are PML-IRIS patients.[40,41] Most PML-IRIS cases occur within 4 to 8 weeks after HAART initiation but may occur as late as 2 years after HAART is commenced[42–45] (Fig. 3). To date five patients with multiple sclerosis who were treated with natalizumab have developed PML. Four of these patients developed PML-IRIS. Each of these patients had clinical and radiological evidence of IRIS 4 to 8 weeks after natalizumab was removed from circulation by plasmaphoresis (Lynda Cristiano, Biogen Idec, personal communication). Differentiating PML versus PML-IRIS can be easily done via MRI. Typically no contrast enhancement is seen in PML, hence the presence of contrast enhancement suggests an inflammatory response and is indicative of PML-IRIS[42,43,45] (Fig. 4). However, some patients may show clinical deterioration despite the

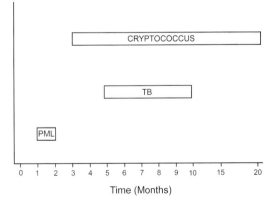

Figure 3. Onset of CNS-IRIS associated with OIs. PML-related CNS-IRIS typically occurs between 1–2 months after the initiation of HAART, although it may also occur much later. Mycobacterial-associated CNS-IRIS most often appears within 5–10 months, whereas cryptococcal-related CNS-IRIS presents between 3–20 months. The difference in timing of the onset of IRIS related to OIs may give insight into the different underlying disease mechanisms.

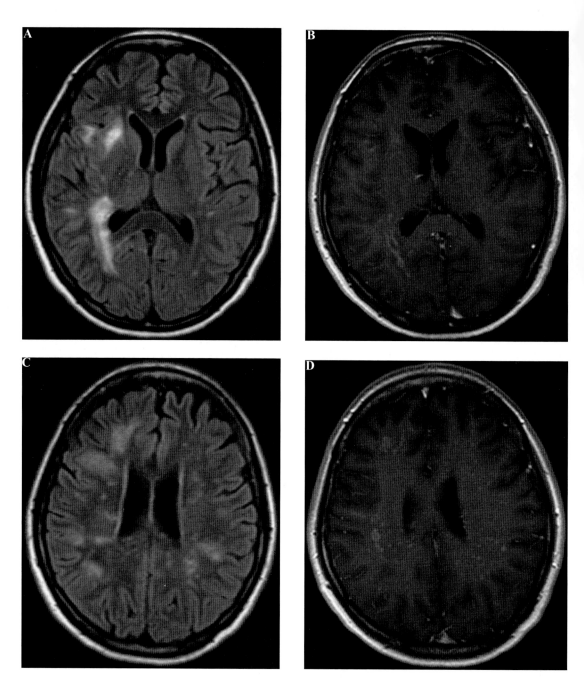

Figure 4. Magnetic resonance imaging features of PML-IRIS. (A) FLAIR image shows multifocal white matter lesions without any mass effect. (B) Corresponding T1 weighted image with gadolinium shows concentric enhancement and other areas of nodular enhancement. (C) FLAIR image from the same patient shows patchy white matter involvement with lesions in the uncinate fibers. (D) Corresponding T1 weighted image with gadolinium shows multiple regions of nodular enhancement.

absence of contrast. While this may be due to progression of the underlying PML, in some it may be due to IRIS, which may not be appreciated on MRI by visual inspection. However a clinical response to steroids confirms the presence of inflammation.[42,43,45,46] Pathology of PML-IRIS revealed macrophages, CD4+ T cells, and CD8+ T cell infiltrates in the perivascular spaces and in some cases parenchymal infiltrates are also present, although CD8+ cells are the predominant cell type.[45,47] A recent retrospective study supported this finding of two forms of PML associated with IRIS, one form that commenced simultaneously with IRIS and one form in which patients known to have PML were started in HAART and then developed IRIS. The disease severity and prognosis of the latter group of patients is worse.[46]

Herpes viruses

Several viruses within the family herpviridae contribute to development of CNS-IRIS. An alpha herpes virus associated with CNS-IRIS is Varicella zoster virus (VZV). VZV is the causative agent of varicella (chicken pox) and zoster (shingles), and once the primary infection has resolved the virus remains in a latent stage within the dorsal root ganglia.[48] VZV is a ubiquitous herpes pathogen seen in approximately 90% of adults above the age of 20 years.[48] This pathogen can be detected in the cerebrospinal fluid (CSF) of patients with both VZV associated encephalitis[49–51] or transverse myelitis,[52] and treatment with intravenous acyclovir improves the clinical condition. VZV can also cause a vasculitis and result in a stroke from a cerebral infarct. In immune-suppressed individuals this may or may not be accompanied with a skin rash, or the history of a skin rash, and the stroke may be separated by several months. If the stroke, however, occurs after initiation of HAART, the possibility that this may be due to a vasculitis resulting from VZV-IRIS needs to be considered.[53]

Cytomegalovirus (CMV) is a betaherpes virus that is the causative agent of CMV retinitis.[54] It is also a fairly common pathogen with seroprevalence rates between 50–80%.[55] Most commonly CMV is associated with CMV-retinitis-IRIS and has only been demonstrated in a few CNS-IRIS cases.[56–59] In these cases ganciclovir was administered successfully and the patients recovered.[56,57,59] CMV can

also cause a radiculitis or ventriculitis in immune-suppressed patients with HIV infection; however, to date IRIS has not been reported with these conditions.

Epstein–Barr virus (EBV) is the causative agent of mononucleosis; however, it may also result in more serious illnesses such as Burkitt's lymphoma, Hodgkin's disease, and neurological complications.[60] There is one reported case of EBV-associated CNS-IRIS in which 6 weeks after HAART initiation the patient presented with vision loss. Imaging demonstrated T2/FLAIR hyperintensities in the optic chiasm, and EBV was detected in the CSF by PCR. This IRIS response resulted in total and permanent vision loss in the patient (Dr. E. Johnson, personal communication).

Herpes simplex viruses (HSV) 1 and 2 are the causative agents of oral and genital lesions respectively, although there is significant cross over among presentation of these viruses.[48] French and colleagues described a case of HSV-associated CNS-IRIS in 2000 in which the encephalitis was resolved with acyclovir therapy although the pathogen was never demonstrated in the CSF.[56]

Herpes viral infections have been much more commonly associated with IRIS when infection occurs outside the CNS. Interestingly, these studies revealed that only 8% of patients that develop herpes-associated IRIS had IL-12β-3′ UT, an anti-inflammatory cytokine polymorphism, whereas 42–54% the non-IRIS or other forms of IRIS carry this polymorphism.[26] Additionally, there appears to be an increased presence of TNFα-308*2 in people who develop herpes-associated IRIS.[26] This suggests that individuals with polymorphisms in the proinflammatory genes may be predisposed to developing IRIS, and potentially CNS-IRIS, although future prospective studies are needed to confirm this.

Other viruses associated with CNS-IRIS

Several other viral pathogens have been associated with CNS-IRIS, including parvovirus,[61] BK virus,[62] and human T lymphotropic virus type-2,[63] although the contributions of these infections appear to be less frequent than the previously described viruses. The descriptions of the pathobiology of these organisms in the role of CNS-IRIS were recently reviewed.[64]

Fungal pathogens associated with CNS-IRIS

Cryptococcus neoformans is a common fungal infection in HIV-infected patients that takes two forms: CNS-associated IRIS, which presents as an aseptic recurrence of meningitis (or rarely as intracranial cryptococcoma), and non-CNS IRIS, which is more common and manifests as lymphadenitis (or rarely as cavitary pneumonia at the site of a cryptococcal nodule or mediastinitis).[14,65–69] This fungal infection remains one of the most important pathogens associated with CNS-IRIS, with an estimated occurrence ranging from 10–30%,[44,70] typically occurring between 3–20 months after the initiation of HAART, although it has been reported as rapidly as 14 days and as long as 2 years after antiretroviral intervention[14] (Fig. 3). Of these cases, upwards of 33–57% result in death.[68,71]

In a patient with cryptococcal meningitis, the presence of acute deterioration characterized by headache, nausea, and vomiting may be mistaken for the development of hydrocephalus. If these symptoms occur soon after starting HAART, the possibility of IRIS should be considered, even in the presence of fever, if there is also sterile inflammation of the CSF, residual cryptococcal antigen, and an absence of viable yeast on culture. Most cases of cryptococcal IRIS are found in patients already diagnosed with cryptococcal infection that are then initiated on HAART after antifungal therapy, but some cases likely represent an emergence of undetectable cryptococcal infection.[18,70] Due to immunosuppression from HIV infection, cellular response in the CSF is not always a reliable indicator; in fact, in one autopsy-proven case, repeated spinal taps failed to show a cellular response. Nonetheless, patients with IRIS-related cryptococcal disease compared to usual HIV-related cryptococcal disease generally had higher opening pressures, white cell counts, and glucose levels.[18,69] In IRIS meningitis, neuroimaging may not be useful either, as pachymeningeal enhancement may occur from the lumbar puncture itself.[72] However, new evidence of meningeal or choroid plexus enhancement or linear perivascular enhancement in the sulci (thought to represent perivascular inflammation) may indicate IRIS meningitis.[73,74]

One important additional risk factor contributing to cryptococcal CNS-IRIS is the initiation of HAART within 1 month of the onset of an antifungal regime.[44] Prospective studies are needed to determine the best course for both antifungal therapies and HAART potentially in conjunction with adjuvant therapies to control inflammation, such as corticosteroids. Patients with cryptococcal meningitis particularly with IRIS are likely to develop a communicating hydrocephalus due to blockage of CSF absorption at the arachnoid villi by cryptococcal antigen and/or the inflammatory cells, which may be a potentially life-threatening complication. Hence CSF pressures need to be monitored in these patients and drained as necessary by repeated lumbar punctures.[75] Understanding the consequences of the timing of these therapies in relation to each other is critical in preventing the onset of CNS-IRIS.

It has been demonstrated that CD4$^+$ T cells activate macrophages to phagocytose *C. neoformans* via INF-γ signaling.[76] The CD4$^+$ T cells also lyse *C. neoformans* using granulysin.[76] This may explain the high occurrence of *Cryptococcus* in individuals who are CD4$^+$ T cells–depleted due to HIV. Therefore, cryptococcal CNS-IRIS may be mediated by CD4$^+$ T cells as opposed to the viral-associated CNS-IRIS, which is dominated by CD8$^+$ T cell infiltration.[45,47]

There has also been a case report of *Candida* meningitis that developed after the onset of HAART. This patient presented with worsening clinical condition despite improvement of laboratory values and undetectable pathogen. Upon histological examination, immune infiltrates, mainly CD8$^+$ T cells, were present, even in regions without *Candida* present, indicating a hyper-responsive immune response.[77]

Bacterial pathogens associated with CNS-IRIS

Mycobacterium infections remain an important complication of HIV infection, and several species of mycobacteria, including *M. tuberculosis*, *M. leprae*, and *M. avium* complex (MAC) contribute to IRIS. Typically most mycobacterial-associated CNS-IRIS cases occur within 5 to 10 months after HAART is commenced,[24,78,79] which is much later than the non-CNS-IRIS-related cases, which occur within 3 months,[80] and present as either simultaneous or delayed CNS-IRIS (Fig. 3). *Mycobacterium tuberculosis* CNS-IRIS presents as tuberculoma or tuberculosis meningitis.[81] Delayed IRIS associated with *M. tuberculosis* occurs in >45% of individuals,[82,83] although estimates for CNS complications are presumed to be much lower. Considering that a third of the world's population has been infected with tuberculosis,[84] CNS-IRIS complications due to mycobacterial species may become more recognizable in regions where tuberculosis and HIV burdens are great. In a recent study that followed a large cohort of tuberculosis/HIV co-infected individuals that were suspected to have IRIS ($n = 80$), none was reported to have CNS-associated complications.[85] Of interest, the authors demonstrated that it was difficult to clinically distinguish tuberculosis-IRIS from drug-resistant tuberculosis infections.[85] This finding is striking in the face of rising drug resistant and multidrug resistant tuberculosis pathogens.

In non-HIV-infected patients, antituberculous therapy has been known to cause clinical deterioration, either in pulmonary or extrapulmonary infection, due to the improved immune function causing pathological inflammation. Paradoxical worsening of *Mycobacterium tuberculosis* disease was described in HIV-infected patients receiving HAART.[86–88] IRIS manifestations included mostly pulmonary symptoms and lymphadenitis, though expansion of intracranial tuberculomas has also been noted.[78] The incidence of IRIS of the CNS in patients with tuberculosis is unclear. In reviews of tuberculosis-associated IRIS, the most common manifestations of IRIS were fever, lymphadenopathy, and worsening respiratory symptoms.[85–88] IRIS occurs in about one third of tuberculosis/HIV co-infected patients who are receiving antituberculous treatment with newly added HAART.[80,82,88,89] The course of tuberculous meningitis in HIV-infected patients is different from HIV-negative patients: cognitive dysfunction is more common, and pathological features demonstrate reduced and atypical inflammatory responses and extensive vasculopathy. Meningeal enhancement is absent or minimal.[90] Hence if the patient develops meningeal signs accompanied by meningeal enhancement on MRI scan and/or a communicating hydrocephalus after the initiation of antitubercular and antiretroviral therapy, the possibility of IRIS should be considered.

Parasitic pathogens associated with CNS-IRIS

The majority of the complications associated with parasitic infections occur in the periphery and do not cause CNS damage; however, there are CNS-associated parasitic infections that can contribute to IRIS. In developed countries parasitic infections contribute only a minor level to CNS-IRIS development; however, these infections represent a significant burden in developing or resource-limited countries. *Toxoplasma gondii*, the causative organism of toxoplasmosis has been reported to cause CNS-IRIS in at least one case report.[91,92] The patient presented with seizure within 1 month of initiating HAART.[92] As the number of HIV-associated parasitic infections treated with HAART rise the complications of parasitic CNS-IRIS may become more prominent and recognizable in areas where these infections are endemic.

Fulminant HIV encephalitis with IRIS

Some patients may develop a severe progressive encephalitis after initiation of HAART therapy resulting in seizures, altered mental status, and eventually coma and death.[16] These patients died at 1–3 months after starting HAART.[16] HIV may be detectable in CSF even when it is undetectable in blood. Alternatively viral load in the CSF is greater that that found in blood. MRI may show diffuse multifocal white matter changes with associated cerebral edema.[51] At autopsy, macrophages and lymphocytes are found diffusely infiltrating the white and gray matter, the leptomeninges, and around blood vessels.[16] Pathological evaluation shows massive infiltration of CD8+ T cells and smaller amounts of CD4+ T cells, macrophages, and B cells. The presence of CD4 cells in the tissue is proportional to the peripheral CD4 cell count.[27,52] Some histopathological studies in HIV encephalitis autopsy and biopsy tissues have demonstrated cytotoxic T cells interacting directly with neurons demonstrating their potential to cause neurotoxicity.[93] Another report of seven patients, five of who had HIV dementia, showed severe neuropathological changes and perivascular inflammatory cells, presumably resulting from immune restoration with HAART.[94] The salient neuropathological changes (myelin loss, lympho-monocytic exudate, axonal injury, and astrocytic gliosis) were considered to be more severe than those observed in the pre-HAART era.[94] These patients may show a dramatic response to treatment with short-term, high-dose intravenous corticosteroids.[51]

Autoimmune diseases of the nervous system as a manifestation of IRIS

Autoimmune responses due to IRIS do occur, although they represent a minor contribution to disease occurrence. While the rates of autoimmune IRIS are low they represent a significant long-term burden, as this type of IRIS may not be resolved by eliminating the offending pathogen driving the immune response. Systemic lupus erythematosus and Guillain–Barre syndrome have been reported in the literature after HAART.[17,95,96] These autoimmune disorders tend to present early after HAART initiation as opposed to Graves' disease which presents much later, as much as 2 years after therapy initiation.[17,97] The difference in timing of the onset of these disorders indicates different underlying immune mechanisms contributing to disease development. This also demonstrates that physicians need to remain vigilant for IRIS complications long-term, although the majority of IRIS cases do occur relatively early in therapy.

Though the burden of autoimmune CNS-IRIS is not clearly understood, there is much interest in the relationship between HIV, IRIS, and multiple sclerosis (MS). Several cases have been reported of HIV patients developing a focal demyelinating leukoencephalopathy comparable with MS.[94,98–100] In one case report a 33-year-old male developed weakness of the right arm and left field visual impairment 2 months after the initiation of HAART. A biopsy was performed, and histology showed demyelination in the absence of JC virus and the presence of perivascular mononuclear infiltrates.[98] Additionally, the cytoplasm of macrophages stained positive for Luxol-fast blue myelin.[98] The patient remains stable 7 years later. It remains unclear if this presentation is truly a relapsing-remitting MS, or resolved PML, although further long-term observations may allow more insight. Similarly, another case report described several patients with severely declining neurological condition associated with demyelination, axonal damage, microgliosis, and astrogliosis, described as more severe than in the pre-HAART era.[94]

Management of CNS-associated IRIS

Optimal management of the various CNS-associated IRIS manifestations remains poorly defined, as there are no randomized treatment trials for these conditions. The heterogeneity of the various IRIS syndromes, lack of standardized definitions for IRIS, and few reported cases make treatment trials challenging.

Differential diagnosis of IRIS

An important step in the management of any IRIS condition is to recognize it as part of the differential diagnosis for patients presenting with a worsening of typical symptoms or new symptoms after HAART initiation. It is imperative to distinguish IRIS from other conditions including drug toxicities, drug interactions, and progression of the underlying disease from resistance, poor adherence, or inadequate drug levels, so that appropriate intervention or treatment can be pursued.[101] Based on a review of the published literature, we provide some guidelines for establishing the diagnosis of CNS-IRIS (Table 1).

Should highly active antiretroviral therapy be discontinued?

HAART and the subsequent boost in the patient's immune system are the proximate causes of IRIS, so stopping HAART may improve the patient's symptoms; however, there is no guarantee that the condition will not recur once HAART is resumed, and stopping therapy also increases the risk both for OIs and for HIV disease progression.[102] Therefore stopping HAART is not recommended, and most conditions will

Table 1. Defining features of CNS-IRIS

1. Worsening of neurological status after initiation of HAART
2. Deterioration of or new neuroradiological findings suggestive of inflammation
3. A decrease in plasma HIV viral load of $\geq 1 \log_{10}$
4. Symptoms not explained by a newly acquired disease or by usual course of previously acquired illness
5. Histopathology demonstrating T cell infiltration

begin to improve after the initial period of deterioration.

When to use corticosteroids?

For the purpose of treatment of CNS-IRIS we have classified CNS-IRIS into three clinical forms.

(a) *Catastrophic CNS-IRIS:* These are patients who have massive inflammation, resulting in impending brain herniation. Despite the absence of any clinical trials, these patients probably need to be treated aggressively with high-dose corticosteroids.[102] The only uncertainty is how long to continue the steroids. Prolonged use of steroids may be favorable for reasons outlined below.

(b) *Symptomatic noncatastrophic CNS-IRIS:* The use of corticosteroids for this group of patients is highly controversial. The management of these patients can only be resolved by a carefully conducted clinical trial. However, in the absence of such information we are faced with the dilemma of making a decision in patients that we currently see. One could make the argument that in the setting of an OI, the inflammation serves the purpose of controlling the infection, hence dampening it would be ill advised. However, several lines of evidence suggest that the inflammatory response often exceeds what is necessary for controlling the infection and results in injury to normal tissue; hence some modulation of these cells may be beneficial. In non-HIV-infected patients such as those with acute bacterial meningitis, tuberculous meningitis, syphilis, and leprosy who develop similar inflammatory syndromes following antimicrobial therapy, clinical trials have shown the efficacy of adjunctive corticosteroid therapy, and the use of steroids in these patients is widely accepted.

In patients with cryptococcal meningitis and IRIS, the inflammatory reaction due to IRIS may lead to raised intracranial pressure due to obstruction of CSF pathways, in which case short-term use of steroids and/or CSF drainage may be necessary.[51]

In patients with HIV dementia/encephalitis and IRIS, the natural course of the illness is death within 1–3 months from the onset of the symptoms of IRIS. In isolated case reports a dra-matic, albeit temporary, improvement in the neurological condition may occur with systemic steroids.[101]

(c) *Asymptomatic IRIS:* These are patients who may show contrast enhancement on MRI, such as patients with PML-IRIS, but these areas of enhancement do not cause any clinical symptoms that can be easily recognized. A wait-and-see approach might be most appropriate here.

How long should corticosteroids be continued?

No consensus exists. While there remains concern that due to the potentially devastating side effects that corticosteroids may have in immunocompromised patients particularly if there is an unrecognized underlying infection, these drugs have been used safely in immune-suppressed patients with HIV infection when used at low dosages for a short duration.[103] In our experience, if steroids are used for only 3–5 days there is often recurrence of symptoms of IRIS upon stopping therapy. This is likely because the OI still persists and when the steroids are removed and the cytotoxic T cells are likely to rebound. The duration of steroid therapy may depend on the types of underlying infection. (1) In the setting of OIs for which effective antimicrobial therapy is available, steroids may be needed for a shorter period until the infection is adequately treated with the antimicrobial. (2) In patients with OI such as PML-IRIS where no specific treatment for the JC virus is present, longer-term treatment may be necessary until the memory T cells recover and a more directed immune response against the JV virus predominates.[46,104] (3) In patients with HIV encephalitis with IRIS, since HIV is resident within the brain and neither HARRT nor the cellular immune responses are able to get rid of the viral reservoir, it is possible that long-term steroids may be necessary. However, that needs to be studied in the context of a clinical trial before any recommendations can be made.

Is there a role for other immunomodulatory drugs?

Pentoxifylline and thalidomide have been successfully used as adjunctive therapy in patients with "leprosy reaction."[105] These drugs attenuate cytokine production from lymphocytes, macrophages, and glial cells. Thalidomide has been successfully used to treat HIV-infected patients with recurrent aphthous ulcers to control the inflammatory reaction.[106] A better understanding of the pathophysiology of IRIS may lead to a more rational approach to treatment. Ideally, the cytotoxic immune responses directed against the infected cells needs to be maintained and those directed against normal tissue need to be muted. Currently available immune modulatory therapies are unable to make that distinction. While recently developed biologic markers are able to distinguish between effector memory T cells and naive T cells, the means by which they cause tissue injury are not understood. Future drug development will require a thorough understanding of these mechanisms.

Chronic inflammation and IRIS

The association between chronic inflammation and disease has been established in such conditions as cancer,[107,108] cardiovascular damage,[109] age-related impairments,[109] and autoimmune disorders.[111] Fulminate CNS-IRIS is readily detectable, albeit not always distinguishable from other conditions; however, there is a distinct possibility that a more moderate, chronic form of IRIS exists. In this case, continuous periods of lower-level inflammation may be preset. High levels of CNS inflammation have been demonstrated, particularly in the hippocampus of patients successfully treated with HAART.[112] Interestingly this inflammation exceeds the level found in the pre-HAART era,[112] and the association between inflammatory markers and HIV cognitive impairment has been revealed.[113,114] It may be revealed that IRIS contributes to higher rates of comorbidities associated with chronic inflammation as HIV has transitioned into a persistent illness.

Conclusion

CNS-IRIS is emerging as a serious complication to HAART. Early recognition of CNS-IRIS is critical in managing the potential neurological complications and ensuing disability. Diagnosis of CNS-IRIS is difficult since the condition has diverse presentations and may be triggered by a wide variety of OIs, HIV, or unknown antigens. As antiretroviral therapy is now becoming available worldwide, incidence of CNS-IRIS may have a major impact on the ability to treat large populations with antiretroviral drugs. Understanding the pathobiology of this syndrome and developing new approaches for diagnosis, prevention, and treatment are critically important in our battle against HIV. Future research into prevention and diagnosis of CNS-IRIS is much needed, as are clinical trials to investigate potential therapeutic regimens.

Acknowledgments

Supported by grants from NINDS, NIH.

Conflicts of interest

The authors declare no conflicts of interest.

References

1. Shelburne, S.A. *et al.* 2002. Immune reconstitution inflammatory syndrome: emergence of a unique syndrome during highly active antiretroviral therapy. *Medicine (Baltimore)* **81:** 213–227.

2. French, M.A., S.A. Mallal & R.L. Dawkins. 1992. Zidovudine-induced restoration of cell-mediated immunity to mycobacteria in immunodeficient HIV-infected patients. *Aids* **6:** 1293–1297.

3. Chan-Tack, K.M. *et al.* 2006. Immune reconstitution inflammatory syndrome presenting as sinusitis with inflammatory pseudotumor in an HIV-infected patient: a case report and review of the literature. *AIDS Patient Care STDS* **20:** 823–828.

4. Corti, M. *et al.* 2007. Soft tissue abscess and lymphadenitis due to Mycobacterium avium complex as an expression of immune reconstitution inflammatory syndrome after a second scheme of highly active antiretroviral therapy. *Rev. Inst. Med. Trop. Sao Paulo* **49:** 267–270.

5. Couppie, P. *et al.* 2006. Increased incidence of genital herpes after HAART initiation: a frequent presentation of immune reconstitution inflammatory syndrome (IRIS) in HIV-infected patients. *AIDS Patient Care STDS* **20:** 143–145.

6. De Lavaissiere, M. *et al.* 2008. Reconstitution inflammatory syndrome related to histoplasmosis, with a hemophagocytic syndrome in HIV infection. *J. Infect.* **58:**(3) 245–247.

7. Domingo, P. *et al.* 2001. Herpes zoster as an immune reconstitution disease after initiation of combination antiretroviral therapy in patients with human immunodeficiency virus type-1 infection. *Am. J. Med.* **110:** 605–609.

8. Feller, L. *et al*. 2008. Human immunodeficiency virus-associated Kaposi sarcoma as an immune reconstitution inflammatory syndrome: a literature review and case report. *J. Periodontol.* **79:** 362–368.

9. Kharkar, V. *et al*. 2007. Type I lepra reaction presenting as immune reconstitution inflammatory syndrome. *Indian J. Dermatol. Venereol. Leprol.* **73:** 253–256.

10. Knysz, B. *et al*. 2006. Graves' disease as an immune reconstitution syndrome in an HIV-1-positive patient commencing effective antiretroviral therapy: case report and literature review. *Viral Immunol.* **19:** 102–107.

11. Leidner, R.S. & D.M. Aboulafia. 2005. Recrudescent Kaposi's sarcoma after initiation of HAART: a manifestation of immune reconstitution syndrome. *AIDS Patient Care STDS* **19:** 635–644.

12. Olalla, J. *et al*. 2002. Paradoxical responses in a cohort of HIV-1-infected patients with mycobacterial disease. *Int. J. Tuberc. Lung Dis.* **6:** 71–75.

13. Skiest, D.J., L.J. Hester & R.D. Hardy. 2005. Cryptococcal immune reconstitution inflammatory syndrome: report of four cases in three patients and review of the literature. *J. Infect.* **51:** e289–e297.

14. French, M.A. 2009. HIV/AIDS: immune reconstitution inflammatory syndrome: a reappraisal. *Clin. Infect. Dis.* **48:** 101–107.

15. Miller, R.F. *et al*. 2004. Cerebral CD8$^+$ lymphocytosis in HIV-1 infected patients with immune restoration induced by HAART. *Acta Neuropathol. (Berl.)* **108:** 17–23.

16. Puthanakit, T. *et al*. 2007. Hospitalization and mortality among HIV-infected children after receiving highly active antiretroviral therapy. *Clin. Infect. Dis.* **44:** 599–604.

17. French, M.A. 2007. Disorders of immune reconstitution in patients with HIV infection responding to antiretroviral therapy. *Curr. HIV/AIDS Rep.* **4:** 16–21.

18. Shelburne, S.A. *et al*. 2005. Incidence and risk factors for immune reconstitution inflammatory syndrome during highly active antiretroviral therapy. *Aids* **19:** 399–406.

19. McCombe, J.A. *et al*. 2009. Neurologic immune reconstitution inflammatory syndrome in HIV/AIDS: outcome and epidemiology. *Neurology* **72:** 835–841.

20. Klotz, S.A. *et al*. 2009. The immune reconstitution inflammatory syndrome in a resource-poor setting. *J. Int. Assoc. Physicians AIDS Care (Chic Ill).* **8:** 122–127.

21. Meintjes, G. *et al*. 2008. Tuberculosis-associated immune reconstitution inflammatory syndrome: case definitions for use in resource-limited settings. *Lancet Infect. Dis.* **8:** 516–523.

22. Services, D.o.H.a.H. Panel on Antiretroviral Guidelines for Adults and Adolescents. Guidelines for the use of antiretroviral agents in HIV-1-infected adults and adolescents. November 3, 2008 [cited January 5, 2009]; 1–139]. Retrieved from http://www.aidsinfo.gov/ContentFiles/AdultandAdolescentGL.pdf

23. Manabe, Y.C. *et al*. 2007. Immune reconstitution inflammatory syndrome: risk factors and treatment implications. *J. Acquir. Immune Defic. Syndr.* **46:** 456–462.

24. Murdoch, D.M. *et al*. 2008. Incidence and risk factors for the immune reconstitution inflammatory syndrome in HIV patients in South Africa: a prospective study. *Aids* **22:** 601–610.

25. Mankowski, J.L. *et al*. 2008. Natural host genetic resistance to lentiviral CNS disease: a neuroprotective MHC class I allele in SIV-infected macaques. *PLoS ONE* **3:** e3603.

26. Price, P. *et al*. 2002. Polymorphisms in cytokine genes define subpopulations of HIV-1 patients who experienced immune restoration diseases. *Aids* **16:** 2043–2047.

27. Riedel, D.J. *et al*. 2006. Therapy Insight: CNS manifestations of HIV-associated immune reconstitution inflammatory syndrome. *Nat. Clin. Pract. Neurol.* **2:** 557–565.

28. Stone, S.F. *et al*. 2002. Levels of IL-6 and soluble IL-6 receptor are increased in HIV patients with a history of immune restoration disease after HAART. *HIV Med.* **3:** 21–27.

29. Kestens, L., N. Seddiki & P.R. Bohjanen. 2008. Immunopathogenesis of the immune reconstitution disease in HIV patients responding to antiretroviral therapy. *Curr. Opin. HIV AIDS* **3:** 419–424.

30. Bonham, S. *et al*. 2008. Biomarkers of HIV immune reconstitution inflammatory syndrome. *Biomark Med.* **2:** 349–361.

31. Bucy, R.P. *et al*. 1999. Initial increase in blood CD4$^{(+)}$ lymphocytes after HIV antiretroviral therapy reflects redistribution from lymphoid tissues. *J. Clin. Invest.* **103:** 1391–1398.

32. Ledergerber, B. *et al*. 2004. Predictors of trend in CD4-positive T-cell count and mortality among HIV-1-infected individuals with virological failure to all three antiretroviral-drug classes. *Lancet* **364:** 51–62.

33. Pakker, N.G. *et al*. 1998. Biphasic kinetics of peripheral blood T cells after triple combination therapy in HIV-1 infection: a composite of redistribution and proliferation. *Nat. Med.* **4:** 208–214.

34. Guadalupe, M. *et al.* 2003. Severe CD4$^+$ T-cell depletion in gut lymphoid tissue during primary human immunodeficiency virus type 1 infection and substantial delay in restoration following highly active antiretroviral therapy. *J. Virol.* **77:** 11708–11717.

35. Kaufmann, G.R. *et al.* 2003. CD4 T-lymphocyte recovery in individuals with advanced HIV-1 infection receiving potent antiretroviral therapy for 4 years: the Swiss HIV Cohort Study. *Arch. Intern. Med.* **163:** 2187–2195.

36. Battegay, M. *et al.* 2006. Immunological recovery and antiretroviral therapy in HIV-1 infection. *Lancet Infect. Dis.* **6:** 280–287.

37. Berard, M. & D.F. Tough. 2002. Qualitative differences between naive and memory T cells. *Immunology* **106:** 127–138.

38. Wyen, C. *et al.* 2004. Progressive multifocal leukencephalopathy in patients on highly active antiretroviral therapy: survival and risk factors of death. *J. Acquir. Immune. Defic. Syndr.* **37:** 1263–1268.

39. Ledergerber, B. *et al.* 1999. AIDS-related opportunistic illnesses occurring after initiation of potent antiretroviral therapy: the Swiss HIV Cohort Study. *JAMA* **282:** 2220–2226.

40. Cinque, P. *et al.* 2003. The effect of highly active antiretroviral therapy-induced immune reconstitution on development and outcome of progressive multifocal leukoencephalopathy: study of 43 cases with review of the literature. *J. Neurovirol.* **9**(Suppl 1): 73–80.

41. Berenguer, J. *et al.* 2003. Clinical course and prognostic factors of progressive multifocal leukoencephalopathy in patients treated with highly active antiretroviral therapy. *Clin. Infect. Dis.* **36:** 1047–1052.

42. Collazos, J. *et al.* 1999. Contrast-enhancing progressive multifocal leukoencephalopathy as an immune reconstitution event in AIDS patients. *Aids* **13:** 1426–1428.

43. Martinez, J.V. *et al.* 2006. Immune reconstitution inflammatory syndrome associated with PML in AIDS: a treatable disorder. *Neurology* **67:** 1692–1694.

44. Torok, M.E., A. Kambugu & E. Wright. 2008. Immune reconstitution disease of the central nervous system. *Curr. Opin. HIV AIDS:* 438–445. Pubmed id: 19373003.

45. Vendrely, A. *et al.* 2005. Fulminant inflammatory leukoencephalopathy associated with HAART-induced immune restoration in AIDS-related progressive multifocal leukoencephalopathy. *Acta Neuropathol.* **109:** 449–455.

46. Tan, K. *et al.* 2009. PML-IRIS in patients with HIV infection. Clinical manifestations and treatment with steroids. *Neurology.* **72:** 1458–1464.

47. Gray, F. *et al.* 2005. Central nervous system immune reconstitution disease in acquired immunodeficiency syndrome patients receiving highly active antiretroviral treatment. *J. Neurovirol.* **11**(Suppl 3): 16–22.

48. Whitley, R.J. 2001. Herpes simplex virus. In *Fields Virology*. Knipe, D.M. & P.M. Howley, Eds.: 2461–2511. Lippincott, Williams, and Wilkins. Philadelphia, PA.

49. Corral, I. *et al.* 2003. Neurological complications of varicella-zoster virus in human immunodeficiency virus-infected patients: changes in prevalence and diagnostic utility of polymerase chain reaction in cerebrospinal fluid. *J. Neurovirol.* **9:** 129–135.

50. De La Blanchardiere, A. *et al.* 2000. Neurological complications of varicella-zoster virus infection in adults with human immunodeficiency virus infection. *Scand J. Infect. Dis.* **32:** 263–269.

51. Venkataramana, A. *et al.* 2006. Immune reconstitution inflammatory syndrome in the CNS of HIV-infected patients. *Neurology* **67:** 383–388.

52. Clark, B.M. *et al.* 2004. Compartmentalization of the immune response in varicella zoster virus immune restoration disease causing transverse myelitis. *Aids* **18:** 1218–1221.

53. Newsome, S.D. & A. Nath. 2009. Varicella-zoster virus vasculopathy and central nervous system immune reconstitution inflammatory syndrome with human immunodeficiency virus infection treated with steroids. *J. Neurovirol.* **15:** 288–291.

54. Zhang, L. *et al.* 1999. Measuring recent thymic emigrants in blood of normal and HIV-1-infected individuals before and after effective therapy. *J. Exp. Med.* **190:** 725–732.

55. Pass, R. 2001. Cytomegalovirus. In *Fields Virology*, Fields, B.N., D.M. Knipe, P.M. Howley, et al., Eds.: 2675–2705. Lippincott-Raven. Philadelphia, PA.

56. French, M.A. *et al.* 2000. Immune restoration disease after the treatment of immunodeficient HIV-infected patients with highly active antiretroviral therapy. *HIV Med.* **1:** 107–115.

57. Janowicz, D.M., R.M. Johnson & S.K. Gupta. 2005. Successful treatment of CMV ventriculitis immune reconstitution syndrome. *J. Neurol. Neurosurg. Psychiatry* **76:** 891–892.

58. Jevtovic, D.J. *et al.* 2005. The prevalence and risk of immune restoration disease in HIV-infected patients treated with highly active antiretroviral therapy. *HIV Med.* **6:** 140–143.

59. Majumder, S. *et al.* 2007. Multiorgan involvement due to cytomegalovirus infection in AIDS. *Braz. J. Infect. Dis.* **11:** 176–178.

60. Robbins, S.L., V. Kumar & R.S. Cotran. 2003. *Robbins Basic Pathology*, 7th edn. Philadelphia: Saunders.

61. Nolan, R.C., G. Chidlow & M.A. French. 2003. Parvovirus B19 encephalitis presenting as immune restoration disease after highly active antiretroviral therapy for human immunodeficiency virus infection. *Clin. Infect. Dis.* **36:** 1191–1194.

62. Vidal, J.E. *et al.* 2007. BK virus associated meningoencephalitis in an AIDS patient treated with HAART. *AIDS Res. Ther.* **4:** 13.

63. Toro, C. *et al.* 2007. Human T lymphotropic virus type 1-associated myelopathy/tropical spastic paraparesis in an HIV-positive patient coinfected with human T lymphotropic virus type 2 following initiation of antiretroviral therapy. *Clin. Infect. Dis.* **45:** e118–e120.

64. Torok, M.E., A. Kambugu & E. Wright. 2008. Immune reconstitution disease of the central nervous system. *Curr. Opin. HIV AIDS* **3:** 438–445.

65. Blanche, P. *et al.* 1998. HIV combination therapy: immune restitution causing cryptococcal lymphadenitis dramatically improved by anti-inflammatory therapy. *Scand. J. Infect. Dis.* **30:** 615–616.

66. Jarvis, J.N. & T.S. Harrison. 2007. HIV-associated cryptococcal meningitis. *Aids* **21:** 2119–2129.

67. Jenny-Avital, E.R. & M. Abadi. 2002. Immune reconstitution cryptococcosis after initiation of successful highly active antiretroviral therapy. *Clin. Infect. Dis.* **35:** e128–e133.

68. Lawn, S.D. *et al.* 2005. Cryptococcal immune reconstitution disease: a major cause of early mortality in a South African antiretroviral programme. *Aids* **19:** 2050–2052.

69. Lortholary, O. *et al.* 2005. Incidence and risk factors of immune reconstitution inflammatory syndrome complicating HIV-associated cryptococcosis in France. *Aids* **19:** 1043–1049.

70. Woods, M.L. *et al.* 1998. HIV combination therapy: partial immune restitution unmasking latent cryptococcal infection. *Aids* **12:** 1491–1494.

71. Kambugu, A. *et al.* 2008. Outcomes of cryptococcal meningitis in Uganda before and after the availability of highly active antiretroviral therapy. *Clin. Infect. Dis.* **46:** 1694–1701.

72. York, J. *et al.* 2005. Raised intracranial pressure complicating cryptococcal meningitis: immune reconstitution inflammatory syndrome or recurrent cryptococcal disease? *J. Infect.* **51:** 165–171.

73. Boelaert, J.R. *et al.* 2004. Relapsing meningitis caused by persistent cryptococcal antigens and immune reconstitution after the initiation of highly active antiretroviral therapy. *Aids* **18:** 1223–1224.

74. King, M.D. *et al.* 2002. Paradoxical recurrent meningitis following therapy of cryptococcal meningitis: an immune reconstitution syndrome after initiation of highly active antiretroviral therapy. *Int. J. STD AIDS* **13:** 724–726.

75. Venkataramana, A. *et al.* 2006. Immune Reconstitution Inflammatory Syndrome in the CNS of HIV infected patients. *Neurology* **67:** 383–388.

76. Zheng, C.F. *et al.* 2007. Cytotoxic CD4$^+$ T cells use granulysin to kill Cryptococcus neoformans, and activation of this pathway is defective in HIV patients. *Blood* **109:** 2049–2057.

77. Berkeley, J.L., A. Nath & C.A. Pardo. 2008. Fatal immune reconstitution inflammatory syndrome with human immunodeficiency virus infection and Candida meningitis: case report and review of the literature. *J. Neurovirol.* **14:** 267–276.

78. Crump, J.A. *et al.* 1998. Miliary tuberculosis with paradoxical expansion of intracranial tuberculomas complicating human immunodeficiency virus infection in a patient receiving highly active antiretroviral therapy. *Clin. Infect. Dis.* **26:** 1008–1009.

79. Ramdas, K. & G.Y. Minamoto. 1994. Paradoxical presentation of intracranial tuberculomas after chemotherapy in a patient with AIDS. *Clin. Infect. Dis.* **19:** 793–794.

80. Lawn, S.D., L.G. Bekker & R.F. Miller. 2005. Immune reconstitution disease associated with mycobacterial infections in HIV-infected individuals receiving antiretrovirals. *Lancet Infect. Dis.* **5:** 361–373.

81. Dhasmana, D.J. *et al.* 2008. Immune reconstitution inflammatory syndrome in HIV-infected patients receiving antiretroviral therapy : pathogenesis, clinical manifestations and management. *Drugs* **68:** 191–208.

82. Breen, R.A. *et al.* 2004. Paradoxical reactions during tuberculosis treatment in patients with and without HIV co-infection. *Thorax* **59:** 704–707.

83. Murdoch, D.M. *et al.* 2007. Immune reconstitution inflammatory syndrome (IRIS): review of common infectious manifestations and treatment options. *AIDS Res. Ther.* **4:** 9.

84. Organization, W.H. 2006. Fact Sheet #104. Global tuberculosis control surveillance, planning, financing. [Cited March 16, 2009]. Available from: http://www.who.int/mediacentre/factsheets/fs104/en/index.html.

85. Meintjes, G. *et al.* 2009. Novel relationship between tuberculosis immune reconstitution inflammatory syndrome and antitubercular drug resistance. *Clin. Infect. Dis.* **48:** 667–676.

86. Kumarasamy, N. *et al.* 2004. Incidence of immune reconstitution syndrome in HIV/tuberculosis-coinfected

patients after initiation of generic antiretroviral therapy in India. *J. Acquir. Immune. Defic. Syndr.* **37:** 1574–1576.

87. Lawn, S.D. 2005. Acute respiratory failure due to Mycobacterium kansasii infection: immune reconstitution disease in a patient with AIDS. *J. Infect.* **51:** 339–340.

88. Narita, M. *et al.* 2002. Short-course rifamycin and pyrazinamide treatment for latent tuberculosis infection in patients with HIV infection: the 2-year experience of a comprehensive community-based program in Broward County, Florida. *Chest* **122:** 1292–1298.

89. Navas, E. *et al.* 2002. Paradoxical reactions of tuberculosis in patients with the acquired immunodeficiency syndrome who are treated with highly active antiretroviral therapy. *Arch. Intern. Med.* **162:** 97–99.

90. Katrak, S.M. *et al.* 2000. The clinical, radiological and pathological profile of tuberculous meningitis in patients with and without human immunodeficiency virus infection. *J. Neurol. Sci.* **181:** 118–126.

91. Lawn, S.D. 2007. Immune reconstitution disease associated with parasitic infections following initiation of antiretroviral therapy. *Curr. Opin. Infect. Dis.* **20:** 482–488.

92. Tsambiras, P.E., J.A. Larkin & S.H. Houston. 2001. Case report. Toxoplasma encephalitis after initiation of HAART. *AIDS Read.* **11:** 608–610, 615–616.

93. Petito, C.K. *et al.* 2006. Brain CD8$^+$ and cytotoxic T lymphocytes are associated with, and may be specific for, human immunodeficiency virus type 1 encephalitis in patients with acquired immunodeficiency syndrome. *J. Neurovirol.* **12:** 272–283.

94. Langford, T.D. *et al.* 2002. Severe, demyelinating leukoencephalopathy in AIDS patients on antiretroviral therapy. *Aids* **16:** 1019–1029.

95. Calza, L. *et al.* 2003. Systemic and discoid lupus erythematosus in HIV-infected patients treated with highly active antiretroviral therapy. *Int. J. STD AIDS* **14:** 356–359.

96. Piliero, P.J. *et al.* 2003. Guillain-Barré syndrome associated with immune reconstitution. *Clin. Infect. Dis.* **36**(Suppl): e111–e114.

97. Crum, N.F. *et al.* 2006. Graves disease: an increasingly recognized immune reconstitution syndrome. *Aids* **20:** 466–469.

98. Corral, I. *et al.* 2004. Focal monophasic demyelinating leukoencephalopathy in advanced HIV infection. *Eur. Neurol.* **52:** 36–41.

99. Berger, J.R. *et al.* 1989. Multiple sclerosis-like illness occurring with human immunodeficiency virus infection. *Neurology* **39:** 324–329.

100. Berger, J.R. *et al.* 1992. Relapsing and remitting human immunodeficiency virus-associated leukoencephalomyelopathy. *Ann. Neurol.* **31:** 34–38.

101. Riedel, D. *et al.* 2006. Screening for human immunodeficiency virus (HIV) dementia in an HIV clade C-infected population in India. *J. Neurovirol.* **12:** 34–38.

102. Lipman, M. & R. Breen. 2006. Immune reconstitution inflammatory syndrome in HIV. *Curr. Opin. Infect. Dis.* **19:** 20–25.

103. McComsey, G.A. *et al.* 2001. Placebo-controlled trial of prednisone in advanced HIV-1 infection. *Aids* **15:** 321–327.

104. Du Pasquier, R.A. & I.J. Koralnik. 2003. Inflammatory reaction in progressive multifocal leukoencephalopathy: harmful or beneficial? *J. Neurovirol.* **9**(Suppl 1): 25–31.

105. Welsh, O. *et al.* 1999. A new therapeutic approach to type II leprosy reaction. *Int. J. Dermatol.* **38:** 931–933.

106. Shetty, K. 2007. Current role of thalidomide in HIV-positive patients with recurrent aphthous ulcerations. *Gen. Dent.* **55:** 537–542.

107. Balkwill, F., K.A. Charles & A. Mantovani. 2005. Smoldering and polarized inflammation in the initiation and promotion of malignant disease. *Cancer Cell* **7:** 211–217.

108. de Visser, K.E. & A. Eichten. 2006. Paradoxical roles of the immune system during cancer development. *Nat. Rev. Cancer* **6:** 24–37.

109. Koh, K.K., P.C. Oh & M.J. Quon. 2009. Does reversal of oxidative stress and inflammation provide vascular protection? *Cardiovasc. Res.* **81:** 649–659.

110. Brinkley, T.E. *et al.* 2009. Chronic inflammation is associated with low physical function in older adults across multiple comorbidities. *J. Gerontol. A Biol. Sci. Med. Sci.* **64:** 455–461.

111. Brown, K.D., E. Claudio & U. Siebenlist 2008. The roles of the classical and alternative nuclear factor-kappaB pathways: potential implications for autoimmunity and rheumatoid arthritis. *Arthritis Res. Ther.* **10:** 212.

112. Anthony, I.C. *et al.* 2005. Influence of HAART on HIV-related CNS disease and neuroinflammation. *J. Neuropathol. Exp. Neurol.* **64:** 529–536.

113. Avison, M.J. *et al.* 2004. Inflammatory changes and breakdown of microvascular integrity in early human immunodeficiency virus dementia. *J. Neurovirol.* **10:** 223–232.

114. Kelder, W. *et al.* 1998. Beta-chemokines MCP-1 and RANTES are selectively increased in cerebrospinal fluid of patients with human immunodeficiency virus-associated dementia. *Ann Neurol.* **44:** 831–835.

Ann. N.Y. Acad. Sci. ISSN 0077-8923

ANNALS OF THE NEW YORK ACADEMY OF SCIENCES

Vertebrobasilar dilatative arteriopathy (dolichoectasia)

Min Lou[1] and Louis R. Caplan[2]

[1]Department of Neurology, the Second Affiliated Hospital of Zhejiang University, School of Medicine, Hangzhou, China.
[2]Department of Neurology, Beth Israel Deaconess Medical Center and Harvard Medical School, Boston, Massachusetts, USA

Address for correspondence: Louis R. Caplan, MD, Harvard Medical School – Department of Neurology, Beth Israel Deaconess Medical Center, 330 Brookline Avenue, Boston, MA 02215, USA. lcaplan@caregroup.harvard.edu

Dolichoectasia (dilatative arteriopathy) describes marked elongation, widening, and tortuosity of arteries. The intracranial vertebral and basilar arteries are preferentially involved. Dolichoectatic arteries usually have an abnormally large external diameter and a thin arterial wall, with degeneration of the internal elastic lamina, multiple gaps in the internal elastica, thinning of the media secondary to reticular fiber deficiency, and smooth muscle atrophy. The most important clinical presentations of dilatative arteriopathy include acute brain ischemia; a progressive course related to compression of cranial nerves, the brain stem, or the third ventricle; and catastrophic outcome caused by vascular rupture. Flow in dilated arteries can become bidirectional, resulting in reduced antegrade flow and thrombus formation. Elongation and angulation of arteries can stretch and distort the orifices of arterial branches, leading to decreased blood flow, especially in penetrating branches.

Keywords: dolichoectasia; intraluminal thrombi; intracranial arteries; brain ischemia

Introduction

Dolichoectasia is a term used to describe marked elongation, widening, and tortuosity of an artery. Because dilatation is the most important feature, the condition is now often referred to as dilatative arteriopathy.[1] Approximately one patient in eight who has intracranial vascular imaging has some increase in the length and diameter of intracranial arteries.[2,3] The prevalence of intracranial dolichoectasia is approximately 0.06–5.8% in the general population.[4,5]

Dilatative arteriopathy is explained by abnormal connective tissue composition and function in large arteries. The intracranial vertebral arteries (VA) and basilar artery (BA) are preferentially involved.[6] Carotid and middle cerebral artery ectasia also occurs, but less often. The clinical findings are quite variable. Many patients have no symptoms and signs. Others have brainstem infarcts and catastrophic subarachnoid hemorrhages. Herein we discuss the present concepts, pathology, pathophysiology, and clinical findings in patients with vertebrobasilar dolichoectasia (VBD).

Vascular imaging diagnosis and criteria

Dolichoectasia is defined as an increased length and diameter of arteries. VBD may not be readily recognized by neurologists or radiologists due to "normal" variations in the course and tortuosity of the vertebral and basilar arteries in healthy individuals. There are no generally accepted quantitative criteria for the diagnosis of VBD. In most reports, the diagnosis was made by consensus of trained neurologists or neuroradiologists who reviewed brain and vascular imaging and had visual impressions that the intracranial arteries were longer and wider than normal.

Recognition of VBD was first based on catheter angiography findings (Fig. 1). With the advent of computed tomography (CT) and magnetic resonance (MRI) brain and vascular imaging, dolichoectasia can be diagnosed noninvasively. Objective criteria for basilar dolichoectasia on CT scans have been proposed that depend on measurements of the diameter of the BA using a graduated 20-diopter lens and analysis of the height of the basilar bifurcation and lateral displacement of the artery.[7] The basilar artery was considered elongated ("dolicho") if at

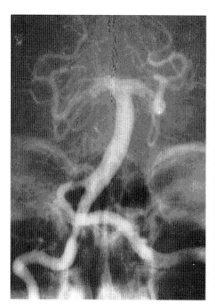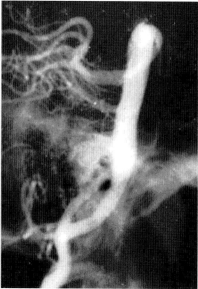

Figure 1. Anteroposterior (*left*) and lateral (*right*) views of the vertebral angiogram showing ectatic (diameter 9.0 mm) and elongated basilar artery. From Ref. 38.

any point throughout its course the artery lay lateral to the margin of the clivus or dorsum sellae, or if its bifurcation was above the plane of the suprasellar cistern. Ectasia was diagnosed if the minimum diameter of the BA was greater than 4.5 mm.

In the "profil GENétique de l'Infarctus Cérébral" (GENIC) case-control study designed to investigate genetic susceptibility for brain infarction, the investigators used diagnostic criteria derived directly from analysis of brain MRI scans.[6] They used a 16-diopter achromatic handheld graduated lens to measure BA diameters at midpons and the two VAs at the V4 segment on T2-weighted axial slices. A vertebral artery diameter >4 mm indicated ectasia. The height of the bifurcation and the transverse position of the BA were also assessed with a semiquantitative 4-point scale for each. The scale for assignment of the height of the BA bifurcation was as follows: 0, at or below the dorsum sella; 1, within the suprasellar cistern; 2, at the level of the third ventricle floor; 3, indenting and elevating the floor of the third ventricle. The rating of BA positioning was based on the most lateral position of the artery throughout its course (0, midline; 1, medial to lateral margin of clivus or dorsum sella; 2, lateral to lateral margin of clivus or dorsum sella; 3, in cerebellopontine angle cistern) (Fig. 2). Patients with segmental,

spindle shaped enlargements of the BA or fusiform enlargement superimposed on dolichoectasia, were not included.

Measurements on magnetic resonance angiography (MRA) source images were used for diagnosis of VBD, prior to three-dimensional time of flight (TOF) arterial reconstruction and direct MRA measurements, which routinely eliminate the neuroanatomical landmarks used in the above CT/MRI criteria[8] (Fig. 3). Volumetric analysis of BA using quantitative MRA was also recommended for accurate vascular measurements because it was considered more sensitive to subtle vasculopathic changes that were missed by qualitative analysis. Some authors utilized multislice CT angiography to derive accurate measurements of vessel length and diameter at multiple points.[9] Although new imaging techniques were developed for the diagnosis of VBD, there are no verified and uniformly accepted angiographic criteria. No study has yet compared the utility of MR angiography plus brain MRI and CT scans and multislice CT angiography (CTA) for the diagnosis of VBD. Strict diagnostic criteria for identifying VBD based on noninvasive neuroimaging studies such as axial slices from brain MRI, MRA, CT, and CTA are needed for future studies.

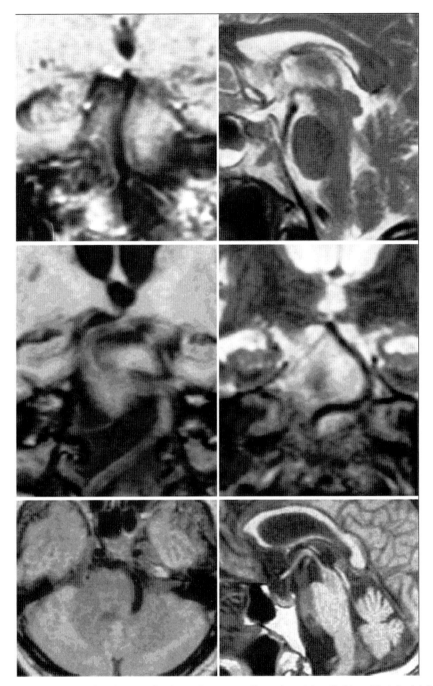

Figure 2. Magnetic resonance (MR) examples for assignment of lateral position (*left*) and height (*right*) of basilar artery: (A) Medial to the lateral margin of clivus or dorsum sellae; (B) lateral to the lateral margin of clivus or dorsum sellae; (C) in the cerebellopontine angle cistern; (D) bifurcation in the suprasellar cistern; (E) bifurcation at the level of the floor of third ventricle; (F) elevating the floor of third ventricle. From Ref. 28.

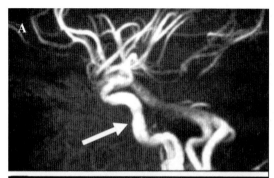

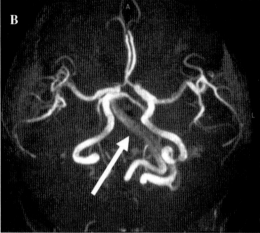

Figure 3. Magnetic resonance angiography showing basilar artery dolichoectasia with enlargement of basilar artery diameter (*arrow*). The ectatic basilar artery measures 7 mm in diameter. From Ref. 57.

Pathology and associations

Unlike atherosclerosis, which primarily involves the intima and endothelia of large- and medium-size arteries, dilatative arteriopathy involves mainly the media of intracranial arteries. Dolichoectatic arteries usually have an abnormally large external diameter with a thin arterial wall; intraluminal thrombi may also be present.[10,11] Histological studies show degeneration of the internal elastic lamina, multiple gaps in the internal elastica, thinning of the media secondary to reticular fiber deficiency, and smooth muscle atrophy[11,12] (Fig. 4). At times, the intima is thickened, and there is severe elastic tissue degeneration and an increase in the vasa vasorum.[13] Although atherosclerosis can be superimposed upon the arterial wall of ectatic basilar arteries, neuropathologic studies show no association between dolichoectasia and large-artery atherosclerosis of brain arteries, except for these basilar artery plaques.[14,15]

The GENIC investigators showed that stroke patients with dolichoectasia also had significantly larger diameters of their thoracic aortas than patients without dolichoectasia.[3] A subsequent report described four patients with concurrent dolichoectasia of basilar and coronary arteries[16] (Fig. 5). These findings suggest that dilatative intracranial arteriopathy is part of a systemic vascular ectatic disease and is not limited to brain-supplying arteries.

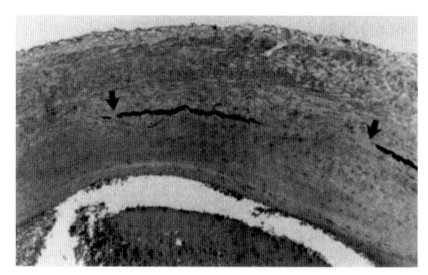

Figure 4. Intraluminal thrombosis and fragmentation of the internal elastic lamina are noted (*arrows*). From Ref. 36.

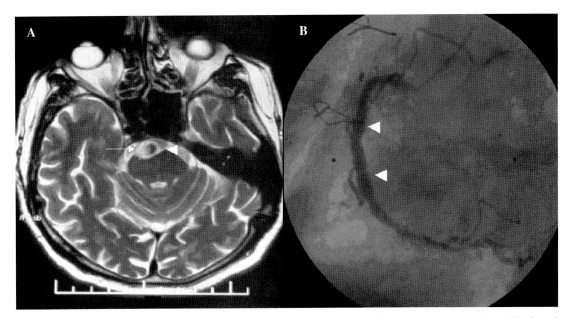

Figure 5. (A) Brain axial T2-weighted MR image: enlarged basilar artery with pons compression (*arrowhead*) and intraluminal thrombus (*arrow*). (B) Coronary angiography: right native coronary arteries with diffuse coronary artery ectasia (arrowhead). From Ref. 16.

Clinical and experimental findings show that biochemical factors such as an imbalance between protease and antiprotease activities in the extracellular matrix lead to loss of elastic fibers, a mechanism that may be important in the formation of abdominal aortic aneurysm and coronary artery ectasia.[17] Recent neuropathologic analysis showed that cerebral small-vessel abnormalities (sclerosis and hyalinosis) were more likely to occur in the small arteries of patients with intracranial dolichoectasia. Both dolichoectasia and small-vessel arteriopathy affect the media of arteries. Abnormal connective tissue within the arterial wall affects biochemical constituents such as matrix metalloproteinases. Dolichoectasia may be a systemic condition that involves the extracellular matrix.

Although VBD is most often recognized in adults, dilatative arteriopathy does occur in children and adolescents. Hereditary factors probably play an important role, especially in the young. Dilative arteriopathy has been found in children and young adults with AIDS, Marfan syndrome, Ehlers-Danlos syndrome, sickle cell disease, and Fabry disease.[18–21] In Fabry disease, VBD and small-artery disease are important causes of stroke.[22] A megadolichobasilar anomaly complicated by thrombosis has recently

been reported in several members of a large family.[23] A recent study reported a prevalence of 2.3% in autosomal dominant polycystic kidney disease (ADPKD) compared with 0% in patients without ADPKD.[24,25] Genetic, infectious, inflammatory, immunological, and degenerative factors are all posited to cause or contribute to the formation and progression of dolichoectasia.

Clinical findings

The most important presentations of dilatative posterior circulation arteriopathy are (1) asymptomatic; (2) acute vertebrobasilar arterial territory ischemia; (3) chronic progressive course related to compression of cranial nerves, the brain stem, or the third ventricle; and (4) catastrophic outcome caused by vascular rupture.

The clinical findings in patients with VBD have been investigated in a number of small series. Among 39 VBD patients over a 6-year period, 22 had brain-stem ischemia. Six patients had symptoms caused by compression of cranial nerves and one had hydrocephalus.[26] In a literature review, among 128 reported VBD patients, Levine and colleagues noted that 58% had cranial nerve compression, in particular, facial spasm (39%) and trigeminal neuralgia (27%), 48% had vertebrobasilar insufficiency or stroke or both, 31% had hydrocephalus, and 24% had symptoms and signs of brain-stem compression.[27] In a prospective study that followed 156 patients with VBD for an average of 11.7 years, 48% patients had stroke (59 ischemic and 21 hemorrhagic), 20% developed new compressive symptoms, and 1% had hydrocephalus.[28]

Posterior circulation ischemia and infarction

Intracranial arterial dolichoectasia is observed in 10% of patients with a first brain infarction.[29] Stroke and transient ischemic attacks (TIA) were the most frequent events in patients with VBD. The relationship between cerebrovascular events and VBD was analyzed in a few reports. The most frequently described ischemic lesion is brain-stem infarction most often located in the pons.[14] Stroke patients with intracranial arterial dolichoectasia often had lacunar brain infarcts on brain imaging.[6,15,29]

In the past, VBD was often posited to be a complication of atherosclerosis. The rationale was the presence of atherosclerotic lesions in some ectatic vessels and that risk factors such as older age, male gender, and arterial hypertension were common to both atherosclerosis and VBD. It is now well accepted that VBD causes posterior circulation infarction independent of atherosclerotic disease; atherosclerotic lesions observed in ectatic arteries are likely the consequence of morphologic and rheologic alterations in these arteries. There are various mechanisms by which VBD provokes transient or persistent vertebrobasilar system ischemia.

Reduced antegrade flow

In patients with VBD, blood flow is often bidirectional antegrade and retrograde within dilated arteries, causing reduced antegrade flow in the vertebrobasilar system.[30,31] Transcranial Doppler studies of dolichoectatic arteries show reduced mean blood flow velocities, with relatively preserved peak flow velocities.[26] The reduced antegrade flow may lead to poor opacification on MRA, even falsely suggesting occlusion of the dolichoectatic artery. Reduced blood flow velocity in the BA correlates with distal lesions involving the thalamus, midbrain, and PCA territory rather than those located in the territory supplied by proximal BA branches.[32] This might ex-

plain the relationship between infarcts located in the PCA territory and severe ectasia and vertical elongation of the BA, which leads to reduced blood flow in the BA.[14] Compensatory flow from either vertebral artery is not sufficient for adequate perfusion distal to the ectatic VAs and BA.

Reduced blood flow also promotes thrombus formation within dilated segments, obstruction of penetrating branches by the thrombus, and embolization of clot fragments into the perforators. Blood flow insufficiency under such circumstances can lead to transient ischemic attacks and explain the transient symptoms seen in some VBD patients. Hemodynamic effects secondary to dolichoectasia and angulation of the BA may also cause brief movement-based vertigo.[33] Alternatively, atherosclerotic plaques may form along the dilated vessel wall and obstruct arterial branches.

Thrombus formation

Reduced flow promotes stagnation of the blood column and thrombus formation within dilated arterial segments. Thrombus formation is often found at necropsy. Sometimes thrombi are visible on high-resolution MRI or CTA of patients with VBD (Fig. 6). Luminal thrombi may obstruct arterial branches, and portions of the clots can embolize distally. When complicated by intraluminal thrombi, VBD patients can become symptomatic even without compression of the brain stem. Repeated intramural hemorrhage and thrombus formation could lead to rapid growth and the progression of small, asymptomatic fusiform aneurysms to symptomatic and giant dolichoectatic aneurysms.[34]

Reduced perfusion in penetrating branches

Elongation and angulation of the vertebrobasilar arteries can stretch and distort the orifices of arterial branches leading to decreased blood flow, especially in penetrating branches of the large arteries, causing BA branch territory infarcts in the pons. This mechanism may explain the observation that the majority of the infratentorial infarcts in the arterial territories supplied by branches of the BA were, in one study, contralateral to the side of the lateral displacement of the BA.[32]

The relationship between dolichoectasia in stroke patients and penetrating artery disease was also noticed in the GENIC study, which showed that dolichoectasia was independently associated with

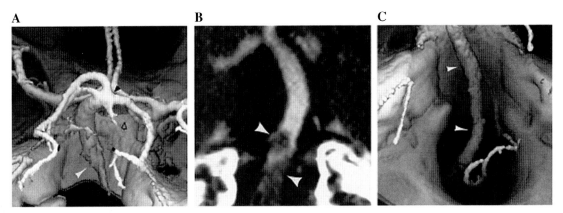

Figure 6. Case 1: 64-year-old man with dolichoectasia of the basilar artery with mural thrombus. (A) Shaded surface display CT angiogram at presentation, viewed from above and behind (patient's right is on the right). The basilar artery is elongated and dilated, with the basilar tip (*solid black arrow*) projecting well above the dorsum sella (open black arrow). The expected locations of the proximal basilar artery and distal left vertebral artery (*white arrowhead*) are not seen because of intraluminal thrombus. (B) Curved reformatted image oriented along the long axis of the vertebrobasilar system, same data set as A. This image approximates an oblique coronal view (patient's left is on the right). Filling defects are visible within the low vertebrobasilar system (*arrowheads*). (C) Repeat CT angiogram, 1 month after treatment. Shaded surface display, seen from similar orientation as in A. The distal left vertebral and proximal basilar arteries (*arrowheads*) now fill normally.

parenchymal manifestations of small vessel disease, including lacunar infarcts, multiple lacunes, severe leukoaraiosis, and severe etat crible (dilated Virchow-Robin spaces around penetrating arteries).[35] Subsequent assessment of the pathology of small intracerebral arteries in dolichoectasic patients with stroke showed evidence of cerebral small-vessel disease, mainly sclerosis and hyalinosis in arteries $< 300\mu$m. The involvement of matrix metalloprointease (MMP) metabolism is one posited mechanism.[15] White matter lesions and lacunes in the cerebral hemispheres are common in patients with posterior circulation dilatative arteriopathy.

Intracranial hemorrhage

Patients with VBD occasionally develop catastrophic bleeding. Pathological changes in the arterial wall, consisting primarily in defects in the internal elastic lamina with thinning of the media secondary to smooth muscle atrophy predispose patients to intracranial bleeding.[25]

Hemorrhagic stroke as a clinical feature of VBD was described in case reports.[36,37] In 2005, Passero and colleagues conducted a prospective study of 156 consecutive VBD patients followed up for an average 9.35 years and reported 32 hemorrhagic strokes

among 28 patients, of which 6 were subarachnoid hemorrhage (SAH) and 26 intraparenchymal hemorrhages (ICH).[38] Most ICHs were located in arterial territories perfused by vessels branching from dolichoectatic parent vessels, and all SAHs were limited to the basal cisterns. The occurrence of hemorrhagic events was associated with the degree of ectasia and elongation of the BA and may be favored by hypertension. Rupture of the dolichoectatic BA is considered rarely (Fig. 7). Hemorrhage might result from damage to vascular beds by VBD coupled with hypertensive atherosclerotic degeneration, causing progressive arteriolar wall damage.[39]

Prescription of antiplatelet and anticoagulant drugs may increase the risk for intracranial bleeding. In VBD patients initially presenting with ischemia, antiplatelet or anticoagulant agents are often prescribed to prevent recurrent brain ischemia. Conventional doses of antithrombotic agents increase the risk of intracranial bleeding.[40,41] Case reports describe VBD patients with ischemic events who were anticoagulated or thrombolysized and subsequently had massive fatal SAH.[36,42] Therefore, caution is warranted in prescribing antiplatelet or anticoagulant agents for patients with severer forms of dolichoectasia.

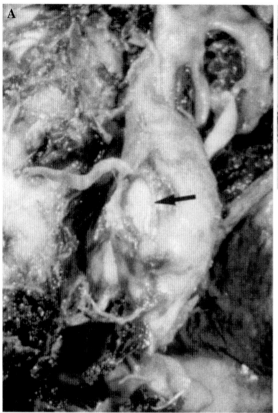
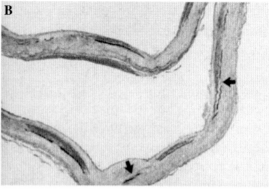

Figure 7. Autopsy findings. (A) Gross views of the basilar artery, with associated rupture site (arrow). (B) Microscopic sections. Fragmentation of the internal elastic lamina is noted (*arrows*). From Ref. 36.

Direct compression

Ectatic, tortuous basilar, or vertebral arteries may exert pressure and displace adjacent structures, the cranial nerves, brain-stem contents, and occasionally the floor of the third ventricle, leading to cranial nerve palsy, brain stem–related signs, or obstructive hydrocephalus.

Dolichoectasia of the BA can cause cranial neuropathies. Most frequently affected are the facial and trigeminal nerves, resulting in hemifacial spasm and trigeminal neuralgia, respectively. Hemifacial spasm is related to vascular compression of the root entry zone of the facial nerve at the brain stem by elongated tortuous vessels of the vertebrobasilar arterial system[43] (Fig 8). In a study involving 648 patients undergoing microvascular decompression for hemifacial spasm, 24% had dolichoectasia of the VA.[44] MRI and MR angiography can document neurovascular contact.

Trigeminal neuralgia may result from demyelination of trigeminal sensory fibers within either the nerve root or the brain stem after compression by marked dolichoectasia of a verterbal artery.[45] Microvascular decompression has been reported to achieve a successful outcome in some of these patients.[46]

Ocular motility disorders can be explained by oculomotor nerve or abducens nerve compression.[47–49] Dolichoectatic basilar artery can cause an abducens nerve paresis. In this setting, the paresis usually is associated with other neurologic deficits; however, isolated abducens nerve paresis caused by BA dolichoectasia has been reported. The anatomic relationship between the sixth cranial nerve root exit zone in the pons and a compressing dolichoectatic artery has been shown by imaging (Fig. 9). Severe BA dolichoectasia rarely causes compression of the optic tract, resulting in homonymous hemianopia and optic atrophy.[50]

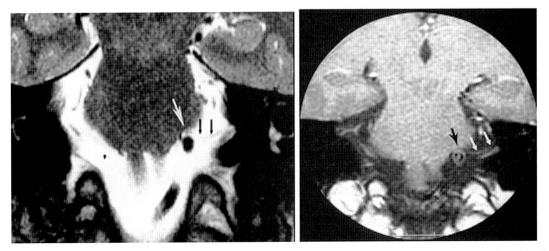

Figure 8. (*Left*) Magnetic resonance imaging (T2-weighted coronal section through pons). An enlarged vertebral artery (black dot) indents the pons and deforms the root of the seventh cranial nerve as it exits the pons (*white arrow*). The subarachnoid course of the seventh cranial nerve is highlighted by black arrows. (*Right*) Magnetic resonance imaging (T1-weighted, contrast-enhanced coronal section through pons).

Occasionally, lingual hemiatrophy is explained by compression of the XIIth nerve in the anterolateral sulcus[51] (Fig. 10). Some patients with VBD describe headaches during exertion; an increase in systemic blood pressure after physical exercise has been posited to lengthen the already elongated vessels and cause stretching pain sensitive fibers around blood vessels.[52]

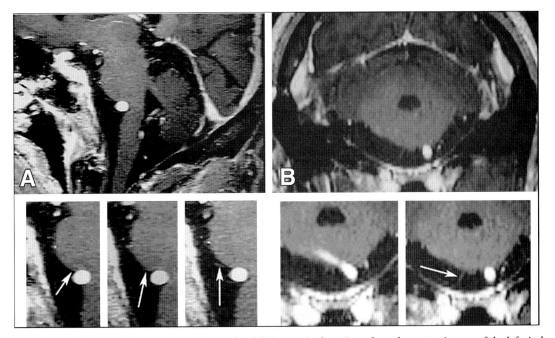

Figure 9. 3-Tesla magnetic resonance angiography. (A) Parasagittal sections show the root exit zone of the left sixth cranial nerve (*white arrows*) and its relation to the dolichoectatic vertebral artery (*white circle*). (B) Axial sections through the caudal pons show the right sixth cranial nerve as it exits the pons (*arrow*); the left sixth cranial nerve exit zone is obscured by the dolichoectatic vessel. From Ref. 49.

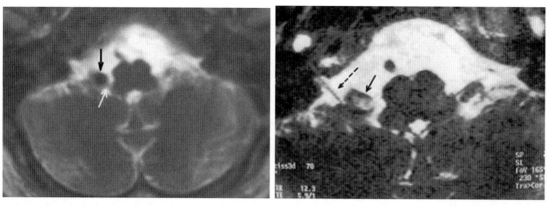

Figure 10. (A) Right lingual hemiatrophy. (B) T2-weighted MR image reveals dolichoectatic right vertebral artery (*black arrow*) with compression of the XIIth nerve (*white arrow*) in the anterolateral sulcus. (C) Millimetric slide of T2-weighted MR image centered on neurovascular conflict (right vertebral artery, *black arrow*, XIIth nerve) (*dashed arrow*). From Ref. 51.

Dilated ecstatic intracranial VAs can directly compress the medulla oblongata causing transient symptoms or persistent deficits (Fig. 11). Compression typically occurs along the anterolateral surface, and motor (ipsilateral or contralateral hemiparesis) and vestibular (vertigo) or cerebellar (gait ataxia) features are the most common resultant signs.[53] Compression may be gradual, allowing for adaptation explaining the poor correlation between symptoms and signs and the extent and severity of compression. Surgical management of the compression has often been unsuccessful and fraught with complications although it may provide temporary symptom relief.

Less often, an elongated BA may provoke hydrocephalus by compression of the floor of the third ventricle[54,55] (Fig. 12). When the basilar artery extends into the floor of the third ventricle, it may

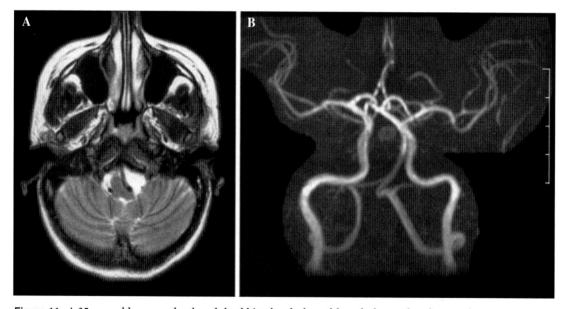

Figure 11. A 35-year-old woman developed throbbing headaches, although the results of a neurologic examination were normal. Magnetic resonance imaging showed impingement of the left anterolateral surface (A) by an angulated left vertebral artery (B). From Ref. 53.

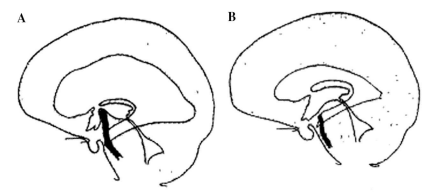

Figure 12. (A) Elongated basilar artery causing impression in the floor of third ventricle and dilatation of lateral ventricles. (B) Normal appearance for comparison. From Ref. 58.

exert a water-hammer cerebrospinal fluid (CSF) pulse pressure that is transmitted to the foramina of Monro, and results in an impaired outflow from the lateral ventricles.

Prognosis

The actuarial survival rate in VBD after 3 years' follow-up was 60% in a small case series without a control group.[56] A retrospective cohort study after a 4–7 year period observed that VBD cases had 36% mortality, with 50% occurring within 34 months of the initial diagnosis.[8] Recently, a prospective study for an average of 11.7 years showed that the cumulative proportion of survivors free of adverse health event was 54.1% at 5 years, 39.5% at 10 years, and 23.5% at 15 years. The long-term prognosis of patients with VBD depends mainly on the severity of the condition at diagnosis (the diameter of BA, height of bifurcation of BA) and on its evolutionary characteristics.[28] VBD may be progressive, and morbidity and mortality increase with the progression. The incidence of recurrent ischemic stroke is high in patients with VBD. This may reflect the evolution of the dolichoectatic process and the limited efficacy of preventive treatment.

The intima and endothelial portions of arteries and plaque formation have received much more attention than the medial and adventitial structures that compose the arterial walls. Although knowledge about VBD is growing, there is still much that is not understood and unsolved. VBD may confer a higher incidence of stroke and mortality rate than expected in affected individuals. Further studies us-

ing new imaging techniques and neuropathologic evidence are needed to clarify mechanisms of brain infarction and guide treatment.

Conflicts of interest

The authors declare no conflicts of interest.

References

1. Caplan, L.R. 2005. Dilatative arteriopathy (dolichoectasia): What is known and not known. *Ann. Neurol.* **57:** 469–471.

2. Smoker, W.R., M.J. Price, W.D. Keyes, *et al.* 1986. High-resolution computed tomography of the basilar artery, 1: normal size and position. *Am. J. Neuroradiol.* **7:** 55–60.

3. Pico, F., J. Labreuche, A. Cohen, *et al.* 2004. Intracranial arterial dolichoectasia is associated with enlarged descending thoracic aorta. *Neurology* **63:** 2016–2021.

4. Dziewas, R., M. Freund, P. Ludemann, *et al.* 2003. Treatment options in vertebrobasilar dolichoectasia: case report and review of the literature. *Eur. Neurol.* **49:** 245–247.

5. Yu, Y.L., I.F. Moseley, P. Pullicino & W.I. McDonald. 1982. The clinical picture of ectasia of the intracerebral arteries. *J. Neurol. Neurosurg. Psychiatry* **45:** 29–36.

6. Pico, F., J. Labreuche, P.J. Touboul & P. Amarenco. 2003. Intracranial arterial dolichoectasia and its association with carotid atherosclerosis and stroke subtype. *Neurology* **61:** 1736–1742.

7. Smoker, W.R., J.J. Corbett, L.R. Gentry, *et al.* 1986. High-resolution computed tomography of the basilar artery, 2: vertebrobasilar dolichoectasia: clinical-pathologic correlation and review. *Am. J. Neuroradiol.* **7:** 61–72.

8. Ubogu, E.E. & O.O. Zaidat. 2004. Vertebrobasilar dolichoectasia diagnosed by magnetic resonance angiography and risk of stroke and death: a cohort study. *J. Neurol. Neurosurg. Psychiatry* **75:** 22–26.

9. Ionita, C.C., A.R. Xavier, J. Farkas & P. Pullicino. 2004. Intracranial arterial dolichoectasia and its relation with atherosclerosis and stroke subtype. *Neurology* **63:** 596; author reply 596.

10. Sacks, J.G. & R. Lindenburg. 1969. Dolicho-ectatic intracranial arteries: symptomatology and pathogenesis of arterial elongation and distention. *Johns Hopkins Med. J.* **125:** 95–106.

11. Gautier, J.C., J.J. Hauw, A. Awada, *et al.* 1988. Dolichoectatic intracranial arteries. Association with aneurysms of the abdominal aorta. *Rev. Neurol. (Paris)* **144:** 437–446.

12. Hegedüs, K. 1985. Ectasia of the basilar artery with special reference to possible pathogenesis. *Surg. Neurol.* **24:** 463–469.

13. Hirsch, C.S. & U. Roessmann. 1975. Arterial dysplasia with ruptured basilar artery aneurysm: report of a case. *Hum. Pathol.* **6:** 749–758.

14. Passero, S. & G. Filosomi. 1998. Posterior circulation infarcts in patients with vertebrobasilar dolichoectasia. *Stroke* **29:** 653–659.

15. Pico, F., J. Labreuche, D. Seilhean, *et al.* 2007. Association of small-vessel disease with dilatative arteriopathy of the brain: neuropathologic evidence. *Stroke* **38:** 1197–1202.

16. Pico, F., Y. Biron, M.G. Bousser & P. Amarenco. 2005. Concurrent dolichoectasia of basilar and coronary arteries. *Neurology* **65:** 1503–1504.

17. Lamblin, N., C. Bauters, X. Hermant, *et al.* 2002. Polymorphisms in the promoter regions of MMP-2, MMP-3, MMP-9 and MMP-12 genes as determinants of aneurysmal coronary artery disease. *J. Am. Coll. Cardiol.* **40:** 43–48.

18. Silverman, I.E., D.M. Berman, G.L. Dike, *et al.* 2000. Vertebrobasilar dolichoectasia associated with Marfan syndrome. *J. Stroke Cerebrovasc. Dis.* **9:** 196–198.

19. Zambrino, C.A., A. Berardinelli, A. Martelli, *et al.* 1999. Dolichovertebrobasilar abnormality and migraine-like attacks. *Eur. Neurol.* **41:** 10–14.

20. Mitsias, P. & S.R. Levine. 1996. Cerebrovascular complications of Fabry's disease. *Ann. Neurol.* **40:** 8–17.

21. Grant Steen, R., J.W. Langston, R.J. Ogg, *et al.* 1998. Ectasia of the basilar artery in children with sickle cell disease: relationship to hematocrit and psychometric measures. *J. Stroke Cerebrovasc. Dis.* **7:** 32–43.

22. Gavazzi, C., W. Borsini, L. Guerrini, *et al.* 2006. Subcortical damage and cortical functional changes in men and women with Fabry disease: a multifaceted MR study. *Radiology* **241:** 492–500.

23. Garzuly, F., L. Maródi, M. Erdös, *et al.* 2005. Megadolichobasilar anomaly with thrombosis in a family with Fabry's disease and a novel mutation in the alpha-galactosidase A gene. *Brain* **128**(Pt 9): 2078–2083.

24. Schievink, W.I., V.E. Torres, D.O. Wiebers & J. Huston, III. 1997. Intracranial arterial dolichoectasia in autosomal dominant polycystic kidney disease. *J. Am. Soc. Nephrol.* **8:** 1298–1303.

25. Graf, S., A. Schischma, K.E. Eberhardt, *et al.* 2002. Intracranial aneurysms and dolichoectasia in autosomal dominant polycystic kidney disease. *Nephrol. Dial. Transplant.* **17:** 819–823.

26. Rautenberg, W., A. Aulich, Rother, *et al.* 1992. Stroke and dolichoectatic intracranial arteries. *Neurol. Res.* **14**(Suppl 2): 201–203.

27. Levine, R.L., P.A. Turski, T.M. Grist. 1995. Basilar artery dolichoectasia: Review of the literature and six patients studied with magnetic resonance angiography. *J. Neuroimaging* **5:** 164–170.

28. Passero, S.G. & S. Rossi. 2008. Natural history of vertebrobasilar dolichoectasia. *Neurology* **70:** 66–72.

29. Ince, B., G.W. Petty, R.D. Brown, Jr., *et al.* 1998. Dolichoectasia of the intracranial arteries in patients with first ischemic stroke: a population-based study. *Neurology* **50:** 1694–1698.

30. Hennerici, M., W. Rautenberg & A. Schwartz. 1987. Transcranial Doppler ultrasound for the assessment of intracranial arterial flow velocity. II. Evaluation of intracranial arterial disease. *Surg. Neurol.* **27:** 523–532.

31. Schwartz, A., W. Rautenberg & M. Hennerici. 1993. Dolichoectatic intracranial arteries: review of selected aspects. *Cerebrovasc. Dis.* **5:** 273–279.

32. Kumral, E., A. Kisabay, C. Ataç, *et al.* 2005. The mechanism of ischemic stroke in patients with dolichoectatic basilar artery. *Eur. J. Neurol.* **12:** 437–444.

33. Welsh, L.W., J.J. Welsh & B. Lewin. 2000. Basilar artery and vertigo. *Ann. Otol. Rhinol. Laryngol.* **109:** 615–622.

34. Nakatomi, H., H. Segawa, A. Kurata, *et al.* 2000. Clinicopathological study of intracranial fusiform and dolichoectatic aneurysms: insight on the mechanism of growth. *Stroke* **31:** 896–900.

35. Pico, F., J. Labreuche, P.-J. Touboul, *et al.* 2005. Intracranial arterial dolichoectasia and small vessel disease in stroke patients. *Ann. Neurol.* **57:** 472–479.

36. Rabb, C.H. & S.L. Barnwell. 1998. Catastrophic subarachnoid hemorrhage resulting from ruptured

vertebrobasilar dolichoectasia: case report. *Neurosurgery* **42:** 379–382.

37. Flemming, K.D., K. Josephs & E.F. Wijdicks. 2000. Enlarging vertebrobasilar dolichoectasia with subarachnoid hemorrhage heralded by recurrent ischemia. Case illustration. *J. Neurosurg.* **92:** 504.

38. Passero, S.G., B. Calchetti & S. Bartalini. 2005. Intracranial bleeding in patients with vertebrobasilar dolichoectasia. *Stroke* **36:** 1421–1425.

39. Peterson, N.T., P.M. Duchesneau, E.L. Westbrook & M.A. Weinstein. 1977. Basilar artery ectasia demonstrated by computed tomography. *Radiology* **122:** 713–715.

40. He, J., P.K. Whelton, B. Vu & M.J. Klag. 1998. Aspirin and risk of hemorrhagic stroke. A meta-analysis of randomized controlled trials. *JAMA* **280:** 1930–1935.

41. Saloheimo, P., S. Juvela & M. Hillbom. 2001. Use of aspirin, epistaxis, and untreated hypertension as risk factors for primary intracerebral hemorrhage in middle-aged and elderly people. *Stroke* **32:** 399–404.

42. De Georgia, M., J. Belden, L. Pao, *et al.* 1999. Thrombus in vertebrobasilar dolichoectatic artery treated with intravenous urokinase. *Cerebrovasc. Dis.* **9:** 28–33.

43. Rahman, E.A., J.D. Trobe & S.S. Gebarski. 2002. Hemifacial spasm caused by vertebral artery dolichoectasia. *Am. J. Ophthalmol.* **133:** 854–856.

44. Barker, F.G. II, P.J. Jannetta, D.J. Bissonette, *et al.* 1995. Microvascular decompression for hemifacial spasm. *J. Neurosurg.* **82:** 201–210.

45. Love, S., D.A. Hilton & H.B. Coakham. 1998. Central demyelination of the Vth nerve root in trigeminal neuralgia associated with vascular compression. *Brain Pathol.* **8:** 1–11.

46. Lye, R.H. 1986. Basilar artery ectasia: an unusual cause of trigeminal neuralgia. *J. Neurol. Neurosurg. Psychiatry* **49:** 22–28.

47. Kasner, S.E., G.T. Liu & S.L. Galetta. 1997. Neuro-ophthalmologic aspects of aneurysms. *Neuroimag. Clin. N. Am.* **7:** 679–692.

48. Goldenberg-Cohen, N. & N.R. Miller. 2004. Noninvasive neuroimaging of basilar artery dolichoectasia in a patient with an isolated abducens nerve paresis. *Am. J. Ophthalmol.* **137:** 365–367.

49. Zhu, Y., K. Thulborn, K. Curnyn, *et al.* 2005. Sixth cranial nerve palsy caused by compression from a dolichoectatic vertebral artery. *J. Neuroophthalmol.* **25:** 134–135.

50. Guirgis, M.F., B.L. Lam & S.F. Falcone. 2001. Optic tract compression from dolichoectatic basilar artery. *Am. J. Ophthalmol.* **132:** 283–286.

51. Castelnovo, G., L. Jomir, A. Le Bayon, *et al.* 2003. Lingual atrophy and dolichoectatic artery. *Neurology* **61:** 1121.

52. Staikov, I.N. & H.P. Mattle. 1994. Vertebrobasilar dolichoectasia and exertional headache. *J. Neurol. Neurosurg. Psychiatry* **57:** 1544.

53. Savitz, S.I., M. Ronthal & L.R. Caplan. 2006. Vertebral artery compression of the medulla. *Arch. Neurol.* **63:** 234–241.

54. Siddiqui, A., N.S. Chew & K. Miszkiel. 2008. Vertebrobasilar dolichoectasia: a rare cause of obstructive hydrocephalus: case report. *Br. J. Radiol.* **81:** e123–e126.

55. Ekbom, K., T. Greitz & E. Kugelberg. 1969. Hydrocephalus due to ectasia of the basilar artery. *J. Neurol. Sci.* **8:** 465–477.

56. Milandre, L., B. Bonnefoi, P. Pestre, *et al.* 1991. Vertebrobasilar arterial dolichoectasia. Complications and prognosis. *Rev. Neurol. (Paris)* **147:** 714–722.

57. Laforêt, P., P. Petiot, M. Nicolino, *et al.* 2008. Dilative arteriopathy and basilar artery dolichoectasia complicating late-onset Pompe disease. *Neurology* **70:** 2063–2066.

58. Breig, A., K. Ekbom, T. Greitz, *et al.* 1967. Hydrocephalus due to elongated basilar artery. A new clinicoradiological syndrome. *Lancet* **1:** 874–875.

Ann. N.Y. Acad. Sci. ISSN 0077-8923

ANNALS OF THE NEW YORK ACADEMY OF SCIENCES

Dermatomyositis and polymyositis
Clinical presentation, autoantibodies, and pathogenesis

Andrew L. Mammen

Department of Neurology, Johns Hopkins University School of Medicine, Baltimore, Maryland, USA

Address for correspondence: Andrew L. Mammen, MD, PhD, Johns Hopkins University School of Medicine, Dept. of Neurology, Johns Hopkins Bayview, Johns Hopkins Myositis Center, Mason F. Lord Building Center Tower, Suite 4100, Baltimore, MD 21224. Voice: 410-550-6962; fax: 410-550-3542. amammen@jhmi.edu

Dermatomyositis (DM) and polymyositis (PM) are autoimmune myopathies characterized clinically by proximal muscle weakness, muscle inflammation, extramuscular manifestations, and frequently, the presence of autoantibodies. Although there is some overlap, DM and PM are separate diseases with different pathophysiological mechanisms. Furthermore, unique clinical phenotypes are associated with each of the myositis-specific autoantibodies (MSAs) associated with these disorders. This review will focus on the clinical features, pathology, and immunogenetics of PM and DM with an emphasis on the importance of autoantibodies in defining unique phenotypes and, perhaps, as clues to help elucidate the mechanisms of disease.

Keywords: myositis; dermatomyositis; polymyositis; autoantibodies; myopathy; autoimmunity

Introduction

The inflammatory myopathies are a group of acquired skeletal muscle diseases that includes polymyositis (PM), dermatomyositis (DM), and inclusion body myositis (IBM).[1–3] Although these disorders share several common features including muscle weakness and inflammatory infiltrates on muscle biopsy, they are a heterogeneous group both in terms of presentation and pathophysiology. For example, PM and DM are characterized by the subacute onset of symmetric proximal muscle weakness, common involvement of other organ systems such as lung and skin, a strong association with autoantibodies, and responsiveness to immunosuppression. Both are widely accepted as having an autoimmune basis. In contrast, patients with IBM typically have slowly progressive weakness in both proximal and distal muscles, rarely have other extramuscular involvement or autoantibodies, and most often do not respond to immunosuppressive therapies. Considerable evidence suggests this disease is a myodegenerative disorder and the pathologic relevance of the inflammatory response is highly controversial.[4]

This review will focus on the diverse presentations of adult-onset DM and PM, emphasizing the association of distinct clinical phenotypes with unique myositis-specific autoantibodies (MSAs). The possible relevance of autoantibodies to the pathophysiology of the disease, including an association between cancer and myositis, will be discussed.

Historical perspective

In 1863, Wagner documented the first case of myositis in a patient who also had significant cutaneous findings.[5] Twenty-four years later, Hepp reported that inflammatory myopathies can also occur in the absence of skin involvement.[1,6] In the same year, Hans Unverricht described a 27-year-old stonemason who developed myalgias and proximal muscle weakness followed by diffuse edema, low-grade fevers, and a blue-tinted rash over his eyelids.[7] Over the ensuing weeks, this patient's condition worsened with the development of dysarthria, dysphagia, dyspnea, and ultimately, pulmonary arrest. A postmortem analysis revealed the presence of a cellular infiltrate within the affected muscles. After describing a second case in 1891, Unverricht coined the term "dermatomyositis" to describe patients with an inflammatory myopathy associated with dermatologic findings.[8] Although

Ann. N.Y. Acad. Sci. 1184 (2010) 134–153 © 2009 New York Academy of Sciences.

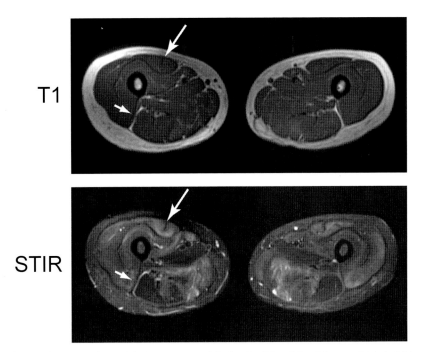

Figure 1. Thigh MRI from a patient with dermatomyositis. In the T1-weighted image, fat is bright and muscle is dark. In the start tau inversion recovery (STIR) sequence, normal muscle is dark and inflamed muscle is bright. The long arrow indicates the inflamed right rectus femoris muscle. The short arrow highlights the right biceps femoris muscle; the bright rim around this muscle is consistent with fascial inflammation, but the body of the muscle appears relatively unaffected.

Eaton,[9] Walton and Adams,[10] Rowland,[11] and Pearson and Rose[12] all contributed to our modern understanding of DM and PM, Bohan and Peter[1] published diagnostic criteria for these diseases in 1975 that, although imperfect, are still widely used today.

Pathology of myositis

Patients with both PM and DM typically experience the onset of symmetric proximal muscle weakness over weeks to months that is usually, but not always, accompanied by high serum creatinine kinase (CK) levels. In both diseases, electromyography often reveals fibrillations, positive sharp waves, and small polyphasic motor units with early recruitment patterns that characterize an irritable myopathy. Skeletal muscle MRI in DM and PM shows areas of T2 hyperintensity in edematous areas as well as fatty replacement of muscle tissue in those patients with chronic disease (Fig. 1). However, despite these clinical similarities, muscle biopsies from DM and PM patients each have distinguishing features. Al-

though there is frequently overlap in pathology, I will emphasize here those disease-specific findings suggesting that different mechanisms underlie DM and PM.

Muscle biopsy findings in dermatomyositis

The hallmark histopathologic feature of DM is the strongly perifascicular distribution of atrophic, degenerating, and regenerating myofibers (Fig. 2A). This striking perifascicular pathology has been proposed to result from the destruction of capillaries populating this region. It is thought that a critical depletion of capillaries here could result in localized hypoxia and subsequent myofiber injury.[3] Indeed, abnormal capillary morphology and capillary loss is an early feature of DM that may occur in the absence of inflammatory infiltrates.[13,14] Even prior to capillary dropout, studies of DM muscle tissue reveal the deposition of the C5b-9 membrane attack complex (MAC) on endothelial cells and the presence of abnormal tuboreticular structures within the smooth endoplasmic reticulum of endothelial

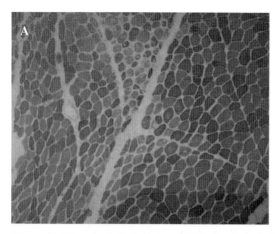 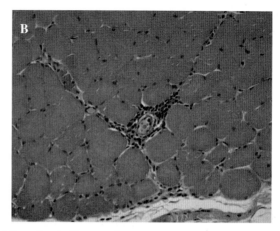

Figure 2. Characteristic features of DM muscle include (A) perifascicular atrophy as seen in this frozen section stained with ATPase pH 9.4 and (B) perivascular inflammation as seen in this paraffin section stained with H&E.

cells.[14,15] Presumably as a consequence of capillary destruction, there is also evidence of neovascularization in DM muscle biopsies, particularly in the juvenile form of the disease.[16] Recent work suggests that neovascularization in myositis muscle may be induced by increased muscle expression and serum concentrations of vascular endothelial growth factor (VEGF), an angiogenic growth factor known to be induced by hypoxia.[17]

Although these findings have led numerous investigators to propose that the immune response in DM is primarily directed against capillaries, no antiendothelial autoantibodies have been identified. Moreover, a recent study demonstrated that capillary number is reduced in both DM and PM muscle biopsies lacking inflammatory infiltrates, indicating that early capillary loss is not disease specific.[17] Finally, animal models of muscle ischemia have demonstrated that the central domains of muscle fascicles are more vulnerable to ischemia than perifascicular regions.[18,19] Taken together, these findings call into question the hypothesis that capillary reduction and subsequent hypoxia underlie the perifascicular atrophy found exclusively in DM.

Another characteristic, though less specific, feature of DM muscle is the presence of perivascular inflammation (Fig. 2B). These collections of lymphocytes are composed primarily of B cells along with a smaller number of CD4+ cells long-thought to be helper T cells.[20] However, recent investigations by Greenberg and colleagues[21] suggest that the ma-

jority of CD4+ cells in DM muscle biopsies are actually plasmacytoid dendritic cells (PDCs). These effector cells of the innate immune system play critical roles in antiviral and antitumor immune responses and are a potent source of interferon (IFN)-α.[22] In this regard, it is noteworthy that genes induced by IFN-α/β are highly expressed in DM muscle biopsies compared with muscle from patients with other inflammatory myopathies.[21] This includes the human myxovirus resistance 1 protein (MxA), which helps defend against a number of RNA viruses by interfering with viral nucleocapsid transport and viral assembly. This protein is selectively upregulated in DM muscle biopsies, where it is frequently localized to perifascicular regions as well as to cytoplasmic inclusions within endothelial cells. As suggested by Greenberg and colleagues, these findings imply a potentially important role for IFN-α and IFN-α-inducible genes in the pathophysiology of DM. This idea has been reinforced by the finding that IFN-α/β-inducible gene expression in the periphery correlates with DM disease activity.[23,24]

Muscle biopsy findings in polymyositis

The presence of autoaggressive inflammatory cells that surround, enter, and destroy morphologically normal appearing myofibers is the characteristic feature of PM (Fig. 3). These inflammatory cells are composed largely of CD8+ T cells and macrophages.[25] In contrast to normal muscle, Major Histocompatability Complex

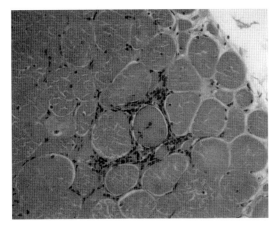

Figure 3. Primary inflammation in PM. Inflammatory cells surround non-necrotic fibers in this paraffin section stained with H&E.

I (MHC)-class I is upregulated on the sarcolemmal membrane of myofibers in PM, even on normal-appearing cells in areas devoid of inflammatory cells.[26–28] Interestingly, targeted overexpression of MHC-I in the muscles of mice results in muscle inflammation and the production of myositis autoantibodies.[29] Moreover, exogenous expression of MHC-I activates endoplasmic reticulum stress response pathways that could also cause muscle damage in PM.[30]

The expression of MHC-I on myositis muscle fibers suggests that these cells may be killed in an human leukocyte antigen (HLA) class I restricted manner by cytolytic T cells. Supporting this concept is the observation that many of the CD8+ T cells include granules containing perforin, a pore-forming protein that mediates the entry of cytotoxic proteases and calcium into target cells. Confocal laser microscopy studies have demonstrated that these perforin-containing granules are selectively oriented toward muscle fibers, consistent with a cytotoxic mechanism of cell death in PM.[31] To date, however, the autoantigens hypothesized to trigger an autoimmune response via this pathway have not been definitively identified.

Although T cells can also kill by inducing apoptosis through a ligand-mediated mechanism (via Fas and the Fas-ligand), apoptotic muscle fibers have not been identified in muscle biopsy specimens from patients with myositis.[32,33] Indeed, muscle seems to be especially resistant to apoptotic cell death, per-

haps through the expression of antiapoptotic factors such as Bcl-2[32,34] and FLIP.[35]

Common pathologic features of DM and PM

In the preceding paragraphs, the unique pathological features of PM and DM have been emphasized. However, there is considerable overlap between these two forms of inflammatory myopathy, and they share many important features.[36] Listed below are several examples:

(i) There is an emphasis on blood vessels as a target of the immune response in DM. However, capillary depletion is characteristic of both DM and PM muscle biopsies, and in both diseases there is evidence supporting a role for VEGF in neovascularization.[17] Furthermore, endothelial cells in muscle biopsy specimens from patients with both DM and PM express high levels of interleukin (IL)-1α, IL-1β, and transforming growth factor (TGF)β1–3.[37]

(ii) Although MHC-I expression is proposed to mediate cytolytic killing in PM, DM patients also express sarcolemmal MHC-I, albeit preferentially on perifascicular fibers.[28]

(iii) Recent work has shown that perivascular infiltrates in DM muscle and endomysial infiltrates in PM muscle both include significant numbers of dendritic cells (DCs), a population of extremely effective antigen presenting cells.[38]

(iv) Numerous studies have revealed very similar cytokine and chemokine profiles in muscle tissue from patients with DM and PM.[37,39–41] This includes IL-17 and IFN-γ, suggesting that activated CD4+ T cells may be involved in both disease processes.[38]

(v) IFN-α/β transcripts are selectively upregulated in DM muscle tissue.[42] However, in the periphery, these transcripts are increased in both DM and PM. Furthermore, their peripheral levels are correlated with disease activity in both diseases.[23]

Skin findings in DM

Cutaneous involvement is the primary clinical feature distinguishing those with DM from those with PM.[43–45] A purplish discoloration around the eyes, especially the upper eyelid, is known as a heliotrope rash and is pathognomonic for DM (Fig. 4). In some patients with DM, this is found in

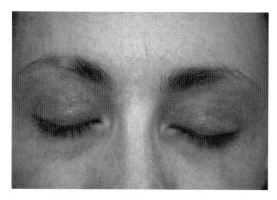

Figure 4. Heliotrope. Violaceous macular erythema on the upper eyelid is often associated with periorbital edema in DM. (Photograph courtesy of Dr. Lisa Christopher-Stine.)

conjunction with periorbital edema. Gottron's sign refers to an erythematous rash over the extensor surfaces of the metacarpophalangeal, proximal interphalangeal, and distal interphalangeal joints. This rash can evolve into a scaly eruption known as Gottron's papules (Fig. 5). Gottron's sign or papules may also occur on the extensor surfaces of the elbows and knees, where they are occasionally misdiagnosed as psoriasis. Like the heliotrope rash, Gottron's papules are specific for DM. It should be noted that the coloration of the heliotrope rash and Gottron's sign may vary depending upon the skin tone of the patient. For example, in African-American patients, these rashes may appear hyperpigmented rather than violaceous or erythematous.[46]

DM patients may also have a combination of atrophy, dyspigmentation, and telangectasias known as poikiloderma. The poikilodermatous rash is commonly found on the upper chest as a V-shaped rash or on the upper back where it is known as a "shawl sign." Facial erythema and scalp involvement are sometimes associated with DM. Nailbed abnormalities are a common feature of DM and may include both periungual telangectasias and cuticular hypertrophy. Although less frequently recognized, the oral mucosa may also have cutaneous manifestations in DM. These include erythema, hemorrhage, vesicles, ulcers, leukokeratosis, and gingival telangectasias.[47,48] Unlike the heliotrope rash and Gottron's sign, these cutaneous features are not necessarily specific for DM. For example, facial erythema may be found in patients with rosacea, and periungual telangectasias are seen in patients with scleroderma.

While not all DM patients report that their rashes are photosensitive, several studies suggest that they are aggravated by exposure to UV light.[49,50]

In a typical DM patient, the cutaneous manifestations may precede, coincide with, or occur after muscle involvement. Occasionally, however, the characteristic skin lesions of DM occur in patients without overt signs of muscle disease.[51–54] Although these patients with amyopathic DM (or dermatomyositis-sine myositis) do not have weakness or elevated CK levels, they may have subtly abnormal magnetic resonance imaging, electromyography, or muscle biopsy findings. Interestingly, a recent analysis of 16 patients initially diagnosed with amyopathic DM and followed longitudinally showed that close to 20% developed overt muscle disease within 5 years.[55]

Diagnostic skin biopsies are often obtained during the evaluation of patients with DM and typically reveal a cell-poor vacuolar interface dermatitis, characterized by a sparse infiltrate of inflammatory cells at the dermoepidermal junction.[56] Pathologic studies have also demonstrated dermal perivascular

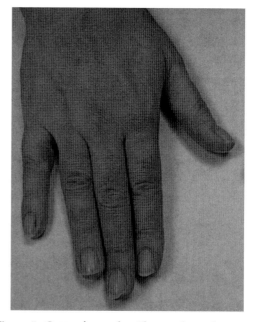

Figure 5. Gottron's papules. These scaly erythematous lesions on the extensor surfaces of the metacarpophalangeal, proximal interphalangeal, and distal interphalangeal joints are pathognomonic for DM. (Photograph courtesy of Dr. Lisa Christopher-Stine.)

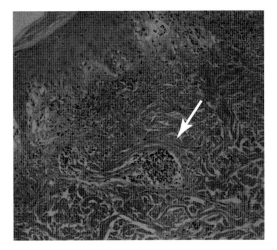

Figure 6. Dermatomyositis skin biopsy. The *arrow* indicates a collection of perivascular inflammatory cells in the dermis (paraffin H&E).

infiltrates consisting of activated T lymphocytes (Fig. 6)[57] and the deposition of membrane attack complex along vessel walls of the dermis.[58,59] These vascular findings, along with the muscle pathology findings discussed below, suggest that blood vessels may be a primary target of the immune response in DM. Furthermore, a recent study showed an increased number of Ki-67 positive keratinocytes and reduced numbers of Bcl-2 positive cells in the basal cell layer of the epidermis, indicating increased proliferation and disrupted apoptotic pathways in DM skin. It should be noted, however, that routine pathologic studies cannot distinguish between the rashes of DM and those of lupus erythematosus. Consequently, a definitive pathological diagnosis of DM can only be made by muscle biopsy (discussed below).

Myosistis-specific autoantibodies and their associated clinical features

As in other systemic autoimmune diseases, a strong association of autoantibodies with distinct clinical phenotypes is found in patients with myositis. These antibodies have classically been divided into myositis-associated autoantibodies (MAAs), which can also be found in patients with other connective tissue diseases, and MSAs. MSAs are found primarily (if not exclusively) in patients with myositis; they are not found in other connective tissue diseases and are virtually absent in patients with muscular

dystrophies, including those, such as facioscapulohumeral dystrophy, which have inflammatory cell infiltrates on muscle biopsy.[60]

This review will focus on the MSAs. Although it remains unclear why they arise and whether they play a pathologic role in the disease process, clues about the pathophysiologic relevance of these antibodies are emerging. I will highlight these along with the important clinical features typically associated with some of these antibodies.

Anti-Jo-1 and other anti-tRNA synthetase autoantibodies

The aminoacyl-tRNA synthetases are ubiquitously expressed cytoplasmic enzymes that catalyze the esterification of a specific amino acid to its cognate tRNA to form an aminoacyl-tRNA. There is a unique tRNA for each of the 20 amino acids. For example, the histidyl-tRNA synthetase attaches histidine to the appropriate tRNA. The aminoacyl-tRNA complex subsequently transfers the appropriate amino acid to an elongating polypeptide chain as the ribosome "reads" the coding sequence of an mRNA.

Autoantibodies against the histidyl-tRNA-synthetase (anti-Jo-1) are the most common MSAs and were first described in 1980.[61] They were subsequently recognized to identify a group of patients with a unique clinical syndrome including myositis, interstitial lung disease (ILD), nonerosive arthritis, fever, and characteristic hyperkeratotic lesions along the radial and palmar aspects of the fingers known as "mechanic's hands."[62,63] This constellation of symptoms has come to be known as the antisynthetase syndrome. Since then, antibodies targeting a number of additional aminoacyl-tRNA synthetases (ARS) have been identified, including those recognizing threonyl-tRNA-synthetase (anti-PL-7),[64] alanyl-tRNA synthetase (anti-PL-12),[65] glycyl-tRNA synthetase (anti-EJ),[66] isoleucyl-tRNA synthetase (anti-OJ),[66] asparaginyl-tRNA synthetase (anti-KS),[67] anti-tyrosyl-tRNA synthetase,[68] and, most recently, anti-phenylalanyl synthetase (anti-Zo).[69]

Anti-Jo-1 is found in approximately 25–30% of myositis patients, and the other anti-ARS autoantibodies occur in about 1–5% of myositis patients.[70] Interestingly, the various antisynthetase antibodies seem to be mutually exclusive in that individual patients do not produce more than one.[71] Although all of the anti-ARS autoantibodies are associated with the antisynthetase syndrome first described for anti-Jo-1, certain differences between patients with the different antisynthetases have been noted. For example, a recent study carefully analyzed the clinical characteristics of 31 patients with anti-PL-12.[72] Ninety percent of these had ILD and 65% presented initially to a pulmonologist. By comparison, only 50–75% of patients with anti-Jo-1 have ILD. Although 90% of the anti-PL-12 patients had some underlying connective tissue disease, only 32% had PM and 19% had DM (the remainder had diagnoses of systemic sclerosis, undifferentiated connective tissue disease, systemic lupus erythematosus, and rheumatoid arthritis). In contrast, 90% of Jo-1 patients have evidence of muscle disease. Compared with Jo-1 patients, PL-12 patients also had much lower rates of arthritis (58% vs. 94%), mechanic's hands (16% vs. 71%), and fever (45% vs. 87%). It should also be noted that ILD occurs in about 30% of myositis patients in the absence of known antisynthetase autoantibodies[73–75]; an intriguing possibility is that these patients may have as yet unidentified autoantibodies.

It is notable that patients with anti-PL-12 and certain other antisynthetases are more likely to have lung disease without clinically detectable muscle disease.[67,72,76,77] In a large study of Japanese patients with antisynthetase antibodies, seven of 88 patients had ILD but did not develop clinically apparent myositis even after more than 6 years.[77] These patients had anti-KS, anti-PL-7, anti-PL-12, anti-EJ, and anti-OJ autoantibodies, but not anti-Jo-1. Interestingly, patients with amyopathic DM may also develop ILD.[55] Whether patients with amyopathic ILD have a separate disease entity or a "forme fruste" of DM or the antisynthetase syndrome remains unclear.

The antisynthetase autoantibodies may be found in patients with either PM or DM, and certain antisynthetases may be more strongly associated with one or the other of these diseases. However, different studies of the same antisynthetase have yielded very different results.[78] For example, in a recent study by Fathi and colleagues, 6/14 (43%) PM and 0/9 (0%) DM patients had anti-Jo-1.[79] Similarly, another study found that only 2/96 (2%) DM patients had anti-Jo-1.[80] On the other end of the spectrum, a third study found anti-Jo-1 in 5/27 (18%) PM

patients and 9/59 (15%) DM patients.[81] Different demographic and referral patterns may account for these differences.

The prognostic significance of ILD has been the subject of several studies. In 1988, Arsura and Greenberg published a report evaluating 67 cases of myositis and ILD described in the literature between 1956 and 1980. This study revealed a mortality rate of 40% after an average follow-up of 31 months for those with lung disease compared with a mortality rate of 24% in 745 PM/DM patients selected without regard for the presence of lung disease.[73] In contrast, a more recent study found that only one of 12 patients (8%) with anti-Jo-1-autoantibodies and the antisynthetase syndrome died after an average follow-up time of 66 months.[82] These conflicting results could be due to different inclusion criteria such as the fact that biopsy-proven lung fibrosis was required for inclusion only in the earlier study. Another contributing factor may be the improved mortality for myositis patients[83]; the 5-year survival rate in the 1960s was 65%[84] and in the last decade has risen to 75–95%.[85–89]

Although the relationship between antisynthetase antibodies and myositis has been studied for almost 30 years, many questions remain about their pathologic significance. Several observations suggest they may play a role in the initiation and/or propagation of disease. For example, the antibody response to the Jo-1 protein (i.e., the histidyl-tRNA synthetase) undergoes class switching, affinity maturation, and spectrotype broadening.[90–93] These features of the immune response suggest that this is a T cell-dependent, antigen-driven process directed against the Jo-1 protein.

Additionally, a number of studies have demonstrated that anti-Jo-1 autoantibody titers are correlated with disease activity.[62,92,94,95] The most recent and extensive of these studies, conducted by Stone and colleagues,[95] included a cross-sectional study of 81 anti-Jo-1 positive patients. This showed that autoantibody titers correlated modestly with CK levels and other measures of both muscle and lung involvement. In 11 patients with serial samples available for study, there were even more dramatic associations of Jo-1 autoantibody titers with indicators of muscle, joint, and lung disease. This included three patients who became anti-Jo-1 negative during periods of disease inactivity. Thus, serial anti-Jo-1 titers followed in an individual patient may be a useful marker of disease activity, particularly in the lung, where this is often difficult to assess. Furthermore, the association of anti-Jo-1 levels with both muscular and extramuscular manifestations of disease activity suggests that there may be a link between the Jo-1 antigen and inflammation in various tissues.

In this regard, Levine and his colleagues have provided some evidence that the immune response against Jo-1 could actually be initiated in the lung.[96] These investigators had previously found that many autoantigens, including Jo-1, are cleaved by granzyme B, a proteolytic enzyme found in the granules of cytolytic T cells.[97] Such cleavage has been proposed to generate "cryptic" epitopes, novel conformations of self-proteins not usually encountered by lymphocytes during their development. Theoretically, lymphocytes that recognize cryptic epitopes within Jo-1 would not be deleted during maturation, should remain in the circulation, and could be activated to drive an autoimmune response.

In a recent paper, Levine and colleagures[96] first identified the granzyme B cleavage site within the Jo-1 protein. Next, they found that Jo-1 exists in two forms, only one of which is susceptible to cleavage by granzyme B. Finally, they demonstrated that this cleavable form of Jo-1 was robustly expressed in the lung relative to other tissues; in muscle, it did not appear to be expressed at all. Taken together, these studies implicate the lung as a likely microenvironment for the generation of cryptic Jo-1 fragments by granzyme B and the subsequent initiation of an anti-Jo-1 immune response. How a lung-initiated anti-Jo-1 response might be redirected to muscle is an open question. It also remains to be determined whether other aminacyl-tRNA synthetases are particularly susceptible to granzyme B cleavage in the lung or elsewhere.

Further evidence that an immune response against the Jo-1 protein may be important event in the initiation of myositis was published recently by Katsumata.[98] In this study, mice were immunized with either human or murine forms of Jo-1 protein emulsified in complete Freund's adjuvant. The anti-Jo-1 immune response was subsequently analyzed at various time points. Although the two proteins are 95% homologous, the immune response was relatively species specific, with antibodies preferentially recognizing the murine form when immunized with the murine form and vice versa. Interestingly, whereas the response to human Jo-1 immunization was uniphasic, mice immunized with the murine protein had evidence of an evolving immune response as evidenced by class switching and epitope spreading. Anti-Jo-1-specific T cells were also found in mice immunized with the murine form of this protein. Moreover, histological studies revealed that some mice immunized with Jo-1 developed inflammation within muscle and lung tissues. Foci of inflammatory cells within muscle tissue were found in a perivascular and endomysial distribution; invasion of myofibers by inflammatory cells was also reported. Within the lung, lymphocytic infiltrates were perivascular and peribronchiolar and also involved the alveoli. It should be noted that a small number of animals immunized with adjuvant alone developed muscle and lung inflammation. Although the relevance of this mouse model to human disease remains to be established, this work, along with the aforementioned studies, suggests that the immune response against Jo-1 may play an important role in the pathogenesis of the antisynthetase syndrome.

Finally, there is evidence that the Jo-1 antigen may have proinflammatory properties in addition to its role in protein synthesis. Specifically, Howard and colleagues[99] have shown that Jo-1 protein can attract lymphocytes, monocytes, and immature dendritic cells through its interaction with chemokine receptor 5. These authors propose that damaged muscle cells could release Jo-1, leading to the recruitment of inflammatory cells which could, in turn, perpetuate autoimmune-mediated muscle destruction.

Anti-Mi-2 autoantibodies

Anti-Mi-2 autoantibodies were first described in a 60-year-old woman with DM (patient Mi), by Reichlin and Mattioli in 1976.[100] The autoantigen recognized by her serum was initially identified only as a nuclear protein, named Mi-2. Characterizations of additional patients with autoimmune myositis showed that 20–30% of DM patients have Mi-2 antibodies. Most studies using immunoprecipitation or immunodiffusion techniques have shown that few, if any, PM patients or normal controls produce Mi-2 autoantibodies.[101–107] However, studies using an ELISA detection assay have found a significant number of Mi-2 positive patients among those with PM, IBM, and even muscular dystrophy.[60,108–110] The ELISA method of detection may simply have a high false positive rate for anti-Mi-2 autoantibodies. Alternatively, the differences in detection between methods may reflect clinically relevant differences in epitope specificities.[103] These issues will require additional studies to resolve.

Almost 20 years elapsed between the description of Mi-2 autoantibodies and the cloning and sequencing of the cognate antigen(s).[111–113] In 1995, Nilasena and colleagues[114] showed that Mi-2 autoantibodies immunoprecipitate a nuclear complex composed of up to eight subunits. A 240 kDa protein was found to be the subunit recognized by Mi-2 autoantibodies. Subsequently, two highly homologous proteins recognized by Mi-2 autoantibodies, Mi-2α and Mi-2β, were cloned and sequenced. Both can be found in the larger complex, but Mi-2β is thought to be the predominant form *in vivo*.

It is now known that Mi-2 is a major component of the nucleosome-remodeling deacetylase, or NuRD, complex. This nuclear complex consists of as many as eight distinct subunits and regulates transcription at the chromosomal level by histone deacetylation and ATP-dependent nucleosome remodeling.[115] Specifically, Mi-2 modifies chromatin structure through its activity as a DNA-dependent, nucleosome-stimulated ATPase.[116] Originally, Mi-2 was thought to function exclusively as a transcriptional suppressor through its association with other members of the NuRD complex including the histone deacetylases HDAC1 and HDAC2, the histone binding proteins RbAp46 and RbAp48, the metastasis-associated proteins MTA1 and MTA2, and the methyl binding domain protein Mbd3. The carboxyl terminus of Mi-2 can mediate this suppression by binding transcriptional repressors such as hunchback, Trk69, and KAP-1 corepressor. However, more recent work indicates that Mi-2 also interacts with transactivating proteins through its amino-terminal domain.[117]

Emerging evidence suggests that Mi-2 and other members of the NuRD complex have specific functions in development.[118] In *Drosophila*, the Mi-2 homolog, dMi-2, functions to repress Hox gene expression and is required for germ cell development.[119] Likewise, in *C. elegans* the Mi-2 homolog, *chd-4*, functions to inhibit ectopic vulval development through Ras-induced pathways.[120] Very recently, the creation of tissue-specific knockout mice has shown that Mi-2 expression is crucial for proper development of the epidermal basal cell layer.[121]

DM patients with anti-Mi-2 autoantibodies tend to have more fulminant cutaneous manifestations, including heliotrope rashes, shawl rashes over the upper back and neck, and cuticular overgrowth. Nonetheless, patients with Mi-2 antibodies have a more favorable prognosis, with better response to steroid therapy, and a diminished incidence of malignancy compared to others with DM.[71,102,104,122,123] These observations suggest that, among individuals with DM, those with anti-Mi-2 antibodies may represent a distinct group.

At least two studies have identified a correlation between latitude and the relative proportion of DM among patients with myositis.[124,125] For example, in Guatemala City 83% of myositis patients have DM and in Glasgow only 27% of patients have DM. A report published by Okada and colleagues demonstrated that increased exposure to ultraviolet (UV) radiation, rather than global gradients in genetic risk factors, is primarily responsible for this gradient.[125] Interestingly, they also observed that the production of Mi-2 autoantibodies occurs more frequently at lower latitudes; in Guatemala City 60% of DM patients are Mi-2 positive and in Glasgow a mere 6.7% of DM patients produce anti-Mi-2 antibodies. Increased surface UV radiation intensity was the single variable identified that increased the odds of developing an immune response against Mi-2.

Given the association of surface UV radiation intensity and the development of an anti-Mi-2 immune response in DM patients, Burd and associates examined the expression of Mi-2 in human keratinocyte cell lines exposed to UV radiation.[126] They found that UV exposure increases Mi-2 protein expression (especially Mi-2α), but not levels of other NuRD complex proteins, in these cells. This upregulation of Mi-2 protein levels occurred rapidly, within 30 min of light exposure, and was regulated through translational and posttranslational mechanisms rather than transcriptionally. Based on their findings, these investigators proposed that the increased expression of Mi-2 protein in UV-induced dermatitis drives the anti-Mi-2 response and explains why this autoantibody is more prevalent at lower latitudes where surface UV radiation intensity is greatest.

In a related prior study by Casciola-Rosen and coworkers,[127] Mi-2 protein levels were found to be relatively low in both normal muscle and in PM muscle biopsy specimens. In contrast, muscle biopsy

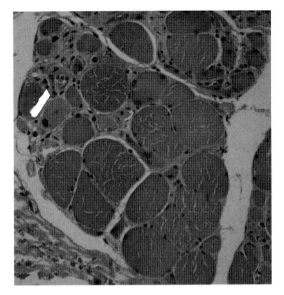

Figure 7. Necrotizing myopathy. In this muscle biopsy from an anti-SRP-positive patient, a fascicle includes numerous degenerating and regenerating myofibers in the absence of inflammatory cells (paraffin H&E).

specimens from many patients with DM had significantly increased expression of Mi-2. These results also support the notion that increased expression of Mi-2 in the DM target tissues serves to drive the anti-Mi-2 immune response.

Anti–signal recognition particle autoantibodies

As discussed above, biopsies from patients with DM and PM are characterized by the conspicuous presence of inflammatory cells. However, about 10% of patients with apparently autoimmune muscle disease have biopsies revealing degenerating, necrotic, and regenerating myofibers with few, if any, infiltrating lymphocytes (Fig. 7). Some of these patients with a "necrotizing myopathy" have autoantibodies targeting components of the signal recognition particle (SRP).

The SRP is a complex of six polypeptides (72, 68, 54, 19, 14, and 9 kDa) and a single 7SL RNA molecule. This cytosolic ribonucleoprotein binds to the endoplasmic reticulum (ER) signal sequences of elongating polypeptide chains during their synthesis and translocates them to the ER membrane. In 1986, Reeves first described the presence of anti-SRP autoantibodies in a "typical polymyositis" patient.[128] Subsequent work has demonstrated that

autoantibodies may be directed to one or more of the six polypeptides as well as to the 7SL RNA.[129] In the first comprehensive analysis of an anti-SRP patient cohort, Targoff identified these autoantibodies in 13/265 (4%) "PM/DM" patients. In this study, it was noted that SRP-positive individuals did not have overlap syndromes or DM rashes.[130] Although they only infrequently had ILD or Reynaud's phenomenon, these patients were noted to have unusually severe muscle disease.

In their 2002 paper, Miller and colleagues reported on the clinical and pathologic features of seven anti-SRP-positive patients.[131] They confirmed that these often have severe and rapidly progressive weakness associated with very high CK levels and respond initially to steroids. Furthermore, they demonstrated that muscle biopsies from these patients reveal abundant necrotic and regenerating fibers, but much less frequent lymphocytic inflammation than seen in patients with DM or PM. As in DM, anti-SRP-positive patients had reduced numbers of capillaries, enlarged capillaries, and capillaries that stained positive for deposition of the membrane attack complex (MAC). However, these patients had neither characteristic rashes nor evidence of perifascicular atrophy as seen in DM.

Subsequently, Kao published a study examining a larger cohort of 19 anti-SRP-positive patients.[132] This confirmed the severity of the initial disease and reported that multiple immunosuppressive medications were frequently required for its control. Despite this, there was no significant difference in 5-year mortality rates between SPR-positive and SRP-negative patients. Like others, these investigators found that muscle biopsies from most of these patients have relatively sparse inflammation, with abundant myofiber degeneration and regeneration; capillary deposition of MAC was observed in 67%. Interestingly, they identified three anti-SRP-positive patients who did not have active muscle disease. Of these, two had systemic sclerosis and one had features of the antisynthetase syndrome, suggesting that these antibodies may not be specific for PM.

Another study of 23 anti-SRP-positive patients confirmed that this antibody is associated with a unique syndrome characterized by a necrotizing muscle biopsy, severe weakness, dysphagia, and high CK levels.[133] Three of these patients had DM. However, myofibers from SRP-positive patients did not stain positive for MHC-I. In contrast to the prior reports, these investigators found MAC deposition only in necrotic muscle fibers, but not on capillaries.

Although patients with anti-SRP autoantibodies have a unique phenotype distinguished by a relative absence of inflammation and abundant myofiber degeneration, the pathologic relevance of these antibodies remains unclear. Future studies will be required to determine what causes their production, whether titers correlate with disease activity, and whether the antibodies play a direct role in mediating muscle damage. It should also be noted that some patients with autoimmune necrotizing myopathies do not have anti-SRP antibodies. Whether these individuals have heretofore unidentified autoantibodies remains to be determined.

Anti-155/140, a DM and cancer-associated MSA

Although the identities of the autoantigens recognized by these antibodies have not been definitively established, two recent papers, one by Kaji and colleagues and another by Targoff and colleagues, reported novel MSAs recognizing 155 and 140 kDA proteins.[134,135] Each group found that the anti-155/140 autoantibody is both highly specific for DM and relatively common, being found in 13–21% of DM patients. Furthermore, each study found that anti-155/140-positive patients had a markedly higher rate of malignancy than seen in DM patients negative for this antibody (e.g., 71% vs. 11%[134]). This was confirmed in another study showing that 8/19 (42%) anti-155/140-positive DM patients had cancer.

Targoff and his associates found a lower frequency of ILD in DM patients with the 155/140 autoantibody compared with other DM patients.[135] Although Kaji and coworkers found that DM patients with anti-155/140 autoantibodies were more likely to have a heliotrope rash and Gottron's papules/sign, Targoff and colleagues found no difference in such clinical features between these groups. This disparity could reflect differences between the Japanese DM population examined by Kaji and the population of subjects studied at the National Institutes of Health in Targoff's study.

Interestingly, these and other researchers have found that anti-155/140 is also found in patients with the juvenile form of DM.[136] This is especially remarkable because the presence of other MSAs in juvenile DM is rare. Further studies will be needed to confirm the identity of the autoantigens recognized by anti-155/140 autoantibodies and to clarify their potential pathologic role.

Epidemiology and genetics

Myositis, including both DM and PM, is a rare disease. Comprehensive epidemiologic data are lacking, but most studies suggest that myositis occurs in about 1 per 100,000 people annually.[3] DM can occur at any age, but there appears to be a peak in the 30–50-year age range. As with many other autoimmune diseases, there is a strong gender bias in myositis, with roughly twice as many women affected as men.

Numerous studies suggest that some individuals may be genetically susceptible to developing inflammatory myopathy, including DM. For example, the immunoglobulin gamma heavy chain Gm 3 23 5,13 phenotype is associated with DM in Caucasian patients,[137] and certain HLA alleles, especially those associated with the 8.1 ancestral haplotype (8.1 AH), may also confer increased risk or protection from DM.[138,139]

Interestingly, the −308A polymorphism in the tumor necrosis factor (TNF) gene promoter is overrepresented in DM patients compared with controls.[140–146] The presence of the TNF-α-308A allele, also associated with systemic lupus erythematosus, leads to increased keratinocyte apoptosis following exposure to UV light[147] and may increase susceptibility to light-induced skin damage. Furthermore, in both DM and lupus, this allele may predispose patients to the characteristic photosensitive rashes through increased production of TNF-α.[142]

Multiple studies have demonstrated a positive relationship between certain MHC Class II alleles and the development of PM.[105,148] Additionally, PM alone is weakly associated with a particular SNP within an intronic region coding for IFN-γ.[149] In contrast, another HLA factor allele (DQA∗0201) is protective for PM; interestingly this allele is also protective for IBM which, like PM, is characterized by T cell infiltrates.[138]

In addition to these positive and negative associations with either DM or PM, numerous studies have demonstrated that some genetic backgrounds, particularly alleles constituting the Caucasian 8.1 AH, are associated with the presence of particular

MSAs and MAAs.[104,105,137–139,150–152] For example, although alleles of the 8.1 AH are risk factors for the development myositis with or without autoantibodies, they are more strongly associated with production of anti-Jo-1. One instance of this is the DRB1*0301 allele, which is a risk factor for myositis irrespective of autoantibody production, with an odds ratio of 3.6; strikingly, the odds ratio associated with this allele in anti-Jo-1 patients is 15.5.[139] In contrast, DRB1*0701 and DQA1*0201 alleles seem to be protective for the development of anti-Jo-1 but significant risk factors for the development of anti-Mi-2.[104,139,151,153,154] As has been pointed out by others, this is consistent with the fact that individual patients may produce either anti-Jo-1 or anti-Mi-2, but not both.

Other noteworthy examples of immunogenetic associations with MSA production include the observation that anti-PL-7 autoantibodies are positively associated with a unique HLA Class I allele (Cw*0304) distinct from the markers associated with other antisynthetase antibodies.[139] In contrast, anti-PL-7 is negatively associated with DQA1*0501. Finally, the production of anti-SRP antibodies is positively associated with HLA-B*5001 and DQA1*0104[139] and, in African-Americans, the GM 6 immunoglobulin gamma heavy chain allotype.[137]

As has been shown in other autoimmune diseases (such as myasthenia gravis), these immunogenetic associations underscore the importance of the 8.1 AH and other immune-related alleles in the development of myositis. However, it should be noted that very few of the many individuals who harbor these alleles will ever develop an autoimmune disease. Presumably, autoimmune disease is only initiated when these predisposing alleles interact with other important genetic and environmental factors. Furthermore, it should be noted that in clinical practice the presence of autoimmune muscle disease in more than one family member is an exceptional occurrence and strongly suggests the presence of an inherited muscular dystrophy or metabolic myopathy.

Myositis and malignancy

Since the first two cases of malignancy-associated DM were reported in 1916,[155,156] multiple studies have confirmed this connection.[157–159] The largest population-based study, utilizing the national databases of Sweden, Denmark, and Finland, identified 618 DM and 914 PM patients.[160] In this cohort, cancer was detected in 32% of DM and 15% of PM patients; this represented an increased risk compared with the rest of the population, with standardized incidence ratios (SIRs) of 3.0 for DM and 1.3 for PM. Although a variety of different tumors were identified, adenocarcinomas were the most common and represented about 70% of these malignancies. Most cancers were detected within 1 year of myositis diagnosis, but DM patients were still at increased risk for malignancy even 5 years later. Cancers were also found at an increased rate in DM patients up to 2 years prior to the development of myositis, suggesting that DM may be a paraneoplastic process in some patients.

A similar study from Australian databases found malignant disease in 104/537 patients with inflammatory myopathies.[161] In about 60% of cases, the cancer was found within 1 week of the diagnosis of myositis. Patients with DM and PM had SIRs of 6.2 and 2.0, respectively, for the presence of malignancy. In another recent publication, 37 cases of malignancy were found in 309 myositis patients seen in Hungarian clinics over a 21-year period.[162] These patients required more aggressive immunosuppression than other patients with myositis. Although successful treatment of the cancer also improved the muscle disease, patients with cancer had worse survival rates than those without cancer.

There is currently no consensus regarding what cancer screening tests should be performed—or how frequently—in patients diagnosed with myositis. However, it is noteworthy that elevated CA-125 levels at the time of myositis diagnosis have been associated with an increased risk for developing a solid malignancy over the next 5 years; this was true even in those who had unrevealing conventional malignancy screening, including pancomputed tomography scans and upper/lower gastrointestinal endoscopy.[163] Furthermore, Chinoy and associates found that patients with most MSAs and MAAs are at a decreased risk for malignancy.[164] For example, out of 66 patients with antisynthetase antibodies, only one had cancer. None of the seven anti-SRP patients and only 2/18 anti-Mi-2-positive patients had cancer. The notable exception, as discussed above, were those DM patients with anti-155/140; of 19 such patients 8 had cancer. Taken together, these findings suggest that patients who are negative for anti-155/140, are positive for one of the other MSAs, and have normal CA-125 levels may not require an extensive malignancy evaluation.

Finally on the topic of cancer and myositis, it should be noted that Cao and colleagues found that 4 of their 16 patients with amyopathic DM had associated malignancies[55]; two of these cases were discovered at the time of diagnosis and two found more than 2 years later. This suggests that these patients, like those with muscle involvement, may require cancer screening at the time of diagnosis and, perhaps, on a routine basis for a number of years following that.

A model of autoimmune muscle disease pathogenesis

Despite concerted efforts over many years, the pathologic mechanisms leading to the initiation and propagation of autoimmune muscle disease remain obscure. For example, what is the pathologic relevance of the MSAs, which, unlike those recognizing the acetylcholine receptor in myasthenia gravis, target ubiquitously expressed intracellular proteins? Why are myositis autoantigens targeted while other muscle proteins are not? Is it significant that virtually all well-characterized myositis autoantigens bind DNA (e.g., Mi-2) or RNA (e.g., aminoacyl-tRNA synthetases and SRP)? What are environmental factors that trigger myositis in genetically susceptible individuals? Why is it that patients with autoimmune myositis are at increased risk for cancer?

While these questions remain unanswered, one recently proposed model attempts to synthesize some of the key findings already summarized in this review. Casciola-Rosen,[127] Levine,[165] Suber,[166] and their respective collaborators have noted that myositis autoantigens such as Jo-1 and Mi-2 are expressed at low levels in normal muscle but at high levels in regenerating muscle fibers.[127] Similarly, myositis autoantigens are expressed at low levels in most normal tissues, but are expressed at high levels in cancerous tissue such as breast and lung adenocarcinomas.[127] These authors have proposed that an anticancer immune response may target myositis autoantigens expressed at high levels in these tumors where atypical processing could generate novel epitopes not recognized as self. Typically, an effective immune response would result in eradication of the tumor prior to its detection with no adverse consequences. However, in a genetically susceptible host with concurrent muscle regeneration (secondary to viral infection or myotoxins, for example), the antitumor response could be redirected to regenerating myofibers that also express high levels of myositis autoantigens. (Since skin cells exposed to UV light also have increased expression of myositis autoantigens,[126] a similar mechanism could potentially underlie the targeting of skin in DM.) Cytokines, produced by infiltrating leukocytes, could upregulate MHC-I expression on muscle and thereby facilitate their killing by cytotoxic T cells. This would initiate further myofiber regeneration and increased production of myositis autoantigens, thus initiating a self-sustaining immune response against muscle. In instances where the immune response was insufficient to destroy the inciting tumor, autoimmune muscle disease and cancer would be found together. Although intriguing, future work will be required to test this model of myositis initiation and propagation.

Acknowledgments

Dr. Mammen is supported by the NIH (grant K08-AR-054783).

Conflicts of interest

The author declares no conflicts of interest.

References

1. Bohan, A. & J.B. Peter. 1975. Polymyositis and dermatomyositis (first of two parts). *N. Engl. J. Med.* **292:** 344–347.

2. Bohan, A. & J.B. Peter. 1975. Polymyositis and dermatomyositis (second of two parts). *N. Engl. J. Med.* **292:** 403–407.

3. Dalakas, M.C. & R. Hohlfeld. 2003. Polymyositis and dermatomyositis. *Lancet* **362:** 971–982.

4. Karpati, G. & E.K. O'Ferrall. 2009. Sporadic inclusion body myositis: pathogenic considerations. *Ann. Neurol.* **65:** 7–11.

5. Wagner, E. 1863. Fall einer seltnen Muskelkrankheit. *Dtsch. Arch. Heilk.* **4:** 282.

6. Hepp, P. 1887. Ueber einen Fall von acuter parenchymatoser Myositis, welche Geschwulste bildete und Fluctuation vortauschte. *Klin. Wochenschr.* **24:** 389.

7. Unverricht, H. 1887. Polymyositis acuta progressive. *Z. Klin. Med.* **12:** 553.

8. Unverricht, H. 1891. Dermatomyositis acuta. *Dtsch. Med. Wochenschr.* **17:** 41.

9. Eaton, L.M. 1954. The perspective of neurology in regard to polymyositis; a study of 41 cases. *Neurology* **4:** 245–263.

10. Walton, J.M. & R.D. Adams. 1958. *Polymyositis.* E & S Livingstone. Edinburgh.

11. Rowland, L.P. 1958. Muscular dystrophies, polymyositis, and other myopathies. *J. Chronic Dis.* **8:** 510–535.

12. Pearson, C.M. & A.S. Rose. 1960. Myositis: the inflammatory disorders of muscle. *Res. Publ. Assoc. Res. Nerv. Ment. Dis.* **38:** 422.

13. Emslie-Smith, A.M. & A.G. Engel. 1990. Microvascular changes in early and advanced dermatomyositis: a quantitative study. *Ann. Neurol.* **27:** 343–356.

14. Kissel, J.T., J.R. Mendell & K.W. Rammohan. 1986. Microvascular deposition of complement membrane attack complex in dermatomyositis. *N. Engl. J. Med.* **314:** 329–334.

15. Kissel, J.T., R.K. Halterman, K.W. Rammohan, *et al.* 1991. The relationship of complement-mediated microvasculopathy to the histologic features and clinical duration of disease in dermatomyositis. *Arch. Neurol.* **48:** 26–30.

16. Nagaraju, K., L.G. Rider, C. Fan, *et al.* 2006. Endothelial cell activation and neovascularization are prominent in dermatomyositis. *J. Autoimmune Dis.* **3:** 2.

17. Grundtman, C., E. Tham, A.K. Ulfgren, *et al.* 2008. Vascular endothelial growth factor is highly expressed in muscle tissue of patients with polymyositis and patients with dermatomyositis. *Arthritis Rheum.* **58:** 3224–3238.

18. Karpati, G., S. Carpenter, C. Melmed, *et al.* 1974. Experimental ischemic myopathy. *J. Neurol. Sci.* **23:** 129–161.

19. Hathaway, P.W., W.K. Engel & H. Zellweger. 1970. Experimental myopathy after microarterial embolization; comparison with childhood x-linked pseudohypertrophic muscular dystrophy. *Arch. Neurol.* **22:** 365–378.

20. Arahata, K. & A.G. Engel. 1984. Monoclonal antibody analysis of mononuclear cells in myopathies. I: Quantitation of subsets according to diagnosis and sites of accumulation and demonstration and counts of muscle fibers invaded by T cells. *Ann. Neurol.* **16:** 193–208.

21. Greenberg, S.A., J.L. Pinkus, G.S. Pinkus, *et al.* 2005. Interferon-alpha/beta-mediated innate immune mechanisms in dermatomyositis. *Ann. Neurol.* **57:** 664–678.

22. Siegal, F.P., N. Kadowaki, M. Shodell, *et al.* 1999. The nature of the principal type 1 interferon-producing cells in human blood. *Science* **284:** 1835–1837.

23. Walsh, R.J., S.W. Kong, Y. Yao, *et al.* 2007. Type I interferon-inducible gene expression in blood is present and reflects disease activity in dermatomyositis and polymyositis. *Arthritis Rheum.* **56:** 3784–3792.

24. Baechler, E.C., J.W. Bauer, C.A. Slattery, *et al.* 2007. An interferon signature in the peripheral blood of dermatomyositis patients is associated with disease activity. *Mol. Med.* **13:** 59–68.

25. Arahata, K. & A.G. Engel. 1986. Monoclonal antibody analysis of mononuclear cells in myopathies. III: Immunoelectron microscopy aspects of cell-mediated muscle fiber injury. *Ann. Neurol.* **19:** 112–125.

26. Dalakas, M.C. 1991. Polymyositis, dermatomyositis and inclusion-body myositis. *N. Engl. J. Med.* **325:** 1487–1498.

27. Appleyard, S.T., M.J. Dunn, V. Dubowitz, *et al.* 1985. Increased expression of HLA ABC class I antigens by muscle fibres in Duchenne muscular dystrophy, inflammatory myopathy, and other neuromuscular disorders. *Lancet* **1:** 361–363.

28. Karpati, G., Y. Pouliot & S. Carpenter. 1988. Expression of immunoreactive major histocompatibility complex products in human skeletal muscles. *Ann. Neurol.* **23:** 64–72.

29. Nagaraju, K., N. Raben, L. Loeffler, *et al.* 2000. Conditional up-regulation of MHC class I in skeletal muscle leads to self-sustaining autoimmune myositis and myositis-specific autoantibodies. *Proc. Natl. Acad. Sci. USA* **97:** 9209–9214.

30. Nagaraju, K., L. Casciola-Rosen, I. Lundberg, *et al.* 2005. Activation of the endoplasmic reticulum stress response in autoimmune myositis: potential role in muscle fiber damage and dysfunction. *Arthritis Rheum.* **52:** 1824–1835.

31. Goebels, N., D. Michaelis, M. Engelhardt, *et al.* 1996. Differential expression of perforin in muscle-infiltrating T cells in polymyositis and dermatomyositis. *J. Clin. Invest.* **97:** 2905–2910.

32. Behrens, L., A. Bender, M.A. Johnson, *et al.* 1997. Cytotoxic mechanisms in inflammatory myopathies. Coexpression of Fas and protective Bcl-2 in muscle fibres and inflammatory cells. *Brain* **120**(Pt 6): 929–938.

33. Schneider, C., R. Gold, M.C. Dalakas, *et al.* 1996. MHC class I-mediated cytotoxicity does not induce apoptosis in muscle fibers nor in inflammatory T cells:

studies in patients with polymyositis, dermatomyositis, and inclusion body myositis. *J. Neuropathol. Exp. Neurol.* **55:** 1205–1209.

34. Vattemi, G., P. Tonin, M. Filosto, *et al.* 2000. T-cell anti-apoptotic mechanisms in inflammatory myopathies. *J. Neuroimmunol.* **111:** 146–151.

35. Nagaraju, K., L. Casciola-Rosen, A. Rosen, *et al.* 2000. The inhibition of apoptosis in myositis and in normal muscle cells. *J. Immunol.* **164:** 5459–5465.

36. Lundberg, I.E. & C. Grundtman. 2008. Developments in the scientific and clinical understanding of inflammatory myopathies. *Arthritis Res. Ther.* **10:** 220.

37. Lundberg, I., A.K. Ulfgren, P. Nyberg, *et al.* 1997. Cytokine production in muscle tissue of patients with idiopathic inflammatory myopathies. *Arthritis Rheum.* **40:** 865–874.

38. Page, G., G. Chevrel & P. Miossec. 2004. Anatomic localization of immature and mature dendritic cell subsets in dermatomyositis and polymyositis: Interaction with chemokines and Th1 cytokine-producing cells. *Arthritis Rheum.* **50:** 199–208.

39. Lundberg, I., J.M. Brengman & A.G. Engel. 1995. Analysis of cytokine expression in muscle in inflammatory myopathies, Duchenne dystrophy, and non-weak controls. *J. Neuroimmunol.* **63:** 9–16.

40. Tews, D.S. & H.H. Goebel. 1996. Cytokine expression profile in idiopathic inflammatory myopathies. *J. Neuropathol. Exp. Neurol.* **55:** 342–347.

41. Lepidi, H., V. Frances, D. Figarella-Branger, *et al.* 1998. Local expression of cytokines in idiopathic inflammatory myopathies. *Neuropathol. Appl. Neurobiol.* **24:** 73–79.

42. Greenberg, S.A., E.M. Bradshaw, J.L. Pinkus, *et al.* 2005. Plasma cells in muscle in inclusion body myositis and polymyositis. *Neurology* **65:** 1782–1787.

43. Callen, J.P. 2000. Dermatomyositis. *Lancet* **355:** 53–57.

44. Dugan, E.M., A.M. Huber, F.W. Miller, *et al.* 2009. Review of the classification and assessment of the cutaneous manifestations of the idiopathic inflammatory myopathies. *Dermatol. Online J.* **15:** 2.

45. Dugan, E.M., A.M. Huber, F.W. Miller, *et al.* 2009. Photoessay of the cutaneous manifestations of the idiopathic inflammatory myopathies. *Dermatol. Online J.* **15:** 1.

46. Bridges, B.F. 1991. The rashes of dermatomyositis in a black patient. *Am. J. Med.* **91:** 661–662.

47. Keil, H. 1942. The manifestations in the skin and mucous membranes in dermatomyositis, with special reference to the differential diagnosis from systemic lupus erythematosus. *Ann. Intern. Med.* **16:** 828.

48. Ghali, F.E., L.D. Stein, J.D. Fine, *et al.* 1999. Gingival telangiectases: an underappreciated physical sign of juvenile dermatomyositis. *Arch. Dermatol.* **135:** 1370–1374.

49. Cheong, W.K., G.R. Hughes, P.G. Norris, *et al.* 1994. Cutaneous photosensitivity in dermatomyositis. *Br. J. Dermatol.* **131:** 205–208.

50. Dourmishev, L., H. Meffert & H. Piazena. 2004. Dermatomyositis: comparative studies of cutaneous photosensitivity in lupus erythematosus and normal subjects. *Photodermatol. Photoimmunol. Photomed.* **20:** 230–234.

51. Euwer, R.L. & R.D. Sontheimer. 1991. Amyopathic dermatomyositis (dermatomyositis sine myositis). Presentation of six new cases and review of the literature. *J. Am. Acad. Dermatol.* **24:** 959–966.

52. Rockerbie, N.R., T.Y. Woo, J.P. Callen, *et al.* 1989. Cutaneous changes of dermatomyositis precede muscle weakness. *J. Am. Acad. Dermatol.* **20:** 629–632.

53. Stonecipher, M.R., J.L. Jorizzo, W.L. White, *et al.* 1993. Cutaneous changes of dermatomyositis in patients with normal muscle enzymes: dermatomyositis sine myositis? *J. Am. Acad. Dermatol.* **28:** 951–956.

54. Cosnes, A., F. Amaudric, R. Gherardi, *et al.* 1995. Dermatomyositis without muscle weakness. Long-term follow-up of 12 patients without systemic corticosteroids. *Arch. Dermatol.* **131:** 1381–1385.

55. Cao, H., T.N. Parikh & J. Zheng. 2009. Amyopathic dermatomyositis or dermatomyositis-like skin disease: retrospective review of 16 cases with amyopathic dermatomyositis. *Clin. Rheumatol.* **28:** 979–984.

56. Crowson, A.N., C.M. Magro & M.C. Mihm Jr. 2008. Interface dermatitis. *Arch. Pathol. Lab. Med.* **132:** 652–666.

57. Dourmishev, L.A. & U. Wollina. 2006. Dermatomyositis: immunopathologic study of skin lesions. *Acta Dermatovenerol. Alp. Panonica Adriat.* **15:** 45–51.

58. Mascaro, J.M., Jr., G. Hausmann, C. Herrero, *et al.* 1995. Membrane attack complex deposits in cutaneous lesions of dermatomyositis. *Arch. Dermatol.* **131:** 1386–1392.

59. Crowson, A.N. & C.M. Magro. 1996. The role of microvascular injury in the pathogenesis of cutaneous lesions of dermatomyositis. *Hum. Pathol.* **27:** 15–19.

60. Hengstman, G.J., L. van Brenk, W.T. Vree Egberts, *et al.* 2005. High specificity of myositis specific autoantibodies for myositis compared with other neuromuscular disorders. *J. Neurol.* **252:** 534–537.

61. Nishikai, M. & M. Reichlin. 1980. Heterogeneity of precipitating antibodies in polymyositis and

dermatomyositis. Characterization of the Jo-1 antibody system. *Arthritis Rheum.* **23:** 881–888.

62. Yoshida, S., M. Akizuki, T. Mimori, *et al.* 1983. The precipitating antibody to an acidic nuclear protein antigen, the Jo-1, in connective tissue diseases. A marker for a subset of polymyositis with interstitial pulmonary fibrosis. *Arthritis Rheum.* **26:** 604–611.

63. Marguerie, C., C.C. Bunn, H.L. Beynon, *et al.* 1990. Polymyositis, pulmonary fibrosis and autoantibodies to aminoacyl-tRNA synthetase enzymes. *Q. J. Med.* **77:** 1019–1038.

64. Mathews, M.B., M. Reichlin, G.R. Hughes, *et al.* 1984. Anti-threonyl-tRNA synthetase, a second myositis-related autoantibody. *J. Exp. Med.* **160:** 420–434.

65. Bunn, C.C., R.M. Bernstein & M.B. Mathews. 1986. Autoantibodies against alanyl-tRNA synthetase and tRNAAla coexist and are associated with myositis. *J. Exp. Med.* **163:** 1281–1291.

66. Targoff, I.N. 1990. Autoantibodies to aminoacyl-transfer RNA synthetases for isoleucine and glycine. Two additional synthetases are antigenic in myositis. *J. Immunol.* **144:** 1737–1743.

67. Hirakata, M., A. Suwa, S. Nagai, *et al.* 1999. Anti-KS: identification of autoantibodies to asparaginyl-transfer RNA synthetase associated with interstitial lung disease. *J. Immunol.* **162:** 2315–2320.

68. Hashish, L., E.P. Trieu, P. Sadanandan, *et al.* 2005. Identification of autoantibodies to tyrosyl-tRNA synthetase in dermatomyositis with features consistent with anti-synthetase syndrome (abstract). *Arthritis Rheum.* **52:** S312.

69. Betteridge, Z., H. Gunawardena, J. North, *et al.* 2007. Anti-synthetase syndrome: a new autoantibody to phenylalanyl transfer RNA synthetase (anti-Zo) associated with polymyositis and interstitial pneumonia. *Rheumatology (Oxford)* **46:** 1005–1008.

70. Hirakata, M. 2005. Autoantibodies to aminoacyl-tRNA synthetases. *Intern. Med.* **44:** 527–528.

71. Targoff, I.N. 2002. Laboratory testing in the diagnosis and management of idiopathic inflammatory myopathies. *Rheum. Dis. Clin. North Am.* **28:** 859–890, viii.

72. Kalluri, M., S.A. Sahn, C.V. Oddis, *et al.* 2009. Clinical profile of anti-PL-12 autoantibody: Cohort study and review of the literature. *Chest* **135:** 1550–1556.

73. Arsura, E.L. & A.S. Greenberg. 1988. Adverse impact of interstitial pulmonary fibrosis on prognosis in polymyositis and dermatomyositis. *Semin. Arthritis Rheum.* **18:** 29–37.

74. Marie, I., E. Hachulla, P. Cherin, *et al.* 2002. Intersti-

tial lung disease in polymyositis and dermatomyositis. *Arthritis Rheum.* **47:** 614–622.

75. Douglas, W.W., H.D. Tazelaar, T.E. Hartman, *et al.* 2001. Polymyositis-dermatomyositis-associated interstitial lung disease. *Am. J. Respir. Crit. Care Med.* **164:** 1182–1185.

76. Friedman, A.W., I.N. Targoff & F.C. Arnett. 1996. Interstitial lung disease with autoantibodies against aminoacyl-tRNA synthetases in the absence of clinically apparent myositis. *Semin. Arthritis Rheum.* **26:** 459–467.

77. Yoshifuji, H., T. Fujii, S. Kobayashi, *et al.* 2006. Anti-aminoacyl-tRNA synthetase antibodies in clinical course prediction of interstitial lung disease complicated with idiopathic inflammatory myopathies. *Autoimmunity* **39:** 233–241.

78. Targoff, I.N. 2008. Autoantibodies and their significance in myositis. *Curr. Rheumatol. Rep.* **10:** 333–340.

79. Fathi, M., J. Vikgren, M. Boijsen, *et al.* 2008. Interstitial lung disease in polymyositis and dermatomyositis: longitudinal evaluation by pulmonary function and radiology. *Arthritis Rheum.* **59:** 677–685.

80. Klein, R.Q., V. Teal, L. Taylor, *et al.* 2007. Number, characteristics, and classification of patients with dermatomyositis seen by dermatology and rheumatology departments at a large tertiary medical center. *J. Am. Acad. Dermatol.* **57:** 937–943.

81. Selva-O'Callaghan, A., M. Labrador-Horrillo, R. Solans-Laque, *et al.* 2006. Myositis-specific and myositis-associated antibodies in a series of eighty-eight Mediterranean patients with idiopathic inflammatory myopathy. *Arthritis Rheum.* **55:** 791–798.

82. Spath, M., M. Schroder, B. Schlotter-Weigel, *et al.* 2004. The long-term outcome of anti-Jo-1-positive inflammatory myopathies. *J. Neurol.* **251:** 859–864.

83. Lundberg, I.E. & C.J. Forbess. 2008. Mortality in idiopathic inflammatory myopathies. *Clin. Exp. Rheumatol.* **26:** S109–S114.

84. Medsger, T.A., Jr, H. Robinson & A.T. Masi. 1971. Factors affecting survivorship in polymyositis. A life-table study of 124 patients. *Arthritis Rheum.* **14:** 249–258.

85. Marie, I., E. Hachulla, P.Y. Hatron, *et al.* 2001. Polymyositis and dermatomyositis: short term and longterm outcome, and predictive factors of prognosis. *J. Rheumatol.* **28:** 2230–2237.

86. Sultan, S.M., Y. Ioannou, K. Moss, *et al.* 2002. Outcome in patients with idiopathic inflammatory myositis: morbidity and mortality. *Rheumatology (Oxford)* **41:** 22–26.

87. Danko, K., A. Ponyi, T. Constantin, *et al.* 2004. Long-term survival of patients with idiopathic inflammatory myopathies according to clinical features: a longitudinal study of 162 cases. *Medicine (Baltimore)* **83:** 35–42.

88. Airio, A., H. Kautiainen & M. Hakala. 2006. Prognosis and mortality of polymyositis and dermatomyositis patients. *Clin. Rheumatol.* **25:** 234–239.

89. Torres, C., R. Belmonte, L. Carmona, *et al.* 2006. Survival, mortality and causes of death in inflammatory myopathies. *Autoimmunity* **39:** 205–215.

90. Raben, N., R. Nichols, J. Dohlman, *et al.* 1994. A motif in human histidyl-tRNA synthetase which is shared among several aminoacyl-tRNA synthetases is a coiled-coil that is essential for enzymatic activity and contains the major autoantigenic epitope. *J. Biol. Chem.* **269:** 24277–24283.

91. Martin, A., M.J. Shulman & F.W. Tsui. 1995. Epitope studies indicate that histidyl-tRNA synthetase is a stimulating antigen in idiopathic myositis. *FASEB J.* **9:** 1226–1233.

92. Miller, F.W., S.A. Twitty, T. Biswas, *et al.* 1990. Origin and regulation of a disease-specific autoantibody response. Antigenic epitopes, spectrotype stability, and isotype restriction of anti-Jo-1 autoantibodies. *J. Clin. Invest.* **85:** 468–475.

93. Miller, F.W., K.A. Waite, T. Biswas, *et al.* 1990. The role of an autoantigen, histidyl-tRNA synthetase, in the induction and maintenance of autoimmunity. *Proc. Natl. Acad. Sci. USA* **87:** 9933–9937.

94. Bernstein, R.M., S.H. Morgan, J. Chapman, *et al.* 1984. Anti-Jo-1 antibody: a marker for myositis with interstitial lung disease. *Br. Med. J. (Clin. Res. Ed.)* **289:** 151–152.

95. Stone, K.B., C.V. Oddis, N. Fertig, *et al.* 2007. Anti-Jo-1 antibody levels correlate with disease activity in idiopathic inflammatory myopathy. *Arthritis Rheum.* **56:** 3125–3131.

96. Levine, S.M., N. Raben, D. Xie, *et al.* 2007. Novel conformation of histidyl-transfer RNA synthetase in the lung: the target tissue in Jo-1 autoantibody-associated myositis. *Arthritis Rheum.* **56:** 2729–2739.

97. Casciola-Rosen, L., F. Andrade, D. Ulanet, *et al.* 1999. Cleavage by granzyme B is strongly predictive of autoantigen status: implications for initiation of autoimmunity. *J. Exp. Med.* **190:** 815–826.

98. Katsumata, Y., W.M. Ridgway, T. Oriss, *et al.* 2007. Species-specific immune responses generated by histidyl-tRNA synthetase immunization are associated with muscle and lung inflammation. *J. Autoimmun.* **29:** 174–186.

99. Howard, O.M., H.F. Dong, D. Yang, *et al.* 2002. Histidyl-tRNA synthetase and asparaginyl-tRNA synthetase, autoantigens in myositis, activate chemokine receptors on T lymphocytes and immature dendritic cells. *J. Exp. Med.* **196:** 781–791.

100. Reichlin, M. & M. Mattioli. 1976. Description of a serological reaction characteristic of polymyositis. *Clin. Immunol. Immunopathol.* **5:** 12–20.

101. Ghirardello, A., S. Zampieri, L. Iaccarino, *et al.* 2005. Anti-Mi-2 antibodies. *Autoimmunity* **38:** 79–83.

102. Targoff, I.N. & M. Reichlin. 1985. The association between Mi-2 antibodies and dermatomyositis. *Arthritis Rheum.* **28:** 796–803.

103. Targoff, I.N. 2006. Myositis specific autoantibodies. *Curr. Rheumatol. Rep.* **8:** 196–203.

104. Love, L.A., R.L. Leff, D.D. Fraser, *et al.* 1991. A new approach to the classification of idiopathic inflammatory myopathy: myositis-specific autoantibodies define useful homogeneous patient groups. *Medicine (Baltimore)* **70:** 360–374.

105. Arnett, F.C., I.N. Targoff, T. Mimori, *et al.* 1996. Interrelationship of major histocompatibility complex class II alleles and autoantibodies in four ethnic groups with various forms of myositis. *Arthritis Rheum.* **39:** 1507–1518.

106. Mierau, R., T. Dick, P. Bartz-Bazzanella, *et al.* 1996. Strong association of dermatomyositis-specific Mi-2 autoantibodies with a tryptophan at position 9 of the HLA-DR beta chain. *Arthritis Rheum.* **39:** 868–876.

107. Hausmanowa-Petrusewicz, I., E. Kowalska-Oledzka, F.W. Miller, *et al.* 1997. Clinical, serologic, and immunogenetic features in Polish patients with idiopathic inflammatory myopathies. *Arthritis Rheum.* **40:** 1257–1266.

108. Hengstman, G.J., W.T. Vree Egberts, H.P. Seelig, *et al.* 2006. Clinical characteristics of patients with myositis and autoantibodies to different fragments of the Mi-2 beta antigen. *Ann. Rheum. Dis.* **65:** 242–245.

109. Brouwer, R., G.J. Hengstman, W. Vree Egberts, *et al.* 2001. Autoantibody profiles in the sera of European patients with myositis. *Ann. Rheum. Dis.* **60:** 116–123.

110. Hengstman, G.J., R. Brouwer, W.T. Egberts, *et al.* 2002. Clinical and serological characteristics of 125 Dutch myositis patients. Myositis specific autoantibodies aid in the differential diagnosis of the idiopathic inflammatory myopathies. *J. Neurol.* **249:** 69–75.

111. Seelig, H.P., I. Moosbrugger, H. Ehrfeld, *et al.* 1995. The major dermatomyositis-specific Mi-2 autoantigen is a presumed helicase involved in transcriptional activation. *Arthritis Rheum.* **38:** 1389–1399.

112. Seelig, H.P., M. Renz, I.N. Targoff, *et al.* 1996. Two forms of the major antigenic protein of the dermatomyositis-specific Mi-2 autoantigen. *Arthritis Rheum.* **39:** 1769–1771.

113. Ge Q., D.S. Nilasena, C.A. O'Brien, *et al.* 1995. Molecular analysis of a major antigenic region of the 240-kD protein of Mi-2 autoantigen. *J. Clin. Invest.* **96:** 1730–1737.

114. Nilasena, D.S., E.P. Trieu & I.N. Targoff. 1995. Analysis of the Mi-2 autoantigen of dermatomyositis. *Arthritis Rheum.* **38:** 123–128.

115. Zhang, Y., G. LeRoy, H.P. Seelig, *et al.* 1998. The dermatomyositis-specific autoantigen Mi2 is a component of a complex containing histone deacetylase and nucleosome remodeling activities. *Cell* **95:** 279–289.

116. Wang, H.B. & Y. Zhang. 2001. Mi2, an auto-antigen for dermatomyositis, is an ATP-dependent nucleosome remodeling factor. *Nucleic Acids Res.* **29:** 2517–2521.

117. Shimono, Y., H. Murakami, K. Kawai, *et al.* 2003. Mi-2 beta associates with BRG1 and RET finger protein at the distinct regions with transcriptional activating and repressing abilities. *J. Biol. Chem.* **278:** 51638–51645.

118. Ahringer, J. 2000. NuRD and SIN3 histone deacetylase complexes in development. *Trends Genet.* **16:** 351–356.

119. Kehle, J., D. Beuchle, S. Treuheit, *et al.* 1998. dMi-2, a hunchback-interacting protein that functions in polycomb repression. *Science* **282:** 1897–1900.

120. Solari, F. & J. Ahringer. 2000. NURD-complex genes antagonise Ras-induced vulval development in Caenorhabditis elegans. *Curr. Biol.* **10:** 223–226.

121. Kashiwagi, M., B.A. Morgan & K. Georgopoulos. 2007. The chromatin remodeler Mi-2beta is required for establishment of the basal epidermis and normal differentiation of its progeny. *Development* **134:** 1571–1582.

122. Hengstman, G.J., W.T. Vree Egberts, H.P. Seelig, *et al.* 2006. Clinical characteristics of patients with myositis and autoantibodies to different fragments of the Mi-2 beta antigen. *Ann. Rheum. Dis.* **65:** 242–245.

123. Roux, S., H.P. Seelig & O. Meyer. 1998. Significance of Mi-2 autoantibodies in polymyositis and dermatomyositis. *J. Rheumatol.* **25:** 395–396.

124. Hengstman, G.J., W.J. van Venrooij, J. Vencovsky, *et al.* 2000. The relative prevalence of dermatomyositis and polymyositis in Europe exhibits a latitudinal gradient. *Ann. Rheum. Dis.* **59:** 141–142.

125. Okada, S., E. Weatherhead, I.N. Targoff, *et al.* 2003. Global surface ultraviolet radiation intensity may modulate the clinical and immunologic expression of autoimmune muscle disease. *Arthritis Rheum.* **48:** 2285–2293.

126. Burd, C.J., H.K. Kinyamu, F.W. Miller, *et al.* 2008. UV radiation regulates Mi-2 through protein translation and stability. *J. Biol. Chem.* **283:** 34976–34982.

127. Casciola-Rosen, L., K. Nagaraju, P. Plotz, *et al.* 2005. Enhanced autoantigen expression in regenerating muscle cells in idiopathic inflammatory myopathy. *J. Exp. Med.* **201:** 591–601.

128. Reeves, W.H., S.K. Nigam & G. Blobel. 1986. Human autoantibodies reactive with the signal-recognition particle. *Proc. Natl. Acad. Sci. USA* **83:** 9507–9511.

129. Satoh, T., T. Okano, T. Matsui, *et al.* 2005. Novel autoantibodies against 7SL RNA in patients with polymyositis/dermatomyositis. *J. Rheumatol.* **32:** 1727–1733.

130. Targoff, I.N., A.E. Johnson & F.W. Miller. 1990. Antibody to signal recognition particle in polymyositis. *Arthritis Rheum.* **33:** 1361–1370.

131. Miller, T., M.T. Al-Lozi, G. Lopate, *et al.* 2002. Myopathy with antibodies to the signal recognition particle: clinical and pathological features. *J. Neurol. Neurosurg. Psychiatry* **73:** 420–428.

132. Kao, A.H., D. Lacomis, M. Lucas, *et al.* 2004. Anti-signal recognition particle autoantibody in patients with and patients without idiopathic inflammatory myopathy. *Arthritis Rheum.* **50:** 209–215.

133. Hengstman, G.J., H.J. ter Laak, W.T. Vree Egberts, *et al.* 2006. Anti-signal recognition particle autoantibodies: marker of a necrotising myopathy. *Ann. Rheum. Dis.* **65:** 1635–1638.

134. Kaji, K., M. Fujimoto, M. Hasegawa, *et al.* 2007. Identification of a novel autoantibody reactive with 155 and 140 kDa nuclear proteins in patients with dermatomyositis: an association with malignancy. *Rheumatology (Oxford)* **46:** 25–28.

135. Targoff, I.N., G. Mamyrova, E.P. Trieu, *et al.* 2006. A novel autoantibody to a 155-kd protein is associated with dermatomyositis. *Arthritis Rheum.* **54:** 3682–3689.

136. Gunawardena, H., L.R. Wedderburn, J. North, *et al.* 2008. Clinical associations of autoantibodies to a p155/140 kDa doublet protein in juvenile dermatomyositis. *Rheumatology (Oxford)* **47:** 324–328.

137. O'Hanlon, T.P., L.G. Rider, A. Schiffenbauer, *et al.* 2008. Immunoglobulin gene polymorphisms are susceptibility factors in clinical and autoantibody subgroups of the idiopathic inflammatory myopathies. *Arthritis Rheum.* **58:** 3239–3246.

138. O'Hanlon, T.P., D.M. Carrick, F.C. Arnett, *et al.* 2005. Immunogenetic risk and protective factors for the idiopathic inflammatory myopathies: distinct HLA-A, -B, -Cw, -DRB1 and -DQA1 allelic profiles and motifs

define clinicopathologic groups in caucasians. *Medicine (Baltimore)* **84:** 338–349.

139. O'Hanlon, T.P., D.M. Carrick, I.N. Targoff, *et al.* 2006. Immunogenetic risk and protective factors for the idiopathic inflammatory myopathies: distinct HLA-A, -B, -Cw, -DRB1, and -DQA1 allelic profiles distinguish European American patients with different myositis autoantibodies. *Medicine (Baltimore)* **85:** 111–127.

140. Hassan, A.B., L. Nikitina-Zake, C.B. Sanjeevi, *et al.* 2004. Association of the proinflammatory haplotype (MICA5.1/TNF2/TNFa2/DRB1*03) with polymyositis and dermatomyositis. *Arthritis Rheum.* **50:** 1013–1015.

141. Chinoy, H., F. Salway, S. John, *et al.* 2007. Tumour necrosis factor-alpha single nucleotide polymorphisms are not independent of HLA class I in UK Caucasians with adult onset idiopathic inflammatory myopathies. *Rheumatology (Oxford)* **46:** 1411–1416.

142. Pachman, L.M., M.R. Liotta-Davis, D.K. Hong, *et al.* 2000. TNFalpha-308A allele in juvenile dermatomyositis: association with increased production of tumor necrosis factor alpha, disease duration, and pathologic calcifications. *Arthritis Rheum.* **43:** 2368–2377.

143. Mamyrova, G., T.P. O'Hanlon, L. Sillers, *et al.* 2008. Cytokine gene polymorphisms as risk and severity factors for juvenile dermatomyositis. *Arthritis Rheum.* **58:** 3941–3950.

144. Werth, V.P., J.P. Callen, G. Ang, *et al.* 2002. Associations of tumor necrosis factor alpha and HLA polymorphisms with adult dermatomyositis: implications for a unique pathogenesis. *J. Invest. Dermatol.* **119:** 617–620.

145. Lutz, J., K.G. Huwiler, T. Fedczyna, *et al.* 2002. Increased plasma thrombospondin-1 (TSP-1) levels are associated with the TNF alpha-308A allele in children with juvenile dermatomyositis. *Clin. Immunol.* **103:** 260–263.

146. Pachman, L.M., T.O. Fedczyna, T.S. Lechman, *et al.* 2001. Juvenile dermatomyositis: the association of the TNF alpha-308A allele and disease chronicity. *Curr. Rheumatol. Rep.* **3:** 379–386.

147. Werth, V.P., W. Zhang, K. Dortzbach, *et al.* 2000. Association of a promoter polymorphism of tumor necrosis factor-alpha with subacute cutaneous lupus erythematosus and distinct photoregulation of transcription. *J. Invest. Dermatol.* **115:** 726–730.

148. Garlepp, M.J. 1993. Immunogenetics of inflammatory myopathies. *Baillieres Clin. Neurol.* **2:** 579–597.

149. Chinoy, H., F. Salway, S. John, *et al.* 2007. Interferon-gamma and interleukin-4 gene polymorphisms in Caucasian idiopathic inflammatory myopathy patients in UK. *Ann. Rheum. Dis.* **66:** 970–973.

150. Franceschini, F. & I. Cavazzana. 2005. Anti-Ro/SSA and La/SSB antibodies. *Autoimmunity* **38:** 55–63.

151. Shamim, E.A., L.G. Rider, J.P. Pandey, *et al.* 2002. Differences in idiopathic inflammatory myopathy phenotypes and genotypes between Mesoamerican Mestizos and North American Caucasians: ethnogeographic influences in the genetics and clinical expression of myositis. *Arthritis Rheum.* **46:** 1885–1893.

152. Shamim, E.A., L.G. Rider & F.W. Miller. 2000. Update on the genetics of the idiopathic inflammatory myopathies. *Curr. Opin. Rheumatol.* **12:** 482–491.

153. Chinoy, H., W.E. Ollier & R.G. Cooper. 2004. Have recent immunogenetic investigations increased our understanding of disease mechanisms in the idiopathic inflammatory myopathies? *Curr. Opin. Rheumatol.* **16:** 707–713.

154. Mierau, R., T. Dick, E. Genth, *et al.* 1999. An update on HLA association of Mi-2 autoantibodies: the association with a tryptophan at position 9 of the HLA-DRbeta chain is strong but not absolute. *Arthritis Rheum.* **42:** 1552–1553.

155. Stertz, G. 1916. Polymyositis. *Berl. Klin. Wochenschr.* **53:** 489.

156. Kankeleit, H. 1916. Uber primaire nichteitrige Polymyositis. *Dtsch. Arch. Klin. Med.* **120:** 335.

157. Williams, R.C., Jr. 1959. Dermatomyositis and malignancy: a review of the literature. *Ann. Intern. Med.* **50:** 1174–1181.

158. Barnes, B.E. & B. Mawr. 1976. Dermatomyositis and malignancy. A review of the literature. *Ann. Intern. Med.* **84:** 68–76.

159. Sigurgeirsson, B., B. Lindelof, O. Edhag, *et al.* 1992. Risk of cancer in patients with dermatomyositis or polymyositis. A population-based study. *N. Engl. J. Med.* **326:** 363–367.

160. Hill, C.L., Y. Zhang, B. Sigurgeirsson, *et al.* 2001. Frequency of specific cancer types in dermatomyositis and polymyositis: a population-based study. *Lancet* **357:** 96–100.

161. Buchbinder, R., A. Forbes, S. Hall, *et al.* 2001. Incidence of malignant disease in biopsy-proven inflammatory myopathy. A population-based cohort study. *Ann. Intern. Med.* **134:** 1087–1095.

162. Andras, C., A. Ponyi, T. Constantin, *et al.* 2008. Dermatomyositis and polymyositis associated with malignancy: a 21-year retrospective study. *J. Rheumatol.* **35:** 438–444.

163. Amoura, Z., P. Duhaut, D.L. Huong, *et al.* 2005. Tumor antigen markers for the detection of solid cancers in

inflammatory myopathies. *Cancer Epidemiol. Biomarkers Prev.* **14:** 1279–1282.

164. Chinoy, H., N. Fertig, C.V. Oddis, *et al.* 2007. The diagnostic utility of myositis autoantibody testing for predicting the risk of cancer-associated myositis. *Ann. Rheum. Dis.* **66:** 1345–1349.

165. Levine, S.M. 2006. Cancer and myositis: new insights into an old association. *Curr. Opin. Rheumatol.* **18:** 620–624.

166. Suber, T.L., L. Casciola-Rosen & A. Rosen. 2008. Mechanisms of disease: autoantigens as clues to the pathogenesis of myositis. *Nat. Clin. Pract. Rheumatol.* **4:** 201–209.

Ann. N.Y. Acad. Sci. ISSN 0077-8923

ANNALS OF THE NEW YORK ACADEMY OF SCIENCES

Advances in the treatment of neurodegenerative disorders employing nanotechnology

Girish Modi,[1] Viness Pillay,[2] and Yahya E. Choonara[2]

[1]Department of Neurology, Division of Neurosciences, University of the Witwatersrand, Johannesburg, South Africa. [2]Department of Pharmacy and Pharmacology, University of the Witwatersrand, Johannesburg, South Africa

Address for correspondence: Prof. Girish Modi, Department of Neurology, Division of Neurosciences, University of the Witwatersrand, Johannesburg, South Africa. Voice: +27836012878; fax: +27114847576. gmodicns@mweb.co.za

Due to limitations posed by the restrictive blood–brain barrier, conventional drug delivery systems do not provide adequate cyto-architecture restoration and connection patterns that are essential for functional recovery in neurodegenerative disorders (NDs). Nanotechnology employs engineered materials or devices that interact with biological systems at a molecular level and could revolutionize the treatment of NDs by stimulating, responding to, and interacting with target sites to induce physiological responses while minimizing side effects. This review provides a concise discussion of the current applications of nano-enabled drug-delivery systems for the treatment of NDs, in particular Alzheimer's and Parkinson's diseases, and explores the future applications of nanotechnology in clinical neuroscience to develop innovative therapeutic modalities for the treatment of NDs.

Keywords: nanotechnology; neuroscience; nanoscience; neurobiology; nanoparticles; nanostructured; nanobiotechnology; blood–brain barrier; engineered nanomaterials; multifunctional nanoparticles; polymers; drug delivery; drug targeting; site-specific; Alzheimer's disease; Parkinson's disease

Introduction

Advances in biotechnology are expected to have a major impact in neurological research leading especially to the development of newer and more directed therapeutic modalities. Nanotechnology is at the core of these advances. Nanotechnology employs engineered polymeric materials to design devices with the smallest functional organization on the nanometer scale (1–100 nm) that are able to interact with biological systems at a molecular level. They may stimulate, respond to, and interact with target cells and tissues to induce desired physiological responses while simultaneously minimizing undesirable side effects. Importantly, nanotechnology may offer ways to manipulate complex biological systems with greater selectivity.

The term *neurodegenerative disorders* (NDs), encompasses conditions that are sporadic and/or familial and characterized by the persistent and progressive loss of neuronal subtypes. The most widely recognized are Alzheimer's disease (AD) and Parkinson's disease (PD), which are among the principal debilitating conditions of the current century.[1–3]

Approximately 24 million people worldwide suffer from dementia, of which 60% is due to AD.[4] AD occurs in 1% of individuals aged 50 to 70 years and dramatically increases to 50% of those over 70 years. AD is typified clinically by learning and memory impairment and pathologically by gross cerebral atrophy, indicative of neuronal loss, with numerous extracellular neuritic amyloid plaques and intracellular neurofibrillary tangles found predominantly in the frontal and temporal lobes, including the hippocampus.[5] The etiology remains elusive, and despite exhaustive searches for clues, the main risk and possible causative factor appears to be the relationship between AD and the Apo Ee4 allele of the Apo E gene family. The Apo Ee4 allele of the Apo E gene, located on chromosome 19, has been associated with an increased risk for and lower age of onset of AD. The role of Apo Ee4 in AD is thought to be related to the formation of amyloid plaques due to its function as a carrier for β-amyloid. Furthermore, it has been suggested that the failure of

Apo Ee4 to bind to tau protein may lead to the failure of phosphorylation of tau and thereby the formation of neurofibrillary tangles. Interestingly, the Apo Ee2 gene appears to confer some protection against sporadic AD. Genetic factors that present as dominant mutations account for less than 1% of the few cases of familial early-onset AD. However, the ultimate cause of AD is unknown and current treatment remains symptomatic. Current treatments for cognitive impairment in AD are based on neurotransmitter or enzyme replacement/modulation, which provide symptomatic benefits and include acetylcholinesterase inhibitors,[6] cholinesterase inhibitors,[7] antioxidants,[8] amyloid-β-targeted drugs, nerve growth factors, c-secretase inhibitors,[9] and vaccines against β-amyloid.[10] However, none of the available therapies appears to be able to cure AD or to attenuate disease progression.

PD is characterized by the sporadic degeneration of midbrain nigrostriatal dopaminergic neurons with resultant reduction in brain dopamine (DA) levels causing the characteristic motor symptoms of bradykinesia, rigidity, and resting tremor.[11] DA is the neural transmitter responsible for transmitting the electrical signals required for normal physical motion. The deficiency of DA that typifies PD results in these abnormal movements. While the etiology of PD is not well known, its pathogenesis is thought to be a multifactorial cascade of deleterious factors. PD affects 1% of the population over the age of 65 years. Genetic factors are decidedly uncommon, with at most 5% of cases being familial or hereditary. A small subset of patients within the hereditary group appears to follow a pattern of autosomal dominant inheritance, although the majority of the hereditary cases do not exhibit a recognizable inheritance pattern. Currently, frontline therapy for PD is the oral administration of dopamine agonists such as levodopa. To complement the pharmacological treatment, deep brain stimulation and transplantation of fetal dopamine neurons have been explored.[12] However, these approaches remain controversial.

Drug delivery to the brain remains the major challenge for the treatment of all NDs because of the numerous protective barriers surrounding the CNS. The bioactive agents that are currently approved by the U.S. Food and Drug Administration have demonstrated modest effects in modifying disease symptoms for relatively short periods in subsets of patients, and none has shown an effect on disease progression. One of the significant facts on neurotherapeutics is the constraint of the blood–brain barrier (BBB) and the drug release kinetics that cause peripheral side effects. Furthermore, contrary to common belief, NDs may be multisystemic in nature, and this presents numerous difficulties for the potential treatment of these disorders. In NDs the death of specific types of neurons is provoked by a cascade of multiple deleterious molecular and cellular events rather than a single pathogenic factor.

The advent of nanotechnology may provide a solution to overcome these diagnostic and neurotherapeutic challenges for AD and PD. Nanotechnology employs engineered materials or devices with the smallest functional organization on the nanometer scale (1–100 nm) that are able to interact with biological systems at the molecular level. Nanoparticles are able to penetrate the BBB of *in vitro* and *in vivo* models.[13–16] Nanotechnology can therefore be used to develop diagnostic tools as well as nano-enabled delivery systems that can bypass the BBB in order to facilitate conventional and novel neurotherapeutic interventions such as drug therapy, gene therapy, and tissue regeneration.[17,18] Nanotechnology is currently being used to refine the discovery of biomarkers, molecular diagnostics, drug discovery, and drug delivery, which could be applicable to the management of AD and PD.

The blood–brain barrier

Transport mechanisms at the BBB can be manipulated for cerebral drug targeting. Studies of kinetic flux have revealed a unidirectional, concentration-dependent movement of compounds across the BBB.[19] The direction of flow was reported to be from the plasma to the brain, or visa versa. Thus the net flux is the difference between the two unidirectional flow rates and is a significant determinant for drugs reaching therapeutic concentrations within the CNS.[27] Small lipophilic molecules pass easily from blood capillaries. Charge-bearing large or hydrophilic molecules require gated channels, ATP, proteins, and/or receptors to facilitate passage across the BBB. Circumvention of the BBB can be achieved through the systemic administration or implantation of nano-enabled drug delivery systems (step 1, Fig. 1) that have the ability to control and target the

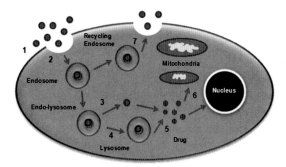

Figure 1. Steps detailing the cytosolic delivery of neurotherapeutic agents via nanoparticles (NPs), 1) cellular association of NPs, 2) internalization of NPs via endocytosis, 3) endosomal escape of NPs or 4) lysosomal degradation of NPs, 5) drug freely diffusing into cytoplasm, 6) cytoplasmic transport of drug to target organelle, 7) exocytosis of NPs.

release of various bioactive agents (step 5, Fig. 1) used in the treatment of NDs.[21–24]

Various potential nanostructures employed for the treatment of neurodegenerative disorders

The majority of nanotechnological drug delivery systems for the treatment of NDs are in the form of polymeric nanoparticles. Polymeric nanoparticles are promising for the treatment of AD and PD as they can pass through tight cell junctions, cross the BBB, achieve a high drug-loading capacity, and be targeted toward the mutagenic proteins in AD and PD. Promising features of these nanosystems in targeted CNS drug delivery are that (1) their chemical properties can be easily modified to achieve organ-, tissue-, or cell-specific and selective drug delivery, (2) the targeted delivery of drugs can be controlled,

(3) they increase the bioavailability and efficacy of incorporated drugs by masking the physicochemical characteristics and thus increase the transfer of drug across the BBB, (4) they protect incorporated drugs against enzymatic degradation, and (5) they have fewer side effects.

Polymeric nanoparticles, nanocapsules, and nanospheres

Polymeric nanoparticles and nanocapsules range from 10–1000 nm.[25] They possess high drug-loading capacities, are able to protect the incorporated drug load against degradation, thus increasing the chances of drug reaching the brain. They are stable and can target the delivery of drugs to the CNS due to their surface properties that can be manipulated in order to evade recognition by macrophages of the reticuloendothelial system.[26] Polymeric nanoparticles have been used for the CNS delivery of several drugs, including doxorubicin.[27–30] Nanospheres are dense polymeric matrices in which drug is dispersed and are prepared by micro-emulsion polymerization.[31] Nanospheres are nanoparticle systems constituted by a solid core with a dense polymeric matrix, whereas nanocapsules are formed by a thin polymeric envelope surrounding an oil-filled cavity.[23,32–34]

Polymeric nanogels and nanosuspensions

Nanogels are networks of cross-linked polymers that often combine ionic and nonionic polymeric chains and are prepared using an emulsification solvent evaporation approach.[35,36] Nanogels swell in water and are able to incorporate molecules such as oligonucleotides, siRNA, DNA, proteins, and low-molecular-mass drugs. The drug-loading capacity is

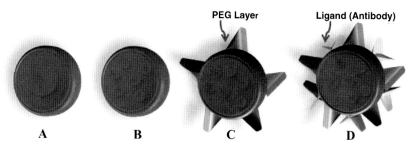

Figure 2. Types of nanoparticles for transport of drugs into the CNS, (A) nanocapsules, (B–D) nanospheres with drug distributed throughout a polymer/lipid matrix, (B) either without a surface coating or coating with a surfactant and/or PEG layer, and (D) additional coating with antibodies and/or ligands.

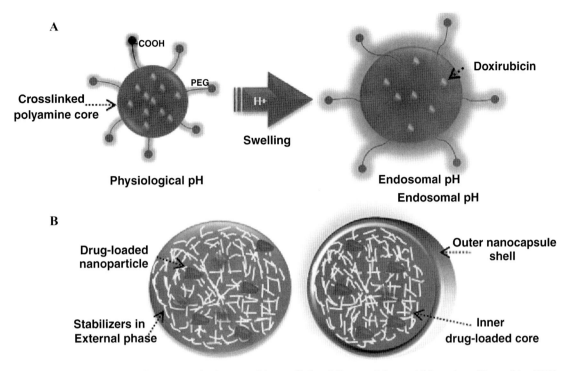

Figure 3. (A) Schematic of endosomal release and intracellular delivery of doxorubicin using pH-sensitive PEG nanogels (adapted from Oishi *et al.*[45]) and (B) illustrations of a functionalized and stable nanosuspension (adapted from Kumar *et al.*[38]).

up to 40–60%.[37] Vinogradov and coworkers[37] have encapsulated oligonucleotides within a cross-linked nanogel for delivery across the BBB. *In vivo* studies suggested that the nanogel increased brain uptake of oligonucleotides while decreasing uptake in the liver and spleen. Drug-loaded nanosuspensions are crystalline drug particles stabilized by nonionic surfactants or mixtures of lipids.[38,39] Major advantages

of nanosuspensions include their simplicity, high drug-loading capacity, and applicability to numerous drugs for CNS delivery.[25,39]

Carbon nanotubes and nanofibers

Carbon nanotubes are being explored to improve chronic CNS electrical stimulation.[40]

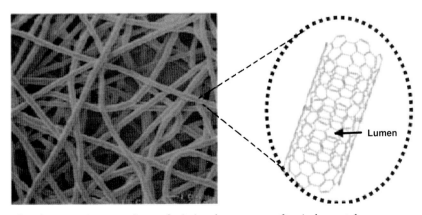

Figure 4. Scanning electron microscope image depicting the structure of typical nanotubes.

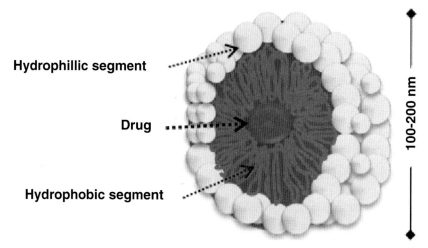

Figure 5. Schematic of the structure of a typical nanomicelle.

Clinically, functional electrical stimulation implants are gaining momentum for the treatment of PD. A significant challenge with the development of recording or stimulating chronic CNS electrodes is device failure associated with the fibrotic response mediated by glial and immune cells.[41] The development of compressed carbon nanofiber–based electrode arrays for CNS neuronal stimulation could be injected at sites of degeneration to provide both a physical substrate and the molecular signals needed to stimulate and support tissue healing in treating NDs.[42] The mechanism involved during carbon nanotube neuronal stimulation may be explicated in terms of an *in vitro* neuronal circuit model that is cultured on nanotube substrates to affect single and multiple synaptic pathway stimulation via the carbon nanotube layers and neuronal–nanotube electrical coupling and adhesion that may facilitate

population firing that is strengthened by the appearance of a fast Na^+ current, taken to constitute an early sign of axonal differentiation. These interactions may also sustain unconventional electrical coupling, thus unveiling new approaches to the basic understanding of the CNS electrophysiology.

Polymeric nanomicelles

Polymeric nanomicelles have a core–shell architecture with a hydrophobic core and a shell of hydrophilic polymer blocks. The core can incorporate up to 20–30% w/w of hydrophobic drugs, thus preventing premature drug release and degradation. The shell stabilizes the nanomicelles and masks the drug from interactions with serum proteins and untargeted cells. Once the target cells are reached drug is released by diffusion. Polymeric nanomicelles are

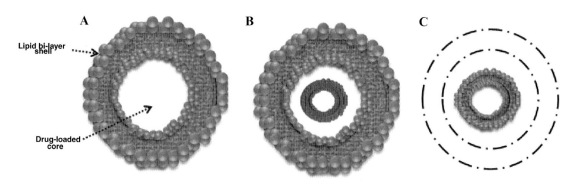

Figure 6. Types of nanoliposomes for transporting drugs across the BBB include (**A**) small unilamellar vesicles (SUV), (**B**) multilamellar vesicles (MLV), and (**C**) stimuli-sensitive nanoliposomes.

versatile and have been shown to efficiently deliver DNA molecules *in vitro* and *in vivo* although no successful study on their delivery to the CNS has been reported thus far.[43–45]

Polymeric nanoliposomes

Nanoliposomes are vesicular structures composed of uni- or multilamellar lipid bilayers surrounding internal aqueous compartments.[46] Relatively large quantities of drug can be incorporated into liposome aqueous compartments or within the lipid bilayers. Extended systemic circulation times can be accomplished with nanoliposomes with modified surfaces that reduce opsonization in plasma and decrease its recognition and removal by the liver and spleen.[46,47] Evaluation of nanoliposomes for targeted CNS drug delivery has been studied for various applications.[48–51]

Nanosystems explored for advanced experimental treatment of Alzheimer's disease

N-butylcyanoacrylate nanoparticles for clioquinol delivery in AD

The quinoline derivative clioquinol (CQ) is a Cu^{2+}/Zn^{2+} chelator known to solubilize β-amyloid plaques *in vitro* and inhibit β-amyloid accumulation in AD induced transgenic mice *in vivo*.[52] (Fig. 7). CQ-encapsulated poly(butylcyanoacrylate) (PBCA) nanoparticles have been prepared as a vector for the *in vivo* brain imaging of β-amyloid se-

nile plaques. Cherney and coworkers[52] showed that CQ-loaded PBCA nanoparticles crossed the BBB at a higher threshold than native CQ and may be a promising prototype for the treatment of AD. Roney and colleagues[53] have also prepared nanoparticles by various polymerization approaches and performed *in vivo* biodistribution studies in order to search for an appropriate candidate for future *in vivo* imaging of β-amyloid plaques. CQ was radio-iodinated and incorporated within PBCA nanoparticles for the *in vivo* biodistribution studies in wild-type mice. The nanoparticles were polymerized as per the modified procedure of Kreuter and coworkers[23] and delivered to the mice intravenously. The nanoparticles were shown to successfully transport CQ across the BBB making it ideal for *in vivo* imaging.

Poly(butyl)cyanoacrylate nanoparticles in AD

PBCA nanoparticles have been used to deliver drugs to the CNS with a good degree of success.[30,33,35] These particles are characteristically 250 nm in diameter and are loaded with drug either by incorporating the drug during the initial particle polymerization process or via absorption onto the surface of the preformed particle. The particles are subsequently coated with polysorbate 80 (Tween 80®) as depicted in Figure 8 . Following intravenous administration the surface of the particle becomes further coated with adsorbed plasma proteins, most prominently apolipoprotein E (Apo-E). It is proposed that the final particle is mistaken for low-density lipoprotein (LDL) particles by the cerebral endothelium and is internalized by the LDL uptake

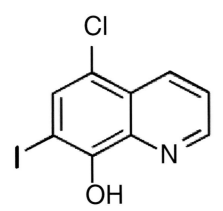

Figure 7. Chemical structure of clioquinol used as a Cu^{2+}/Zn^{2+} chelator that is able to solubilize β-amyloid plaques *in vitro* and inhibit β-amyloid accumulation in Alzheimer's disease.

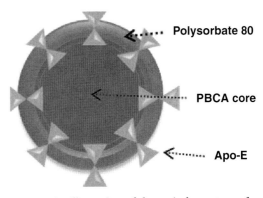

Figure 8. An illustration of the typical structure of an immuno-nanoliposome.

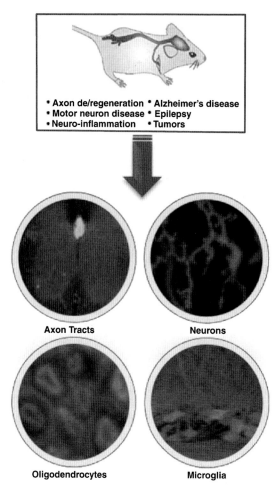

Figure 9. *In vivo* imaging of encapsulated *ThT* poly(butylcyanoacrylate) nanocapsules delivered to the mouse brain by direct intrahippocampal injection.

system.[29,34] Transactivating-transduction (TAT) peptide may also be attached to the surface of both liposomes[54] and nanoparticles. This modification facilitates internalization by cells.[55]

Thioflavin-T nanocapsules for β-amyloid detection in AD

Thioflavin-T (*ThT*) has been previously described as a probe for the detection of β-amyloid in senile plaques of AD.[56] Hartig and colleagues[57] delivered the *ThT*-loaded nanocapsules comprising PBCA into the brains of mice by direct intrahippocampal injection, and followed the photoconversion of *ThT* from the nanocapsules in fixed tissues, post injection (Fig. 9). The nanocapsules were prepared by emul-

sion polymerization of styrene in a water–ethanol mixture containing *ThT*. The brains were fixed 3 days postinjection, and the nanocapsules were localized by photoconversion of the *ThT* in a closed chamber enriched with oxygen. Light microscopy localized the photoconverted nanocapsules in the dentate gyrus, and vacuoles were found in the cytoplasm near the aggregated latex nanocapsules. Transmission electron microscopy verified the presence of the nanocapsules in microglia and neurons. Furthermore, confocal microscopy demonstrated that *ThT* was delivered from the nanocapsules. As a result, the authors suggested that *ThT* nanocapsules may be used to probe the synthesis of β-amyloid, which is an extracellular cleavage product of the amyloid precursor protein (APP).[58] They have not delivered the nanocapsules to the brain through the systemic circulation. However, the chemical similarity of the nanocapsules to PBCA, which has been shown to cross the BBB after intravenous administration, suggests that this approach has potential as a β-amyloid detection method for AD.[32]

D-penicillamine nanoparticles for the treatment of AD

The concentration of metal ions in the brain increases with age, and this imparts lethal effects on the AD brain.[59] An increase in the concentration of copper ions (Cu^{2+}) initiates oxidative stress that generates toxic hydroxyl radicals that disrupt DNA and modify proteins and lipids.[60] It is known that amyloid plaques contain elevated levels of Cu^{2+} and Zn^{2+} compared to the healthy brain.[24] These findings have formed the basis of new therapeutic approaches for AD, which involves iron-chelating compounds with limited neurotoxicity. Iron-chelating compounds have been recently incorporated in the form of nanoparticles to facilitate BBB penetration.[61] In an *in vitro* study of the chelation therapy for the possible treatment of AD, Cui and coworkers[24] conjugated the Cu (I) chelator D-penicillamine to nanoparticles to reverse the metal-induced precipitation of the β-amyloid protein. Nanoparticles were prepared from micro-emulsion precursors. The sodium salts of 1,2-dioleoyl-sn-glycero-3phosphoethanolamine-N-[4-(p-maleimidophenyl) butyramide] (MPB-PE) or 1,2 dioleoyl-sn-glycero-3-phosphoethanolamine-N-[3-(2-pyridyldithio)-propionate] (PDP-PE)

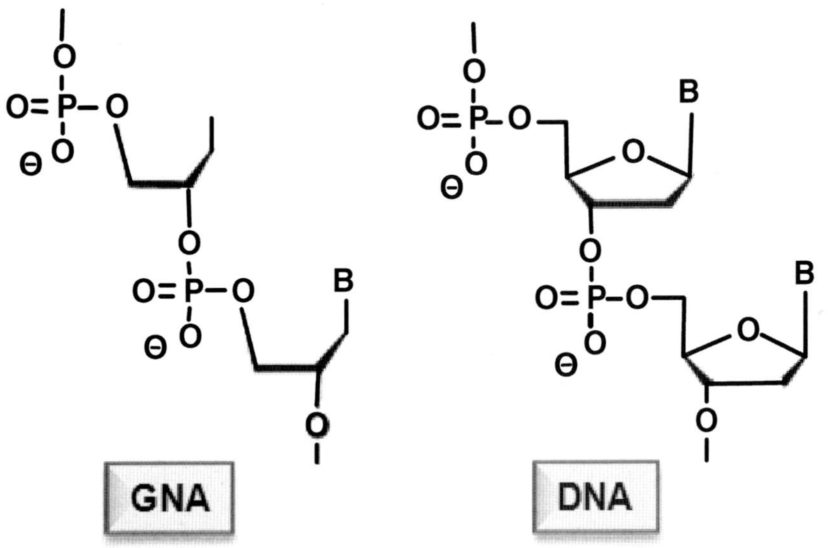

Figure 10. Molecular structures of GNA and DNA (adapted from Chaput[72]).

were added and the sulfhydryl moiety of d-penicillamine was coupled to the MPB-PE or PDP-PE nanoparticles. Cui and coworkers[24] have shown that the nanoparticles together with the partially released D-penicillamine resolubilized plaques under reducing conditions. At equimolar concentrations, the resolubilization of β-amyloid was 80% with EDTA and 40% with D-penicillamine, but at higher concentrations of D-penicillamine, resolubilization was just as effective and they concluded the significant role of nanoparticles in the *in vivo* investigation of AD through Cu^{2+} chelation.

Gold nanoparticles employed to destroy β-amyloid plaques in AD

A recently identified approach to the treatment of AD has the potential to destroy β-amyloid fibrils and plaques contributing to mental decline through a type of "molecular surgery" involving the use of gold nanoparticles to halt or slow the progression of AD without harming healthy brain cells. Attempts have been made to attach gold nanoparticles to a group of β-amyloid fibrils, incubating the resulting mixture for several days, and then exposing it to weak microwave fields for several hours. The energy levels of the fields were found to be six times smaller than those of conventional cell phones and thus unlikely to harm healthy cells.[62] The fibrils subse-

quently dissolved and remained dissolved for at least 1 week after being irradiated. This indicated that the treatment was not only effective at breaking up the fibrils but also reduced the tendency of the proteins to reaggregate. A similar approach holds promise for treating other neurodegenerative diseases that involve protein aggregation, including PD. The approach is similar to an experimental technique that uses metallic nanoparticles to label and destroy cancer cells.[40]

Self-assembling biomolecular nanostructures in AD

Self-assembly of biological molecules is a basic principle in the formation of complex biological structures. Numerous proteins and peptides have been emerging as nano-biomaterials due to their ability to self-assemble into nanoscale structures such as nanotubes, nanovesicles, helical ribbons, and three-dimensional fibrous scaffolds.[63] For instance Stupp and colleagues[64] managed to have paralyzed lab mice with spinal cord injuries regain the ability to walk using their hind limbs 6 weeks after an injection of a nanomaterial designed for the purpose. By injecting molecules that were designed to self-assemble into nanostructures in the spinal tissue, they were able to rescue and regenerate damaged neurons.[64] Nanofibers are pivotal for stimulating the body into regenerating lost or damaged cells. In

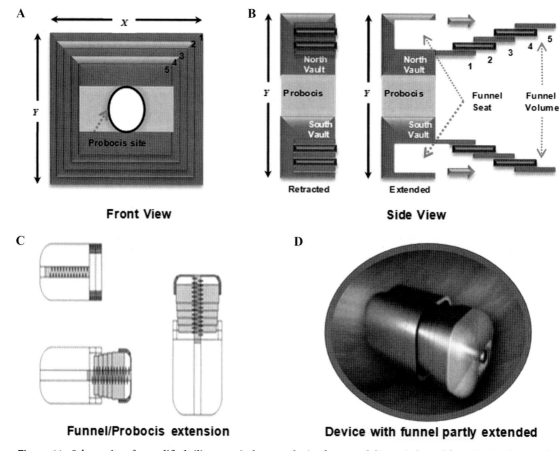

Figure 11. Schematics of a modified silica nonviral vector device for gene delivery (adapted from Freitas Jr., 2007).

addition, they play a role in preventing the formation of scar tissue, which inhibits spinal cord healing. When the nanofibers form they can be immobilized in an area of tissue where it is necessary to activate a biological process, for example regenerating differentiated cells from stem cells. This has significant implications for the treatment of AD and PD, in which key brain cells stop functioning.[63,64]

Glycerol nucleic acid: A nano-based DNA chemical analogue in AD

DNA has being utilized to produce nano-sized elements for potential application in the treatment of AD. DNA is an ideal building block for nanotechnology due to its ability to self-assemble and bind into various shapes based on the natural chemical rules of attraction.[65–71] Chaput[72] has produced a self-assembled nanostructure comprising glycerol nucleic acid (GNA), a synthetic analog of DNA

(Fig. 10). The only chemical difference between DNA and GNA is the polysaccharide molecule. GNA uses the 3-carbon polysaccharide glycerol rather than the 5-carbon deoxyribose used in DNA. The polysaccharide provides the chemical backbone for nucleic acid polymers, anchoring a phosphate molecule and nitrogenous base (Fig. 10). GNA nanostructures possess additional properties not found in DNA, including the ability to have anti-amyloid activity and form mirror image structures.[67,71,72] GNA is an oligonucleotide. GNA can therefore be used to inhibit undesirable gene expression or to synthesize therapeutic proteins that can play a vital role in the *in vivo* gene delivery of AD treatments.

Inhibition of β-amyloid plaque formation using nanogels in AD

The formation of fibrils by β-amyloid is considered a key step in the pathology of AD.

Inhibiting the aggregation of β-amyloid is a promising approach for AD therapy. Biocompatible nanogels have been developed comprised of polysaccharide pullulan backbones with hydrophobic cholesterol moieties (cholesterol-bearing pullulan, CHP) as artificial chaperones to inhibit the formation of β-amyloid (1–42) fibrils with marked amyloidgenic activity and cytotoxicity. The CHP-nanogels are able to incorporate up to 6–8 β-amyloid (1–42) molecules per particle and induce a change in the conformation of β-amyloid from a random coil to an alpha-helix- or β-sheet-rich structure. The structure is stable over 24 h (at 37°C), and the aggregation of β-amyloid (1–42) can be suppressed. Furthermore, the dissociation of the nanogel caused by the addition of methyl-β-cyclodextrin released monomeric β-amyloid molecules. Nanogels composed of amino-group-modified CHP (CHPNH$_2$) with positive charges under physiological conditions have a greater inhibitory effect than CHP nanogels, suggesting the importance of electrostatic interactions between CHPNH$_2$ and β-amyloid for inhibiting the formation of fibrils. In addition, CHPNH$_2$ nanogels protected PC12 cells from β-amyloid toxicity. *Ex vivo* studies showed that biocompatible nanogels 20–30 nm in diameter can prevent aggregation of proteins associated with AD and inhibit amyloid fibers from forming.

Nanosystems explored for advanced experimental treatment of Parkinson's disease

Brain-targeted delivery of dopamine using nanosystems in PD

Various approaches of delivering dopamine (DA) to the brain with particular focus on the use of redox-based delivery systems for the targeted delivery and localized release of DA in the brain have been performed.[73] Results have shown that DA can be successfully delivered into the brain, accompanied by localized release and metabolism, which allows the execution of appropriate pharmacological responses. These results open the possibility of treating a variety of NDs, since normally the BBB restricts the entry of polar compounds such as DA into the brain parenchyma.[73]

Convection-enhanced drug delivery in PD

The intravascular administration of neuroactives has been confounded by the BBB, which prohibits the entry of molecules based on size, lipid solubility, and ionic charge, thus limiting the entry of charged small molecules or larger compounds such as proteins, genes, or viral particles.[74] Osmotic disruption of the BBB has been used clinically to temporarily infiltrate the BBB and allow a greater quantity and variety of intravascular neuroactives to access the brain parenchyma, including monoclonal antibodies and radio-immunoconjugates.[75,76] Unfortunately, despite selective opening of unilateral or bilateral vertebrobasilar or carotid cerebrovascular distributions via the arterial approach, controlling the site of treatment through this technique remains complicated and limited to a major vascular distribution.[74] In addition, repeated treatment adds to patient discomfort and potential morbidity, ultimately narrowing the clinical use of osmotic BBB disruption therapy. However, convection-enhanced delivery (CED) technology is able to deliver neuroactives at a larger and more consistent treatment volume than standard diffusion-based technologies.[74] CED employs bulk flow of the neuroactives through the extracellular space of the tissue.[77] Bulk flow distributes neuroactives homogeneously within a controlled brain volume, regardless of molecular size, with a steep concentration drop at the advancing margin of the bulk flow. This allows for the convection of viral particles (for gene therapy) and large macromolecules such as growth factors into the brain. The volume in which a neuroactive (such as a drug, virus, gene, or growth factor) distributes in the brain with CED is primarily a function of the infusion rate and specific tissue characteristics. CED has been modeled in animals and has recently been evaluated in human brain tumor trials.[78–80] CED of neuroactives within the brain is becoming a more frequent experimental treatment option in the management of brain tumors, and more recently in Phase I trials for gene therapy in PD.[74]

Nonviral vectors for the safe and efficient delivery of genes in PD

Gene therapy for PD may become clinically relevant upon the development of viral and nonviral gene-transfer vectors. Viral vectors are able to deliver a gene to the nucleus of a cell and have it expressed through its integration into the genome or as an episomal vector.[81] A critical concern for any form of gene therapy is the safety of the vector, as there is a risk of excessive immune response as well as insertional mutagenesis when viruses are used as transfection vectors. Actual death has occurred in human trials, leading to a halt in further use of viral vectors for gene transfection. In addition, the approach of using viral vectors suffers from inherent challenges in the pharmaceutical processing, scale-up, immunogenicity, and reversion of an engineered virus.[82] A focus in nanotechnology is the development and use of nonviral vectors for the safe and efficient delivery of genes.[83] The potential for the treatment of PD has advanced based on the ability to identify specific defective or absent genes responsible for PD. Specifically designed therapeutic genes, if successfully delivered into the appropriate cells, may provide a significant advancement in the therapy of PD.[83] *In vivo* gene delivery involves the use of genetic materials such as DNA, RNA, and oligonucleotides that are able to inhibit undesirable gene expression or synthesize therapeutic proteins.[81,82] However, for effective gene therapy, a genetic payload must be delivered to the targeted cell or tissue and thereafter be transported to the nucleus of the cell to achieve expression.[83] Amino-functionalized organically modified silica (ORMOSIL) nanoparticles as a nonviral vector have been shown to bind and protect plasmid DNA from enzymatic digestion and to effect cell transfection *in vitro*.[84] ORMOSIL nanoparticles are able to overcome the limitations of "unmodified" silica nanoparticle. The presence of both hydrophobic and hydrophilic groups on the precursor alkoxy organosilane assists self-assembly of both normal and reverse micelles under appropriate conditions. ORMOSIL nanoparticles are prepared from oil-in-water micro-emulsions that avoid corrosive solvents and follow a complex purification process (Fig. 3). Organic groups can be further modified for the attachment of biodegradable targeting molecules that can also impart a degree of flexibility to the rigid silica matrix, enhancing the stability of the particles in aqueous systems.[85]

Nanoparticle-based gene therapy for PD

Yurek and coworkers[86] have assessed the feasibility of employing novel technology to condense DNA

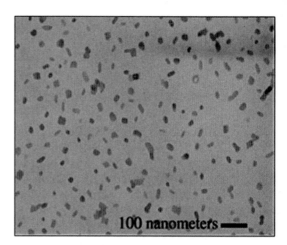

Figure 12. An electron micrograph depicting the size of DNA-compacted nanoparticles (adapted from news.uky.edu/news/Media/2007).

plasmids into nanoparticles for delivery to the brain in order to halt or prevent neurodegeneration in an animal model of PD (Fig. 12). They explored a relatively new gene-therapy approach for the treatment of PD and established that the strategy has the potential to repair defective genes. Yurek and coworkers used transduction, a technique for expressing a particular gene in a cell by delivering DNA into the cell and making the cell synthesize the protein that corresponds to that DNA. Furthermore, by capitalizing on the fact that neurotrophic factors are neuroprotective, it is possible to utilize neurotrophic factors to revive dormant brain cells and assist them to produce DA, thereby prompting a dramatic improvement of symptoms in animal models.[86] A study conducted by Kaplitt and During[87] in advanced PD patients showed that there was lack of side effects related to gene therapy. In addition, there were statistically significant improvements from baseline in both clinical symptoms and abnormal brain metabolism as measured by tomography.[87] Their study represents not only an encouraging first step in the development of a promising new approached to PD therapy, but also provides a platform to translate a variety of new gene-therapy agents into human clinical trials for numerous NDs.

Nanofibers as stem cell therapy in PD

Polymer-based biodegradable nanofibers have been engineered to prepare a scaffold that could

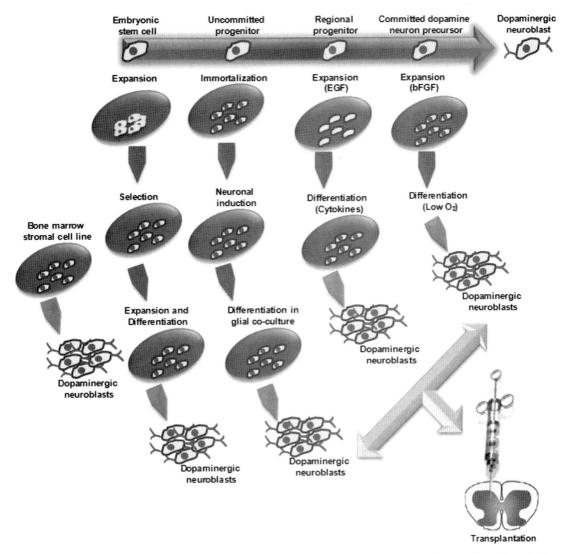

Figure 13. A schematic showing the use of stem cells and immature progenitors in producing dopaminergic-like neurons for the treatment of Parkinson's disease (adapted from Lindvall and Hagell[89]).

potentially allow stem cells to repair damaged nerves rapidly and effectively.[88] This was achieved by utilizing a combined process of electrospinning and chemical treatment to customize the nanofiber structure into a scaffold that can then be located within the body.[88] The scaffold is injected into the body at the site that requires nerve regeneration. The stem cells can be imbedded into the scaffold externally or once the scaffold is implanted. The nerve cells adhere to the scaffold, which forms a bridge in the brain or spinal cord. As time progresses, the scaffold erodes and is naturally eliminated from the body, leaving the newly regenerated nerves intact.[88] This approach may lead to a cure for PD. In another endeavor using stem cells for treating PD, Lindvall and Hagell[89] revealed the genes that initiate and control the DA-producing nerve cells within the brain. They managed to develop embryonic stem cells into DA-producing nerve cells in chicken and mouse models (Fig. 13). However, a significant challenge was that they could not succeed in producing pure samples of the DA-producing cells as they also produced 10–20% of unwanted stem cells.

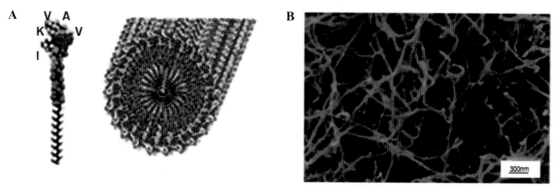

Figure 14. (**A**) Molecular schematic of an IKVAV-loaded peptide amphiphile molecule and its self-assembly into nanofibers and (**B**) scanning electron micrograph of an IKVAV nanofiber network formed by adding cell media to a peptide amphiphile aqueous solution.

Nanorobots as stem cell therapy in PD

The potential of stem cell therapy for NDs has been demonstrated on implantation of different types of stem cells in animal models of PD.[90] Transplantation of stem cells into the rat brain has demonstrated the reinnervation of striatal neurons and the partial recovery of motor deficit associated with DA deficiency.[91] Similar results have been obtained after transplantation of fetal dopaminergic neurons in clinical trials. Thus, it is possible to employ various types of stem cells to generate dopaminergic neurons. Currently, the process of dopaminergic neuron differentiation from embryonic stem cells *in vitro* is most effective.[92] Recent progress in human therapeutic cloning allows this approach of generating neurons to be more attractive.[93] Approaches for therapy may include *in vitro* processing of stem cells before implantation, supporting and guiding the cells after implantation with the help of nanorobots, and the *in vivo* creation of molecular scaffolds for stimulating their growth in the correct direction.[94] Nanorobots are controllable biomachines that algorithmically respond to stimuli and are capable of actuation, sensing, signaling, information processing, intelligence, and swarm behavior in order to interact and influence cells at the molecular level. Nanorobot actuators are also designed to be biocompatible and to have sufficient dimensions to transport and guide cells and other biomolecules. The potential for neural stem cells to establish appropriate long-distance axonal projection after region-specific differentiation has been demonstrated.[95] Unfortunately, the adult brain when compared to the neonatal brain has unfavorable conditions for axon growth in the

sense that growth does not occur in the correct direction. Thus the stimulation of new neuron growth along the surface of neurons in the zone of progressive degeneration is necessary.[94] This therapeutic strategy may be possible after the development of technology for the controlled growth of neurons along the surface of target (dysfunctional) neurons with the help of nanorobots. It is evident that using dysfunctional neurons as a "niche for growth" is one way of ensuring accurate and safe regeneration of neuronal circuits. With gradual replacement of the dysfunctional or apoptotic neurons, new neurons will be integrated into the existing cellular structure and therefore be involved in the intended processes without any obvious mental degeneration.[94,95]

Carbon nanotube and nanowire biosensors in PD

Through the use of nanotechnology, wireless implantable biosensors that may help in treating patients with PD have been developed.[96] The biosensors comprise carbon nanotubes and nanowires that are hollow, light weight, and chemically inert and have superior mechanical strength (Fig. 15). They are grown and organized into arrays that are combined to make nanochips similar to those found in electronic devices. Carbon nanochips are biocompatible and are not rejected by the human body as a foreign object. Once inside the body, nanochips perform several functions, such as sensing and monitoring the release of DA produced by the brain. The carbon nanotube–based biosensor that was developed by Li and colleagues[96] records the loss of DA and stimulates activity between neurons and

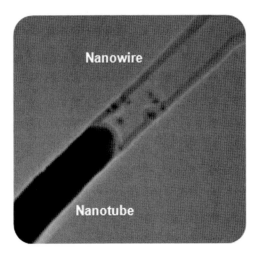

Figure 15. Hybrid structure of a carbon nanotube and nanowire.

neurites (immature developing neurons). Thus, they generally monitor and control DA levels in the brain. In addition to sensing the release of DA and contributing to the growth of healthy DA-producing neurons, the biosensor also communicates with an organic, polymer-based sensor attached to an area of the body in which a tremor occurs. The signal from the implanted sensor can control and direct the motion of the area of the body on which the exterior sensor is attached.[96] This exterior sensor can be easily placed under a wristwatch. Essentially, the implanted carbon nanotube–based sensor detects the sensor attached to the watch, controls the trembling, and directs the hand or prosthetic limb movement.[96]

Deep brain stimulation in PD

Deep brain stimulation (DBS) has been shown to be effective for PD, though with a few limitations.[97] The limitations include the large size of current microelectrodes (~1 mm diameter), lack of monitoring of local brain electrical activity and DA levels, and the open-loop nature of the stimulation.[97] It has been demonstrated that reducing the size of the monitoring and stimulating electrodes to the nanoscale allows a remarkable improvement in both the monitoring (spatial resolution, temporal resolution, and sensitivity) and the stimulation.[97] Carbon nanofiber nano-electrode technology (Fig. 16) offers the possibility of trimodal arrays for monitoring electrical activity, monitoring DA levels, and precise stim-

ulation.[98] DBS can then be guided by changes in brain electrical activity and/or DA (i.e., closed-loop DBS).[99] Thus, there is a need for thoroughly understanding the basic manufacturing techniques of prototype nano-electrodes used in DBS, their electrical characteristics, and the electro-conductive polymers that can be used to optimize DBS *in vivo*. Such an approach may offer a generic electrical-neural interface for use in various NDs such as PD and AD.

Surgical intervention in the treatment of PD

Femtosecond laser systems, nanoneedles, and nanotweezers are currently emerging nanotechnologies that have the potential to revolutionize the practice of neurosurgery in PD.[100] Surgery for PD was popularized in the mid-20th century before the advent of effective medical therapies.[100] Early lesioning treatments contributed to the understanding of the functional anatomy of PD. Observations of the limitations and long-term complications of established pharmacological therapies for PD, together with major contributions from animal research to elucidate the roles of the basal ganglia in movement disorders, inspired a recent renaissance in neurosurgical interventions for PD, including DBS.[100] The development of potentially restorative treatment modalities, such as gene therapy, neural transplantation, and nanotechnology, hold much promise for surgery, both therapeutically and in revealing further insights into the pathophysiology of PD.

Conclusions

Nanotechnology has proven to have great potential for providing neurotherapeutic modalities to limit and reverse the neuropathology of AD and PD by supporting and promoting functional regeneration of damaged neurons, providing neuroprotection, and facilitating the delivery of neuroactives such as drugs, genes, and cells across the BBB. It may contribute significantly toward the development of nano-enabled drug delivery systems for the treatment of NDs, taking advantage of the nanoscale structures of neural cells. Several novel approaches, inspired by recent advances in nanotechnology are already applicable to the treatment of AD and PD. Nanoscale classes of neuroactives will widen the scope of therapeutic action beyond merely modifying transmitter function to include

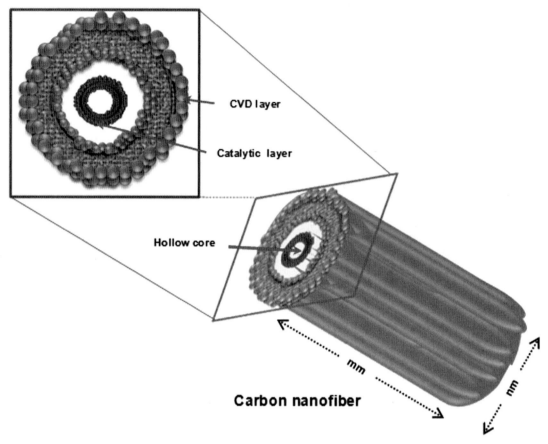

Figure 16. A schematic diagram of prototype carbon nanofibers (adapted from Silva[94]).

stem cell and gene therapies that could offer a more selective mode of targeting. However, in order for nanotechnology applications directed toward NDs to be fully exploited, it would be important for neurosurgeons, neurologists, and neuroscientists to participate and contribute to the scientific process along with pharmaceutical scientists and biomedical engineers to develop technological advancements in conjunction with advancements in basic and clinical neuroscience.

Conflicts of interest

The authors declare no conflicts of interest.

References

1. McArthur, J.C. 2004. HIV dementia: An evolving disease. *J. Neuroimmunol.* **157:** 3–10.

2. Flachenecker, P. 2006. Epidemiology of neuroimmunological diseases. *J. Neurol.* **253:** 2–8.

3. Kabanov, A.V. & H.E. Gendelman. 2007. Nanomedicine in the diagnosis and therapy of neurodegenerative disorders. *Prog. Polym. Sci.* **32:** 1054–1082.

4. Ferri, C.P., M. Prince, C. Brayne, *et al.* 2005. Global prevalence of dementia: A delphi consensus study. *Lancet* **366:** 2112–2117.

5. Popovic, N. & P. Brundin. 2006. Therapeutic potential of controlled drug delivery systems in neurodegenerative diseases. *Int. J. Pharm.* **314:** 120–126.

6. Coyle, J. & P. Kershaw. 2001. *Biol. Psych.* **49:** 289.

7. Marder, K. 2004. *Curr. Neurol. Neurosci. Rep.* **4:** 349.

8. Zandi, P.P., J.C. Anthony, A.S. Khachaturian, *et al.* 2004. *J. Arch. Neurol.* **61:** 82.

9. Selkoe, D.J. 2001. *Physiol. Rev.* **81:** 741.

10. Nash, J.M. 2001. *Time* **157:** 85.

11. Singh, N., V. Pillay & Y.E. Choonara. 2007. Advances in the treatment of Parkinson's disease. *Prog. Neurobiol.* **81:** 29–44.

12. Freed, C.R., P.E. Greene, R.E. Breeze, *et al.* 2001. Transplantation of embryonic dopamine neurons for

severe Parkinson's disease. *N. Engl. J. Med.* **344:** 710–719.

13. Kostarelos, K. & A.D. Miller. 2005. Synthetic, self-assembly ABCD nanoparticles; a structural paradigm for viable synthetic non-viral vectors. *Chem. Soc. Rev.* **34:** 970–994.

14. Born, P.J.A. & D. Muller-Schulte. 2006. Nanoparticles in drug delivery and environmental exposure: same size, same risks? *Nanomedicine* **1:** 235–249.

15. Xu, Z.P., Q.H. Zeng, G.Q. Lu & A.B. Yu. 2007. Inorganic nanoparticles as carriers for efficient cellular delivery. *Chem. Eng. Sci.* **61:** 1027–1040.

16. Foged, C. & H.M. Nielsen. 2008. Cell-penetrating peptides for drug delivery across membrane barriers. *Expert Opin. Drug Deliv.* **5:** 1435–1342.

17. Leary, S.P., C.Y. Liu & M.L.J. Apuzzo. 2006. Toward the emergence of nanoneurosurgery: Part III-nanomedicine: Targeted nanotherapy, nanosurgery, and progress toward the realization of nanoneurosurgery. *Neurosurg.* **58:** 1009–1026.

18. Gaur, A., A. Midha & A.L. Mbatia. 2008. Applications of nanotechnology in medical sciences. *Asian J. Pharm.* **2:** 80–85.

19. Ma, S.H., L.A. Lepak, R.J. Hussain, *et al.* 2005. An endothelial and astrocyte co-culture model of the blood-brain barrier utilizing an ultra-thin, nanofabricated silicon nitride membrane. *Lab Chip.* **5:** 74–85.

20. Miller, G. 2002. Drug targeting: breaking down barriers. *Science* **297:** 1116–1118.

21. Calvo, P., B. Gouritin, H. Villarroya, *et al.* 2002. Quantification and localization of pegylated polycyanoacrylate nanoparticles in brain and spinal cord during experimental allergic encephalomyelitis in the rat. *Eur. J. Neurosci.* **15:** 1317–1326.

22. Gupta, A.K., C. Berry, M. Gupta & A. Curtis. 2003. Receptor-mediated targeting of magnetic nanoparticles using insulin as a surface ligand to prevent endocytosis. *IEEE Trans. Nanobiosci.* **2:** 255–261.

23. Kreuter, J. 2004. Influence of the surface properties on nanoparticle-mediated transport of drugs to the brain. *J. Nanosci. Nanotechnol.* **4:** 484–488.

24. Cui, Z., P. Lockman, R. Atwood, *et al.* 2005. Novel d-penicillamine carrying nanoparticles for metal chelation therapy in Alzheimer's and other CNS diseases. *Eur. J. Pharm. Biopharm.* **59:** 263–272.

25. Muller, R.H. & C.M. Keck. 2004. Drug delivery to the brain-realization by novel drug carriers. *J. Nanosci. Nanotechnol.* **4:** 471–483.

26. Behan, N., C. Birkinshaw & N. Clarke. 2001. Poly n-butyl cyanoacrylate nanoparticles: a mechanistic study of polymerization and particle formation. *Biomat.* **22:** 1335–1344.

27. Calvo, P., B. Gouritin, H. Chacun, *et al.* 2001. Long-circulating pegylated polycyanoacrylate nanoparticles as new drug carrier for brain delivery. *Pharm. Res.* **18:** 1157–1166.

28. Alyaudtin, R.N., A. Reichel, R. Lobenberg, *et al.* 2001. Interaction of poly(butylcyanoacrylate) nanoparticles with the blood-brain barrier *in vivo* and *in vitro*. *J. Drug Target.* **9:** 209–221.

29. Kreuter, J., P. Ramge, V. Petrov, *et al.* 2003. Direct evidence that polysorbate-80-coated poly(butylcyanoacrylate) nanoparticles deliver drugs to the CNS via specific mechanisms requiring prior binding of drug to the nanoparticles. *Pharm. Res.* **20:** 409–416.

30. Steiniger, S.C., J. Kreuter, A.S. Khalansky, *et al.* 2004. Chemotherapy of glioblastoma in rats using doxorubicin-loaded nanoparticles. *Int. J. Cancer* **109:** 759–767.

31. Hyuk, I.M.S., U. Jeong & Y. Xia. 2005. Polymer hollow particles with controllable holes in their surfaces. *Nat. Mater.* **4:** 671–675.

32. Kreuter, J., R. Alyautdin, D. Kharkevich & A. Ivanov. 1995. Passage of peptides through the blood-brain barrier with collodial polymer particles (nanoparticles). *Brain Res.* **674:** 171–174.

33. Kreuter, J. 2001. Nanoparticulate systems for brain delivery of drugs. *Adv. Drug Deliv. Rev.* **47:** 65–81.

34. Kreuter, J., D. Shamenkov, V. Petrov, *et al.* 2002. Apolipoprotein-mediated transport of nanoparticle-bound drugs across the blood-brain barrier. *J. Drug Target.* **10:** 317–325.

35. Bronich, T.K., S. Bontha, L.S. Shlyakhtenko, *et al.* 2006. Template-assisted synthesis of nanogels from pluronic-modified poly(acrylic acid). *J. Drug Targeting* **14:** 357–366.

36. Bontha, S., A.V. Kabanov & T.K. Bronich. 2006. Polymer micelles with cross-linked ionic cores for delivery of anticancer drugs. *J. Control. Rel.* **114:** 163–174.

37. Vinogradov, S.V., A.D. Zeman, E.V. Batrakova & A.V. Kabanov. 2005. Polyplex nanogel formulations for drug delivery of cytotoxic nucleoside analogs. *J. Control. Rel.* **107:** 143–157.

38. Kumar, R.M., M. Sameti, *et al.* 2003. Polymeric nanoparticles for drug and gene delivery. In *Encyclopedia of Nanoscience & Nanotechnology*. Nalwa, H.S., Ed.: 1–19. American Scientific Publishers.

39. Friedrich, I., S. Reichl & C.C. Muller-Goymann. 2005. Drug release and permeation studies of nanosuspensions based on solidified reverse micellar solutions (SRMS). *Int. J. Pharm.* **305:** 167–175.

40. Kabanov, A.V. & H.E. Gendelman. 2007. Nanomedicine in the diagnosis and therapy of neurodegenerative disorders. *Prog. Polym. Sci.* **32:** 1054–1082.

41. McKenzie, J.L., M.C. Waid, R. Shi & T.J. Webster. 2004. Decreased functions of astrocytes on carbon nanofiber materials. *Biomat.* **25:** 1309–1317.

42. du Toit, L.C., V. Pillay, Y.E. Choonara, *et al.* 2007. Patenting of nanopharmaceuticals in drug delivery: No small issue. *Recent Patents on Drug Deliv. Form.* **1:** 131–142.

43. Nguyen, H.K., P. Lemieux, S.V. Vinogradov *et al.* 2000. Evaluation of polyether-polyethyleneimine graft copolymers as gene transfer agents. *Gene Ther.* **7:** 126–138.

44. Harada-Shiba, M., K. Yamauchi, A. Harada, *et al.* 2002. Polyion complex micelles as vectors in gene therapy-pharmacokinetics and *in vivo* gene transfer. *Gene Ther.* **9:** 407–414.

45. Oishi, M., H. Hayashi, M. Iijima & Y. Nagasaki. 2007. Endosomal release and intracellular delivery of anticancer drugs using pH-sensitive pegylated nanogels. *J. Mater. Chem.* **17:** 3720–3725.

46. Shi, N., W. Zhang, C. Zhu, *et al.* 2001. Brain-specific expression of an exogenous gene after i.v. administration. *Proc. Natl. Acad. Sci. USA* **98:** 12754–12759.

47. Voinea, M. & M. Simionescu. 2002. Designing of 'intelligent' liposomes for efficient delivery of drugs. *J. Cell Mol. Med.* **6:** 465–474.

48. Mora, M., M.L. Sagristá, D. Trombetta, *et al.* 2002. Design and characterization of liposomes containing long-chain N-acylpes for brain delivery: penetration of liposomes incorporating GM1 into the rat brain. *Pharm. Res.* **19:** 1430–1438.

49. Schmidt, J., J.M. Metselaar, M.H.M. Wauben, *et al.* 2003. Drug targeting by long-circulating liposomal glucocorticosteroids increases therapeutic efficacy in a model of multiple sclerosis. *Brain* **126:** 1895–1904.

50. Gosk, S., C. Vermehren, G. Storm & T. Moos. 2004. Targeting anti-transferrin receptor antibody (OX26) and OX26-conjugated liposomes to brain capillary endothelial cells using in situ perfusion. *J. Cereb. Blood Flow Metab.* **24:** 1193–1204.

51. Chekhonin, V.P., Y.A. Zhirkov, O.I. Gurina, *et al.* 2005. Pegylated immunoliposomes directed against brain astrocytes. *Drug Deliv.* **12:** 1–6.

52. Cherney, R.A., C.S. Atwood, M.E. Xilinas, *et al.* 2001. Treatment with a copper-zinc chelator markedly and rigidly inhibits B-amyloid accumulation in Alzheimer's disease transgenic mice. *Neuron* **30:** 665–676.

53. Roney, C., P. Kulkarn, V. Arora, *et al.* 2005. Targeted nanoparticles for drug delivery through the blood–brain barrier for Alzheimer's disease. *J. Control. Rel.* **108:** 193–214.

54. Torchilin, V.P. 2002. Peg-based micelles as carriers of contrast agents for different imaging modalities. *Adv. Drug Deliv. Rev.* **54:** 235–252.

55. Begley, D.J. 2004. Delivery of therapeutic agents to the central nervous system: The problems and the possibilities. *Pharmacol. Ther.* **104:** 29–45.

56. Ritchie, C.W., A.I. Bush & C.L. Masters. 2004. Metal-protein attenuating compounds and Alzheimer's disease. *Expert Opin. Invest. Drugs* **13:** 1585–1592.

57. Hartig, W., B. Paulke, C. Varga, *et al.* 2003. Electron microscopic analysis of nanoparticles delivering thioflavin-T after intrahippocampal injection in mouse: implications for targeting h-amyloid in Alzheimer's disease. *Neurosci. Lett.* **338:** 174–176.

58. Dong, J., C. Atwood, V. Anderson, *et al.* 2003. Metal binding and oxidation of amyloid-beta within isolated senile plaque cores: raman microscopic evidence. *Biochem.* **42:** 2768–2773.

59. Liu, C.Y., M.L. Apuzzo & D.A. Tirrell. 2003. Engineering of the extracellular matrix: working toward neural stem cell programming and neurorestoration-concept and progress report. *Neurosurg.* **52:** 1154–1165.

60. Lovell, M., J. Robertson, W. Teesadale, *et al.* 1998. Copper, iron and zinc in Alzheimer's disease senile plaques. *J. Neurol. Sci.* **158:** 47–52.

61. Mandel, S.A., T. Amit, M. Machluf & M.B.H. Youdim. 2007. Nanoparticles: A step forward for iron chelation in the brain. *Future Neurol.* **2:** 265–269.

62. Kogan, M.J., N.G. Bastus, R.D. Grillo-Bosch, *et al.* 2006. Nanoparticle-mediated local and remote manipulation of protein aggregation. *Nano Lett.* **6:** 110–115.

63. Subramani, K., A. Khraisat & A. George. 2008. Self-Assembly of proteins and peptides and their applications in bionanotechnology. *Curr. Nanosci.* **4:** 201–207.

64. Stupp, S.I. 2007. Nanotechnology offers hope for treating spinal cord injuries, diabetes and Parkinson's disease. Nanowerk, http://www.nanowerk.com/news/newsid=1816.php. Accessed on 2.20.2009.

65. Yan, H., S.H. Park, G. Finkelstein, *et al.* 2003. DNA-templated self-assembly of protein arrays and highly conductive nanowires. *Science* **301:** 1882–1884.

66. Ke, Y., S. Lindsay, Y. Chang, *et al.* 2008. Self-assembled water-soluble nucleic acid probe tiles for label-free RNA hybridization assays. *Science* **319:** 180–183.

67. Seeman, N.C. 2005. From genes to machines: DNA nanomechanical devices. *Trends Biochem. Sci.* **30:** 119–125.

68. Niemeyer, C.M. 2000. Self-assembled nanostructures based on DNA: Towards the development of nanobiotechnology. *Curr. Opin. Chem. Biol.* **4:** 609–618.

69. Liu, H., J. Gao, S.R. Lynch, *et al.* 2003. A four-base paired genetic helix with expanded size. *Science* **302:** 868–871.

70. Yang, Y.W., S. Zhang, E.O. McCullum & J.C. Chaput. 2007. Experimental evidence that GNA and TNA were not sequential polymers in the prebiotic evolution of RNA. *J. Mol. Evol.* **65:** 289–295.

71. Zhang, R.S., E.O. McCullum & J.C. Chaput. 2008. Synthesis of two mirror image 4-helix junctions derived from glycerol nucleic acid. *J. Am. Chem. Soc.* **130:** 5846–5847.

72. Chaput, J. 2008. GNA: DNA chemical cousin is a nanotechnology building block. *Sci. Blog. Sci.* 2, http://www.scientificblogging.com/news releases/. Accessed on 2.20.2009.

73. Simpkins J.W. & N. Bodor. 1994. Brain-targeted delivery of dopamine using a redox-based chemical delivery system. *Adv. Drug Deliv. Rev.* **14:** 243–249.

74. Fiandaca, M.S., J.R. Forsayeth, P.J. Dickinson & K.S. Bankiewicz. 2008. Image-guided convection-enhanced delivery platform in the treatment of neurological diseases. *Neurother.* **5:** 123–127.

75. Neuwelt, E.A. 2004. Mechanisms of disease: the blood-brain barrier. *Neurosurg.* **54:** 131–140.

76. Nowakowski, G.S. & T.E. Witzig. 2006. Radioimmunotherapy for B-cell non-Hodgkin lymphoma. *Clin. Adv. Hematol. Oncol.* **4:** 225–231.

77. Bobo, R.H., D.W. Laske, A. Akbasak, *et al.* 1994. Convection-enhanced delivery of macromolecules in the brain. *Proc. Natl. Acad. Sci. USA* **91:** 2076–2080.

78. Krauze, M.T., J. Forsayeth, J.W. Park & K.S. Bankiewicz. 2006. Real-time imaging and quantification of brain delivery of liposomes. *Pharm. Res.* **23:** 2493–2504.

79. Lidar, Z., Y. Mardor & T. Jonas, *et al.* 2004. Convection-enhanced delivery of paclitaxel for the treatment of recurrent malignant glioma: A phase I/II clinical study. *J. Neurosurg.* **100:** 472–479.

80. Kioi, M., S.R. Husain, D. Croteau, *et al.* 2006. Convection-enhanced delivery of interleukin-13

receptor-directed cytotoxin for malignant glioma therapy. *Technol. Cancer Res. Treat.* **5:** 239–250.

81. Anderson, W.F. 1998. Human gene therapy. *Nature* **392:** 25–30.

82. Davis, S.S. 1997. Biomedical applications of nanotechnology-implications for drug targeting and gene therapy. *Trends Biotechnol.* **15:** 217–224.

83. Luo, D. & W.M. Saltzman. 2000. Synthetic DNA delivery systems. *Nat. Biotechnol.* **18:** 33–37.

84. Klejbor, I., E.K. Stachowiak, D.J. Bharali, *et al.* 2007. ORMOSIL nanoparticles as a non-viral gene delivery vector for modeling polyglutamine induced brain pathology. *J. Neurosci. Meth.* **165:** 230–243.

85. Jain, K.K. 2005. The role of nanobiotechnology in drug discovery. *Drug Discov. Today* **10:** 1435–1442.

86. Yurek, D. 2007. Nanoparticle gene therapy for Parkinson's disease. Nanotechwire.com. http://nanotechwire.com/news.asp?nid=4393&ntid=183&pg=8. Accessed on 2.20.2009.

87. Kaplitt, M.G. & M.J. During. 2008. Gene therapy study shows safety and statistically significant improvement in Parkinson's disease. *Biomed.* http://www.bio-medicine.org/biology-news/Gene-therapy-study-shows-safety-and-statistically-significant-improvement-in-Parkinsons-disease-5440-1/. Accessed on 2.20.2009.

88. Nisbet, D.R., K.E. Crompton, M.K. Horne, *et al.* 2007. Neural tissue engineering of the CNS using hydrogels. *J. Biomed. Mat. Res. Part B: App. Biomat.* **1:** 251–263.

89. Lindvall, O. & P. Hagell. 2002. Role of cell therapy in Parkinson's disease. *Neurosurg. Focus.* **13:** e2.

90. Parati, E.A., A. Bez, D. Ponti, *et al.* 2003. Neural stem cells: Biological features and therapeutic potential in Parkinson's disease. *J. Neurosurg. Sci.* **47:** 8–17.

91. Kim, J.H., J.M. Auerbach, J.A. Rodríguez-Gómez, *et al.* 2002. Dopamine neurons derived from embryonic stem cells function in an animal model of Parkinson's disease. *Nature* **418:** 50–56.

92. Barberi, T., P. Klivenyi, N.Y. Calingasan, *et al.* 2003. Neural subtype specification of fertilization and nuclear transfer embryonic stem cells and application in parkinsonian mice. *Nat. Biotech.* **21:** 1200.

93. Woo, S.H. 2004. Evidence of a pluripotent human embryonic stem cell line derived from a cloned blastocyst. *Science* **303:** 1669–1674.

94. Silva, G.A., C. Czeisler, K.L. Niece, *et al.* 2004. Selective differentiation of neural progenitor cells by high-epitope density nanofibers. *Science* **303:** 1352–1355.

95. Englund, U., A. Bjorklund, K. Wictorin, *et al.* 2002. Grafted neural stem cells develop into functional

pyramidal neurons and integrate into host cortical circuitry. *Proc. Natl. Acad. Sci. USA* **99:** 17089–17094.

96. Li, J., H.T. Ng & H. Chen. 2008. Protein nanotechnology protocols, instrumentation, and applications. In *Methods in Molecular Biology*, Vol. 300. Vo-Dinh, T., Ed.: 191–223. Humana Press Inc. Totowa, NJ, USA.

97. Li, J. & R.J. Andrews. 2007. Trimodal nanoelectrode array for precise deep brain stimulation: prospects of a new technology based on carbon nanofiber arrays. *Operative Neuromod.* **97:** 537–545.

98. Nguyen-Vu, T.D.B., H. Chen, A.M. Cassell, *et al.* 2006. Vertically aligned carbon nanofiber arrays; an advance toward electrical-neural interfaces. *Small* **2:** 89–94.

99. Lovat, V., D. Pantarotto, L. Lagostena, *et al.* 2005. Carbon nanotubes substrates boost neuronal electrical signaling. *Nano Lett.* **5:** 1107–1110.

100. Pereira, E.A.C. & T.R. Aziz. 2006. Surgical insights into Parkinson's disease. *J. Royal Soc. Med.* **99:** 238–244.

Ann. N.Y. Acad. Sci. ISSN 0077-8923

Neurologic Wilson's disease

Matthew T. Lorincz

Department of Neurology, University of Michigan Health Systems, Ann Arbor, Michigan, USA

Address for correspondence: Matthew T. Lorincz, M.D., Ph.D., Assistant Professor, University of Michigan Health Systems, Department of Neurology, 1500 E. Medical Center Drive, SPC 5316, Ann Arbor, MI 48109-5316. Voice: 734-615-8234; fax: 734-615-4991. Lorincz@umich.edu

Despite a long history, Wilson's disease, an autosomal recessive disease caused by mutations in the ATP7B gene, remains a commonly misdiagnosed import disease. Mutations in ATP7B result in abnormal copper metabolism and subsequent toxic accumulation of copper. Clinical manifestations of neurologic Wilson's disease include variable combinations of dysarthria, dystonia, tremor, and choreoathetosis. Among neurodegenerative diseases, it is unusual in that misdiagnosis and delay in treatment are clinically relevant because treatments can prevent and cure Wilson's disease, if they are given appropriately. If left untreated, Wilson's disease progresses to hepatic failure or severe neurologic disability and death, while those adequately treated have normal life spans. This review focuses on the neurologic features of Wilson's disease, its diagnosis, and treatment options.

Keywords: ceruloplasmin; copper; dysarthria; dystonia; tremor; Parkinsonism; movement disorders

The history of neurologic Wilson's disease

The landmark paper in this disease was written in 1912 by Samuel Alexander Kinnier-Wilson, an American neurologist working at The National Hospital at Queen Square in London.[1] He described a neurologic disorder associated with progressive lenticular degeneration of the brain and cirrhosis of the liver that came later to be known as Wilson's disease, or hepatolenticular degeneration. Prior to Wilson's description, Kayser in 1902 had described pigmented corneal rings, later to bear his name, in a patient believed affected by Wilson's disease. Wilson did not initially believe the connection of Kayser-Fleischer rings or liver pathology to the disease that bears his name. The disease described by Wilson was one dominated by juvenile age at onset with dystonia and contrasts to the form of disease described by Westpahl in 1883 as pseudosclerotic, having a young-adult age of onset and symptomatically consisting principally of tremor and dysarthria. Only later was parkinsonism recognized as a major clinical feature of Wilson's disease.

A connection to copper metabolism may have first been described in 1913 and was strengthened by observations of sunflower cataracts in Wilson's disease. This type of cataract had been recognized as being produced by copper-containing foreign bodies. Subsequently, in 1929 and 1930 excess brain and liver copper was described.[2] In 1952 ceruloplasmin was demonstrated to be low in Wilson's patients.[3] From 1963 through the mid 1970s use of radiocopper tracing by Walshe and colleagues demonstrated that in presymptomatic disease the liver is able to sequester injected copper. In symptomatic patients, injected copper was unable to be bound in the liver and was found in other tissues including the brain.[4,5] A low biliary excretion of copper was later shown to be responsible for a failure to regulate copper balance. An autosomal inheritance pattern was delineated by Hall in 1921 and was confirmed by Bearn in 1960.[6] The molecular era of medicine brought the chromosomal localization of the Wilson's disease gene to chromosome 13q14.3 and identification of the causative gene, ATP7B a copper transporting P-type transmembrane ATPase.[7–9]

Cumings, who was the first to postulate an etiologic role for copper, suggested that chelation therapy with British antilewisite (BAL or dimercaprol) might be of benefit.[10] The agent had been used during World War II as an agent to treat lewisite, an arsenic poison. By 1951, Cumings, Denny-Brown, and Porter described benefits of BAL in treatment of Wilson's disease.[11,12] Alleviation of the painful BAL injections and their associated toxicity became possible with the description by Walshe in 1956 of the potential use of penicillamine to chelate copper in Wilson's disease.[13] Early in the 1960s use of zinc as a decoppering agent was first undertaken by Schouwink and Hoogenrand, findings that have subsequently been borne out by larger trials.[14,15] Seeking an alternate to penicillamine therapy, in 1969 Walshe began using trientine and has subsequently reported its beneficial effects in those refractory to penicillamine.[16] As had been observed with zinc, molybdenum was know to induce copper deficiency in sheep. This observation eventually lead Walshe, in 1986, to consider its use in Wilson's disease. The effectiveness of tetrathiomolybdate as a treatment of Wilson's disease has now been confirmed.[17–20]

Epidemiology

Wilson's disease appears to be typical of rare autosomal recessive diseases in that it is present at a low frequency in all populations. An estimate for the disease frequency in most populations is about 17 per million, which would lead to a carrier frequency of 1 in 122.[21] As with most autosomal recessive diseases, there may be pockets of excess Wilson's disease produced by founder effects, particularly if consanguity is common in the population.[22]

Clinical manifestations

During early life, the patient is presymptomatic but is accumulating copper, which invariably causes subclinical liver disease. Then, between early childhood and the fifth or sixth decade of life, but with a peak incidence of around 17 years, the patient presents with hepatic, neurologic, and psychiatric manifestations.[23] It has been suggested that the hepatic, neurologic, and psychiatric presentations of Wilson's disease occur in roughly equal proportions. An accurate estimate of the presenting proportions is challenging because many of the large case series have ascertainment bias based on clinical specialty, and likely underrepresent the psychiatric presentation. Those with a primarily hepatic presentation appear to have an earlier age at presentation than those with the primarily neurologic presentation.[23,24] Although Wilson's disease usually presents

in childhood into early adulthood, a wider range of age at onset is recognized. Generally, is extremely rare for Wilson's disease to present after age 35, but late-onset cases continued to be reported.[25] This review deals primarily with neurologic Wilson's disease, and hepatic manifestations will be briefly considered. Excellent descriptions of hepatic Wilson's disease can be found elsewhere.[22,23,26]

Neurologic manifestations

Neurologic subtypes

Walshe, who introduced penicillamine, trientine, and tetrathiomolybdate therapy, stated that "no two patients are ever the same, even in a sibship," and that there is no such thing as a typical picture of Wilson's disease.[27] Mean age at onset of neurologic symptoms from large case series range from about 15–21 years of age.[24,27–33] Neurologic manifestations at initial presentation have been reported in approximately 18–68%.[27,29–31,34] The main clinical categories of neurologic Wilson's disease have been variably divided by neurologic presentation and signs. The clinical categories that encompass the majority of neurologic Wilson's disease are, dysarthric, dystonic, tremor, pseudosclerotic (tremor +/– dysartrria), or parkinsonian.[24,27–33,35–37] It is not uncommon for a single manifestation such as tremor, dysarthria, dystonia, or less frequently parkinsonism to be present at the initiation of the symptomatic period. As the disease progresses, it is typical for complex combinations of neurologic symptoms and signs to coexist in a single patient, with a small subset of features predominating. During the course of the disease, other neurologic features include, chorea, athetosis, myoclonus, seizures, ataxia, pyramidal signs, drooling, and eye movement abnormalities.[27]

Neurologic features

Dysarthria
Dysarthria is probably the most common neurologic manifestation of Wilson's disease. In large series that delineate dysarthria as a feature of Wilson's disease, it has been found in 85–97% of those with neurologic Wilson's disease.[29,31,37] Dysarthria in Wilson's disease is most frequently of the mixed type with varying spastic, ataxic, hypokinetic, and dystonic components.[30,31,38] Speech involvement is

frequently concordant with the neurologic involvement in individual patients. In those with dystonia, speech frequently will have dystonic qualities with a strained or harsh quality. In those with parkinsonism, the speech quality may have hypokinetic properties.[39] Ataxic dysarthria, with variation in word spacing and volume, is often found in association with other types of dysarthria and may be more common in those with tremor.[31]

Dystonia

Dystonia can be focal, segmental, multifocal, or generalized and ranges in severity from mild to debilitating.[38] Dystonia is a common finding in Wilson's disease, reported to be present in about 11–65%.[29–31,33,34,38] A common focal dystonic manifestation of Wilson's disease is the dystonic facial expression known as risus sardonicus. This type of dystonia inflicts the patient with a forced, often exaggerated, smile.[38] Focal dystonia of the vocal cords, muscle of articulation, and swallowing frequently results in dysphonia, dysarthria, and dysphagia. Focal dystonia of the vocal cords, muscle of articulation, and swallowing can be an initial isolated feature or part of a generalized dystonia. Other focal dystonias include blepharospasm, cervical dystonia (torticollis), and writer's cramp. As the disease progresses focal dystonia can progress to segmental, multifocal, hemidystonia, and generalized dystonia. Dystonia, like many neurologic features of Wilson's disease, typically has a unilateral onset or predominance, but can progress to bilateral or generalized involvement. Severe dystonia may lead to extreme posturing of the trunk, neck, or extremities. As in other forms of dystonia, sensory tricks can often lead to temporary improvement. The presence of dystonia has been demonstrated to correlate with MRI signal abnormalities in the putamen.[31,38]

Tremor

Wilsonian tremor has been reported to be present in 22–55% and can occur at rest, upon assumption of a posture, or with action.[27,29,30,32,34] Although widely known, the wing-beating tremor of Wilson's disease does not appear to be the most frequent tremor type. Early in the neurologic presentation of Wilson's disease, the tremor can be identical to the tremor of essential tremor, with the arms most frequently involved but also involving the head and legs. Persistence of tremor asymmetry and absence of voice tremor may differentiate this type of Wilsonian tremor from essential tremor, which is typically symmetric and frequently involves the voice. As the disease progresses, Wilsonian tremor may take on characteristics atypical of essential tremor. It is not uncommon to encounter a tremor with multiple position- and task-dependent characteristics in an individual patient.[32] The kinetic tremor is most frequently a distal upper extremity, low amplitude, medium-to-high frequency tremor. The classical posture-induced wing-beating tremor, thought to be associated with lesions of the dentadorubrothalamic pathway, is a less frequently observed, lower frequency higher amplitude proximal upper extremity tremor elicited by holding the arms extended laterally or with the arms held in front with flexed elbows and palms facing downward. The wing-beating tremor is typified by increasing amplitude with increased duration of posture holding.[2] A unilateral isolated rest tremor is atypical in Wilson's disease. When rest tremor is present it is usually accompanied by postural and kinetic tremor, which may be more severe than the rest tremor.[29]

Parkinsonism

In series in which parkinsonism has been considered as a separate symptom category, it has been reported in 19–62%.[27,31,33,34] Bradykinesia, imbalance, and cogwheel rigidity are the more common parkinsonian features. Unilateral rest tremor and parkinsonism are rarely isolated clinical feature of Wilson's disease, but like idiopathic Parkinson's disease, rigidity, and tremor are typically asymmetric.

Choreoathetosis

Chorea and athetosis have been reported to occur in 6–16% of those with neurologic Wilson's disease.[29–31,33,34,37] Chorea is characterized by involuntary irregular rapid movements of the face, head, trunk, and extremities that are superimposed on and interrupt normal movement. Choreic movements can be subtle and small, occurring distally in the fingers resembling piano playing movements, and may also resemble fidgetiness and be incorporated into apparently purposeful movements. In an extreme form, they can manifest as disabling uncontrolled flailing movements of the extremities, termed ballism. Chorea is frequently accompanied by athetosis, a slow writhing movement of the limbs, trunk, or neck, and this combination is referred to as choreoathetosis. When present in Wilson's disease, chorea is more common in young onset disease (16 years of age and younger), where it has been reported in 20%. In contrast, chorea was reported in only 3% of adult onset (17 years of age and older).[27] Chorea can have many causes[40] and is not usually present in isolation in neurologic Wilson's disease.

Ataxia

Ataxia has been reported as a common feature in Wilson's disease, present in around 30%,[29,33] but it has not been observed or reported in other large case series.[27,31,32,34] Cerebellar findings are rarely clinically relevant and are not found in isolation; on exam, frank limb ataxia is infrequent. Cerebellar signs, other than extremity dysmetria, such as overshoot dysmetria of the eyes and limbs, or ataxic dysarthria can be found.[31]

Cognition

Cognitive impairment in Wilson's disease can be subtle, masked by affective involvement and recognized only in retrospect by the family or patient. When present, cognitive impairment falls into two main, not mutually exclusive, categories, a frontal lobe syndrome, or a subcortical dementia.[41,42] The frontal syndrome may manifest as impulsivity, promiscuity, impaired social judgment, apathy, decreased attention, executive dysfunction with poor planning and decision making, and emotional lability, at an extreme having pseudobulbar features. The subcortical dementia is characterized by slowness of thinking, memory loss, and executive dysfunction, without cortical signs of aphasia, apraxia, or agnosia.[41,42] Others have suggested that cognitive involvement in Wilson's disease may be primarily related to psychiatric and motor manifestations.[43,44]

Other neurologic features

Seizures are not an uncommon feature, occurring in approximately 6% (exceeding the general population frequency by 10-fold), are rarely the presenting feature, and have been associated with initiation of chelating therapy.[45] Hyperreflexia, unusual stereotyped movements, and tics have also been reported.[29]

Ophthalmologic manifestations

Copper deposits in the limbic region of the cornea known a Kayser-Fleischer (KF) rings are seen in nearly 100% of those with neurologic Wilson's disease, Figure 1.[23,33,46] In hepatic and presymptomatic Wilson's disease KF rings are present in about 50%.[23] KF rings are often evident by unaided visual inspection, but slit-lamp evaluation should be performed to verify their presence. KF rings are typically brown to brownish-green in color and are usually more prominent in the superior and inferior regions of the cornea. KF rings are not exclusive to Wilson's disease and can uncommonly be found in other obstructive liver disease.[47] Sunflower cataracts are seen less commonly than KF rings, present in about 17%.[46] Sunflower cataracts do not impair vision, cannot be seen with the unaided eye or with an ophthalmoscope, and require slit-lamp evaluation for detection. With treatment, KF rings and sunflower cataracts become less prominent and can disappear.[46] Other less common ophthalmologic findings include slowing of saccades, impaired upgaze, and strabismus. The absence of nystagmus in Wilson's disease can also be diagnostically useful.[46]

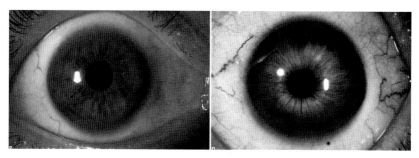

Figure 1. KF rings with prominence at the upper and lower corneal pole in an individual with brown eyes (*left panel*). Prominent full-circle KF rings in an individual with blue eyes (*right panel*).

Initial neurologic features

Knowledge of the ways neurologic Wilson's disease first manifests is critical to early diagnosis and prompt initiation of treatment. Unfortunately, Wilson's disease is often misdiagnosed, and the average time from symptom onset to diagnostic treatment is long, about 12 months.[27,29,31] Initial misdiagnosis in Wilson's disease includes over 100 different entities.[48] Highlighting the diagnostic challenge, initial neurologic misdiagnosis was found to span a spectrum from "no diagnosis," to "neurological problem," and included many common and rare entities.[48]

Diagnostic delay appears clinically significant, as treatment outcomes have been demonstrated to be better in those with a short diagnostic delay.[16] In patients who made a "very good" recovery, becoming free of neurologic symptoms, 21/57 (37%) had initiated therapy in less than 1 month. When delay in diagnosis increased to 1–6 months only 7/36 (19%) were able to achieve a "good" outcome, defined as minor disability.[16] It has also been shown that a delay in diagnosis increases the likelihood of a poor response to treatment. Walshe and Yealland demonstrated an increasing likelihood of a "poor" response to treatment as delay in diagnosis increased. Poor response was defined as being left with major disability. In those diagnosed in less than 1 month 12% had a poor outcome, diagnosis in 1–6 months lead to 21% with poor recovery, a diagnostic delay of 7–18 months led to 19% with poor outcome, while a greater than 18-month delay resulted in 38% with major disability.[16]

The true initial neurologic manifestations of Wilson's disease are illusive, but symptoms and signs at diagnosis have been reported in a number of large case series (Table 1).[27,29–31,34] In studies that categorize initial manifestations, dysarthria is the most common (57.6%), followed by dystonia (42.4%), abnormal gait (37.8%), tremor (36.2%), parkinsonism (17.3%), chorea or athetosis (15.3%), and seizures (4.7%). Ataxia was described as a separate category in only one study.[29] In these studies, investigations did not use the same criteria to define signs, studies did not use the same categorization, and the proportion of the time symptoms were present in isolation was not specified. Dysarthria, dystonia, tremor, and parkinsonism can be sole initial disease manifestations.

Psychiatric features

Psychiatric manifestations may be present as often as 30–50% of the time prior to a diagnosis of Wilson's disease.[43,44] Because psychiatric symptoms are often ill defined and attributed to other causes, diagnosis of Wilson's disease is rarely made during the period in which psychiatric symptoms are the sole manifestation. This aspect of Wilson's disease is likely a factor in diagnostic and treatment delay. At diagnosis, the most common psychiatric symptoms

Table 1. Initial clinical features of neurologic Wilson's disease

	35[a](%)	30[b]	28[c]	31[d]	32[c]	Total or (%Average)
Number of patients	48	119	136	27	31	361
Age at onset (years)		19.6	16.2	20.9	21	
Diagnostic delay (months)		~12	12.8		~12	
Dysarthria	46	91	39	15	97	(57.6)
Dystonia	38	69	29	11	65	(42.4)
Abnormal gait	24	75	10		42	(37.8)
Tremor	22	55	35	37	32	(36.2)
parknisonism	12	58[e]	21		19	(17.3)
Chorea or athetosis	6	30			10	(15.3)
seizures	6	4.2		4		(4.7)
Ataxia/cerebellar		28				

[a]first manifestations, [b]at time of diagnosis, [c]initial signs of neurologic presentation, [d]initial symptoms of neurologic presentation, [e]bradykinesia.

have been reported to be personality change, incongruous behavior, irritability, and depression.[44] During the course of disease, in addition to persistence of the presenting psychiatric symptoms, other features that can develop include impulsivity, dysinhibition, irritability, reckless behavior, anxiety, substance abuse, catatonia, emotionality, and mania.[43,44,49] Depression has been estimated to occur in 20–30% of those affected by Wilson's disease. It has been suggested that depression in Wilson's disease may be reactive, but this does not account for those presenting with depression. Psychotic features do not appear to be a common manifestation of Wilson's disease.[44,49] Psychiatric manifestations of Wilson's disease appear to be more common with neurologic involvement and are uncommon in the hepatic presentation.[44,50]

Hepatic features of Wilson's disease

The hepatic presentation can be divided into four main presentations, acute hepatitis, chronic active hepatitis, cirrhosis, and acute fulminant hepatic failure.[51] Other hepatic presentations include clinical pictures indistinguishable from alcoholic liver disease and autoimmune hepatitis.[26] A younger onset is seen in those whose symptoms are first hepatic: 11–15 years of age.[22,24] Because separating hepatitis, cirrhosis, or liver failure due to Wilson's disease from other etiologies is clinically challenging, screening for Wilson's disease should be performed in the appropriate clinical setting. Patients who present with hepatic failure may have mild failure with jaundice, low blood albumin, and edema, but not be in an acute, rapidly deteriorating, fulminant liver failure. Other patients may present with acute fulminant hepatic failure with Coombs-negative hemolytic anemia, coagulopathy, renal failure, and encephalopathy.[52] Hemolysis is believed to occur secondary to large copper release by acute hepatic necrosis. The occurrence of hemolysis in hepatic disease should always trigger a search for Wilson's disease because it is by far the most likely diagnosis. Patients with a neurologic presentation frequently have subclinical liver disease with a mild-to-moderate cirrhosis. For those with further interest, excellent reviews regarding hepatic features of Wilson's disease are available.[24,26,53]

In addition to the neurologic, psychiatric, and hepatic features, patients with Wilson's disease may have a variety of other clinical manifestations. These include abnormalities of renal tubular function, including Fanconi syndrome. Renal stones and gallstones are not uncommon. Patients may have osteoporosis or osteomalacia, or they may have joint disorders such as arthritis or arthralgias. Female patients frequently have oligomenorrhea or amenorrhea. Abnormalities of the heart include interstitial fibrosis and myocarditis. Electrocardiographic abnormalities and orthostatic hypertension are not uncommon. Pancreatic disease, parathyroidism, and skin abnormalities may be present.[23]

Natural history

Neurologic Wilson's disease most frequently becomes symptomatic in late childhood through early adulthood with a mean age of onset between 15 and 21 years of age.[27,29–33] It is unusual for Wilson's disease to become symptomatic after age 55, but a small number have neurologic onset over age 55 (Ref. 54, personal observation). Like the variable combinations of disease manifestations, the clinical course of Wilson's disease is highly variable. Although symptoms are typically gradual in their progression, sudden worsening, both with and without treatment, occurs. Day-to-day fluctuations of symptom severity is observed. It has been suggested that those with tremor-predominant symptoms may have a slower course than those with the predominantly dystonic form.[37] Younger-onset patents are more likely to have chorea and dystonia, and less likely to have a tremor predominant manifestation, whereas as those with an older onset tend to have tremor as the predominant sign.[27] Prior to the treatment era, the medial survival following development of neurologic symptoms was approximately 2–5 years, but Wilson's disease can progress slowly over more than 25 years.[16,55] In the absence of treatment, neurologic symptoms were progressive and resulted in a severely dystonic akinetic mute state with relative preservation of cognition; untreated Wilson's disease was inevitably fatal.[23] Experience and detailed investigations convincingly demonstrate the benefit of treatment, with chelation therapy normalizing life expectancy.[16–20,24,33]

Neuropathology

Wilson described softening of the lenticular nuclei, but it is now realized that brain pathology can be widespread and include the thalamus, subthalamic nuclei, brainstem, and frontal cortex. Grossly, the brain often demonstrates atrophy and increased ventricular size. The putamen and caudate can be brown and shrunken. Cavitation and cyst formation in the putamen, and frontal lobes is seen in advanced disease. Spongy degeneration of the cerebral cortex and subcortical white matter, particularly in the frontal lobes, occurs. Microscopic evaluation of affected areas demonstrates neuronal loss, pigment- and lipid-containing macrophages, and gliosis; Opalaski cells in the globus pallidus are a distinctive feature.[22,56]

Molecular genetics and pathogenesis

The Wilson's disease gene was mapped to chromosome 13q14.3, and the causative gene identified as ATP7B.[7–9] ATP7B is a 1411–amino acid, copper-transporting, P-type transmembrane ATPase that is highly expressed in the liver, kidney, and placenta.[7] Humans, including Wilson's disease patients, take in about 1.0 mg of copper per day in their diet and have a requirement for only about 0.75 mg. Thus, the extra 0.25 mg must be eliminated. The normal mechanism for elimination of excess copper is excretion in the bile for loss in the stool. Dietary copper is absorbed in the stomach and duodenum and transported via the portal vein to the liver, the main organ controlling copper regulation. Copper is absorbed into hepatocytes by copper transporter 1, then ATOX1, a copper-specific chaperone protein, transports copper to ATP7B. The normal function of ATP7B appears to be incorporation of copper into ceruloplasmin and secretion of copper into bile. As a result of the mutation in the ATP7B gene, the liver is not capable of excreting excess copper into the bile, and a positive copper balance, averaging about 0.25 mg/d, is established. Copper accumulates over time, first in the liver and then in other parts of the body, such as in the brain. The damage from excessive copper appears to be oxidant in nature.[23,53]

Wilson's disease is an autosomal recessive disease that occurs when a patient carries mutations in both copies of his/her ATP7B gene. Mutational analysis has identified over 300 different mutations throughout the ATP7B gene. A much smaller number of mutations is seen in the majority of patients, and individual mutations have been associated with different ethnic populations. The H1069Q substitution is the most common mutation in white populations representing approximately 40–60% of identified mutations.[57] The H1069Q is not prominent in Chinese or Indian populations, in whom other mutations, including R778G, occur at higher frequency.[58,59] The H1069Q mutation, particularly when homozygous, has been associated with a later onset neurologic disease.[60,61] Other consistent genotype–phenotype correlations have been elusive. Because of the large number of disease-causing mutations, most patients are compound heterozygotes (have two different mutations). It is not know how the same mutation is able to cause hepatic disease in some, but neurologic in others. A combination of environmental, genetic, and epigenetic factors is likely responsible.

Differential diagnosis

Neurologic Wilson's disease must be distinguished from other common and rare neurologic diseases. Because Wilson's disease is treatable, it should be considered as a possible diagnosis in every young person with a movement disorder. The more common neurologic disorders that can mimic Wilson's disease include essential tremor, young-onset Parkinson's disease, and generalized dystonia. Rare juvenile genetic extrapyramidal disorders including Huntington disease, Hallervorden-Spatz disease, idiopathic torsion dystonia, chorea-acanthocytosis, and benign familial chorea can at times mimic Wilson's disease. Neither chorea nor ataxia is typically found in isolation, and although Wilson's disease can be considered, diagnostic consideration for other causes of primarily choreic and ataxic diseases should be undertaken. The psychiatric abnormalities may be mistaken for a psychological abnormality, affective disorder, early schizophrenia, or drug abuse. The presence of Kayser-Fleischer rings and the coexistence of liver disease provide important clues.

Diagnostic workup

The most common screening method for Wilson's disease is a blood ceruloplasmin determination, although this is inadequate for either ruling in or ruling out Wilson's disease. The ceruloplasmin value is usually low in Wilson's disease, but in approximately 10% of patients it may be normal or near normal. About 10% of heterozygous carriers who will never have clinical problems will also demonstrate low ceruloplasmin values. The most useful screening procedure is a 24-h urine copper test.[22,23] In symptomatic Wilson's disease 24-h urine copper is always elevated to a value greater than 100 μg per 24 h (normal is 50 or less). The 24-h urine sample must be collected in a container free of trace elements. A laboratory capable of measuring copper in low concentrations is required to do the assay. If these difficulties can be overcome, this test is quite reliable in screening for Wilson's disease.

Another common screening procedure is a slit-lamp examination for KF rings. Visual inspection is not adequate. KF rings are invariably present in the psychiatric and neurologic presentations; however, they are present in only about 50% of patients who present with liver disease. In a patient with classical clinical disease, KF rings, and elevated urine copper, the diagnosis can be made with certainty. If any question remains, the gold standard for diagnosis is a measure of quantitative copper in a percutaneous liver biopsy. The hepatic copper value in untreated Wilson's disease is above 200 μg/g dry weight of tissue, with normal being 50 μg/g or less. Carriers of the Wilson's disease gene may have mild elevations of hepatic copper, but never to 200 μg/g. It is important not to rely on the stain for copper, for if the copper is still diffusely cytoplasmic, the copper stain may be negative in the face of very great elevations of hepatic copper. Radiocopper studies have been suggested for the diagnosis of Wilson's disease, but their usefulness is questionable. While these tests are abnormal in Wilson's disease, they are also abnormal in carriers of the disease and thus are fraught with the risk of misdiagnosis.[23]

The gene for Wilson's disease has been cloned,[7–9] fostering hope for the development of a direct DNA test. This approach is not practical because more than 300 different mutations that may cause Wilson's disease have been identified.[53,57] However, if a mutation is identified in a proband, then search for this mutation in relatives can provide crucial information for the identification of as yet asymptomatic relatives and of heterozygotes, and provides the opportunity for preventive therapy and genetic counseling.

Central nervous system imaging can be helpful in the diagnosis, Figure 2. MRI scans generally demonstrate abnormalities in patients with neurologic or psychiatric symptoms but are often normal in patients with only liver disease. In neurologically in-

volved patients, the most common findings are areas of high T2 signal in the lentiform and caudate nuclei, thalamus, brain stem, and white matter.[31,62,63] High signal T1 images, like those in portal-systemic encephalopathy may also be observed.[64] Dopamine D2 receptor binding and regional cerebral glucose metabolism are reduced in the striatum and have been shown to return to almost normal levels after penicillamine therapy.[65]

Treatment

Wilson's disease is a condition that can be effectively treated. Treatment can be divided into initial therapy, maintenance therapy, and treatment of the presymptomatic patient.[23,26] Available pharmacologic agents include penicillamine, trientine, zinc acetate, and tetrathiomolybdate. The aim of treatment is to reduce the amount of toxic free copper. Free copper is toxic whereas copper bound to ceruloplasmin or metallothionein is not.

Although penicillamine demonstrated clear therapeutic advantages over BAL, initial neurologic worsening following initiation of penicillamine therapy is a concern. In their retrospective study, Brewer and colleagues found that the risk for neurologic worsening was about 50% when penicillamine was used as initial treatment of neurologic Wilson's disease and that 50% of those who deteriorated never recovered to their prepenicillamine baseline.[66] The majority of patients observed to have deteriorated did so within 4 weeks of beginning penicillamine therapy. It has been suggested that mobilization of large hepatic copper stores raises blood free-copper levels leading to increased toxic copper exposure to the brain and subsequent worsening.[66]

Others have investigated the efficacy and toxicity of penicillamine treatment of neurologic Wilson's disease.[24,32,67] In a description of their experience Walshe and colleagues described outcomes following treatment of neurologic Wilson's disease with penicillamine. In this study if toxicity developed while using penicillamine, therapy was switched to trientine. In some patients in this series, trientine was used as first-line therapy, and in a small number zinc, BAL, or tetrathiomolybdate was used following penicillamine.[16] In all, 137 patients were followed, 57 (41%) became symptom free, 36 (26%) were left with minor neurologic deficit, 24 (18%) were left disabled, and 20

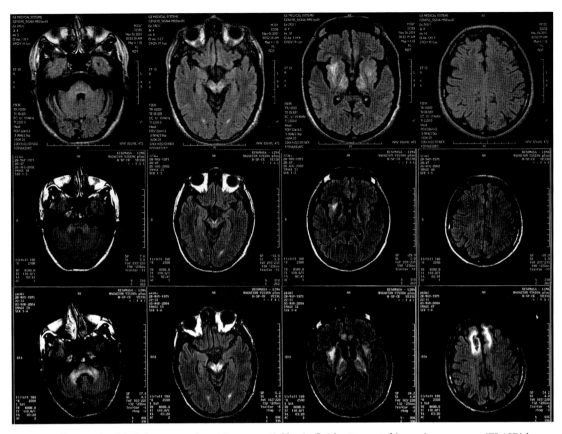

Figure 2. Progressive MRI changes as shown in sequential brain fluid–attenuated inversion-recovery (FLAIR) imaging in an individual with untreated Wilson's disease. Representative images are shown at the level of the superior cerebellar peduncle (*first column*), the midbrain (*second column from the left*), the basal ganglion (*third column from the left*), and at the level of the cerebral cortex (*right-most column*). Images in the top, middle, and bottom rows were obtained in 2001, 2002, and 2004, respectively.

(15%) died.[16] Most patients who improved began to do so in 3–6 months. Thirty (22%) had increased symptom severity after initiation of treatment. In those who had initial worsening, 11 (37% of those who worsened) eventually became symptom free, 9 (30%) were left with minor neurologic deficit, and 10 (33%) were left disabled.[16] No features were identified that were able to predict those who worsened. Of individuals who died despite treatment, no factors could be identified to predict who would die. These patients were not more likely to present with a dystonic phenotype, but most had become severely dystonic prior to death.[16] In this study penicillamine was associated with toxicity requiring discontinuation of its use in around 20%.[16] In another study of largely neurologic Wilson's disease 44% discontinued penicillamine secondary to

side effects.[68] Complications of penicillamine include rash, immune complex nephropathy, systemic lupus erythematosus, thrombocytopenia, and leucocytopenia.[16,68]

This study is additionally notable because neurologic features were examined for an association with treatment outcome. The pseudosclerotic (tremor and dysarthric) form of neurologic Wilson's disease was found to be associated with the best chance of a favorable outcome.[16] Patients with the pseudosclerotic form of neurologic Wilson's disease were found to have an 82% chance of becoming symptom free or having minor neurologic deficit. Those with chorea had a 75% chance, those with parkinsonism a 63% chance, and those with dystonia a 53% chance of becoming symptom free or having minor neurologic deficit.[16]

Stremmel and colleagues described their experience with penicillamine in a total of 51 patients, 31 with neurologic Wilson's disease.[32] In this study neurologic and hepatic Wilson's were often considered together. Improvement in neurologic features was described following penicillamine therapy. No description of initial neurologic worsening was reported, but penicillamine-induced adverse reactions occurred in 25%.[32] Stremmel and colleagues further described treatment of Wilson's disease in 163 additional Wilson's disease patients, 58 with neurologic Wilson's disease.[24] In the neurologic group, 54% improved, 22% were stable, and 24% worsened. Of all the patients 70.3% developed side effects to penicillamine and 31% experienced severe side effects including neurologic worsening. Neurologic worsening occurred early after initiation of therapy and in some did not improve.[24]

Because of concern for neurologic worsening in those treated with penicillamine, use of other agents has been recommended for initial treatment of neurologic Wilson's disease.[14,20,24,69] If penicillamine is used, the standard starting dose is 250 mg four times a day or 500 mg twice a day. It has been suggested that starting with lower doses, 250–500 mg per day for a few weeks may lessen side effects.[26] When initiated, the patient should be carefully monitored for toxicities including to the bone marrow and kidney. An acute hypersensitivity reaction occurs in about 25% of patients, which may respond to corticosteroid therapy or withdrawal of the drug and readministration in very low doses.

Trientine has often been used as an alternative or second-line therapy, but like penicillamine it can cause neurologic worsening in approximately 25%.[20,26] Trientine is a chelator that, like penicillamine, promotes urinary excretion of copper. Trientine is used in doses of 750–1500 mg for initial therapy and 750 mg to 1000 mg for maintenance therapy, divided into two or three doses per day. It should be given 1 h before or 2 h after meals. Although trientine has fewer side effects than penicillamine it shares a common mechanism of action and can cause neurologic worsening. In a double-blind study comparing tetrathiomolybdate to trientine, 24% of those treated with trientine experienced neurologic worsening and in those who initially worsened 50% died.[20] While on trientine, urine copper is a reflection of enhanced urinary copper excretion and total body copper load. Upon initial treatment

with trientine, 24-h urinary copper excretion may be 1000–3000 μg (normal is 20–50 μg/24 h). After a few weeks urinary copper decreases to 500–1000 μg per 24 h, and after approximately 1 year of therapy it should decrease to 200–500 μg per 24 h. Nonceruloplasmin-bound copper, free copper, is a useful measure for monitoring efficacy of trientine and can be calculated by the formula: (Total serum copper in μg/mL × 100) – (ceruloplasmin in mg/dL × 3) = free copper (normal range is 5–15 μg/dL). Another way that free copper can be accurately estimated is by subtracting 3 μg for every 1 mg/dL of ceruloplasmin from the serum copper, expressed as μg/dL. During the maintenance phase of trientine therapy keeping free copper below 25 mg is the goal.

Zinc acetate therapy has been used successfully as a preventative therapy in presymptomatic patients, as initial treatment for neurologic Wilson's disease, and as maintenance therapy following an initial course of decoppering.[69,70] Zinc induces intestinal cell metallothionein, a protein that complexes intestinal food copper or endogenously secreted copper in saliva and gastric secretions. The complex cannot be absorbed in to the blood, and as intestinal cells die they, along with the complex, are sloughed into the stool resulting in a negative copper balance. The net effect of zinc therapy is an intestinal blockade of zinc absorption. Zinc has the additional effect of inducing hepatocyte metallothionein production, which may reduce the toxic effect of free copper in these cells.[22,70]

The decoppering effect of zinc is slow: a period of 4–8 months of treatment is required to reduce copper to nontoxic levels. In symptomatic individuals, the natural course of disease continues during this period and can lead to permanent worsening. To avoid potential toxicities of trientine and penicillamine, some have successfully used zinc in the initial treatment of neurologic Wilson's disease.[15,69,71–75] An advantage of zinc is its lack of serious significant side effects and safety in long-term use.[71,76] Approximately 10% experience gastric discomfort or nausea upon initiation of zinc therapy. The use of the zinc acetate compared to zinc sulfate reduces gastric discomfort. Generally, gastric symptoms subside within days to weeks. For maintenance and prophylactic therapy in adults, 50 mg of zinc three times a day is recommended.[69,70,76] It is important to separate the zinc from food by at least an hour. For maintenance therapy zinc is favored over penicillamine or trientine, because while all three drugs are effective, zinc has a superior side-effect profile and does not appear to cause neurologic worsening.[23,69] Because zinc therapy does not induce urinary excretion of copper, as do trientine or penicillamine, urine copper is an accurate reflection of body copper stores. Following a year of zinc therapy, a 24-h copper of around 125 μg is a reflection of good copper control. Compliance with zinc can be assessed by monitoring 24-h urine zinc excretion, which should be above 2 mg.[22]

For the initial treatment of patients presenting with neurologic or psychiatric disease, the use of tetrathiomolybdate (TM) followed by zinc maintenance therapy has been suggested to provide a good best balance of efficacy and side effects, but TM is not yet FDA approved.[20] TM acts by forming a tripartite complex with copper and protein. Given with food, TM binds food copper and endogenously secreted copper preventing copper absorption. Given between meals, TM is absorbed into the blood and forms a complex with free copper and albumin. Free copper in the blood is in equilibrium with tissue copper so that binding of serum copper to TM shifts the equilibrium to mobilize copper from tissue stores into serum where it is bound by TM and excreted into bile. The result is a rapid removal of tissue copper, which is then bound in the serum by TM, reducing potential copper toxicity, and significantly less neurologic worsening compared to penicillamine or trientine.[17–20] In a double-blind study 48 patients were randomized to TM or trientine for the initial treatment of neurologic Wilson's disease. TM, 20 mg three times a day with meals and 20 mg three times a day between meals, or trientine, 500 mg two times per day, were given for 8 weeks with zinc, 50 mg twice daily, followed by zinc maintenance therapy. Both trientine and TM were found to improve neurologic and speech function, but TM was significantly less likely to be associated with neurologic worsening than trientine.[20] In the trientine arm 6 of 23 (26%) patients worsened neurologically, and 3 of those who worsened died. In the TM arm 1 of 25 (4%) patients developed neurologic deterioration, a statistically significant difference. In an earlier open-label study of TM in initial treatment of neurologic Wilson's disease 2 of 55 (3.6%) patients treated with TM worsened.[19] Serious adverse effects from TM were not observed. TM was associated with reversible increases in transaminase levels and

anemia in about 15%.[19,20] Anemia and transaminase elevations responded to temporary suspension of TM without subsequent abnormalities following reinitiation of TM at half dose.[19,20] 24-h urine copper monitoring during treatment with TM can be used to monitor therapy. In untreated Wilson's disease, 24-h urinary excretion always exceeds 100 μg per 24 h. The goal of treatment following an initial course of TM followed by maintenance therapy with zinc is a 24 h urine copper excretion of 50–100 μg. A study evaluating lower doses of TM is ongoing (G.J. Brewer, personal communication, 2008). It is anticipated that TM will be FDA approved, and more widely available.

Some have reported that individuals with decompensated liver disease treated with orthotopic liver transplant demonstrated improvement of neurologic symptoms.[77,78] Other studies have not demonstrated a benefit, and orthotopic liver transplant is not recommended as a treatment for neurologic Wilson's disease.[22,79] In those studies reporting on the effect of treatment, the largest degree of improvement was observed between 6 months and 2 years of adequate copper control, with some benefit reported to occur for up to 3 years.[20,24,32,43,44,67] The response to treatment is variable. Few studies have systematically investigated or reported the effect of treatment on individual neurologic signs or symptoms. Currently no reliable predictors exist to differentiate those who will make an excellent recovery from those whose symptoms will stabilize but not improve. It has been suggested that tremor may be more treatment responsive than dystonia and dysarthria.[16,36] Those who did not respond to treatment tended to have a more severe neurologic disease, with more frequent dysarthria and dystonia.[16,44] In those severely impaired by neurologic Wilson's disease, attempts to determine factors associated with a good recovery were not found.[67]

Symptomatic treatment of the movement disorders found in Wilson's patients has not be carefully studied, and response to treatment is inconsistent.[16] There are no good studies that have investigated dopamine agonists for treatment of parkinsonism in Wilson's disease. L-dopa and dopamine agonists do not appear to provide reliable relief of parkinsonism. β-blockers and primidone, medications used to treat essential tremor, can be tried in those with limiting essential tremor-like tremor, but their benefit is limited. Artane, baclofen, and valium can be used in symptomatic therapy of dystonia. Speech and physical therapy can provide a great deal of benefit.

Psychiatric manifestations of Wilson's disease also have a variable response to treatment. Incongruous behavior and cognitive impairment were reported to be more treatment responsive than irritability or depression. Improvements tended to occur relatively early in the course of treatment, before 3.5 years, and then reach a plateau.[44] Others have suggested that the most prominent improvement occurs between 6 and 18 months following initiation of therapy and then plateaus after 2 years of copper-level normalization.[43]

In patients who present with liver disease, if the disease if fulminant, hepatic transplant may be the only way to save the patient's life. However, in cases of mild hepatic failure, a picture of chronic cirrhosis, or a picture of mild hepatitis, medical treatment can be quite effective. The prognostic index of Nazer is useful in differentiating which patients will likely do well with medical therapy.[80] The combination of trientine followed by zinc maintenance may represent the best medical treatment for hepatic Wilson's disease. The trientine is given to obtain a rather robust negative copper balance. Zinc is given to induce hepatic metallothionein and allow that metallothionein to complex copper in the liver in a nontoxic form. This combination is used for 4 months and then the trientine is discontinued.

Over the years, considerable attention has been paid to diet in Wilson's disease. In the United States only liver and shellfish are high enough in copper to be of concern.[22,23] Because animals are fed high levels of minerals, the liver can be very high in copper and should not be ingested during the decoppering period (first 4 months) and after that only in small amounts. Shellfish are intermediately high in copper and should not be ingested during the decoppering period and not ingested more often than once a week during maintenance therapy. Other foods are not restricted because the content of copper is not high enough to be of concern. Occasionally, drinking-water samples will be found to be high in copper. If the level is higher than about 0.1 ppm the patient should use an alternative source of drinking water.

Prevention

Identification and treatment of presymptomatic Wilson's disease patients can prevent development of symptoms. Aggressive screening measures in clinic populations at risk are critical. An important target population is the siblings of the newly diagnosed patient. Each sibling has a 25% risk of being in the presymptomatic disease stage. Because prophylactic therapy will prevent the onset of the disease, these patients should be examined and disease status determined. All full siblings should be screened for blood ceruloplasmin, and 24-h urine copper levels. A 24-h urine copper in presymptomatic siblings with a value of 100 is diagnostic of Wilson's disease. If it is less than 50 in an adult patient, it essentially excludes the diagnosis. If it is intermediate, it is compatible either with the carrier state, since some of these patients have mild elevations of urine copper, or the presymptomatic affected state, since some of these patients do not have diagnostic levels of urine copper. The patients in this intermediate zone should have a liver biopsy to make the diagnosis. The liver copper level in such a patient is diagnostic. Because the risk of Wilson's disease is significantly elevated in nieces and nephews (1/600) and cousins (1/800), compared to the general population, these relatives can be screened for ceruloplasmin and 24-h urine copper levels.

Conclusion

The history of Wilson's disease is remarkable in many aspects. Like other well known neurodegenerative diseases such as Alzheimer's or Parkinson's disease, pioneering individuals contributed seminal observations regarding disease features and etiology. Unlike other neurodegenerative diseases this work has lead to treatment that can essentially cure the disease. Unfortunately, neurologic Wilson's disease continues to suffer from clinically significant diagnostic delay. Currently available therapies have had a major positive impact on the outcome of neurologic Wilson's disease, but have limitations. Future studies promise to delineate optimal therapeutic regimes and improved clinical outcomes.

Acknowledgments

The author would like to thank Dr. Wayne Cornblath for providing the KF ring images. The author would also like to acknowledge Dr. George Brewer for his continued commitment to Wilson's disease patients and for providing me the opportunity to be involved in his research.

Conflicts of interest

The author declares no conflicts of interest.

References

1. Wilson, S. 1912. Progressive lenticular degeneration: A familial nervous disease associated with cirrhosis of the liver. *Brain* **34:** 295–509.

2. Walshe, J.M. 1988. Wilson's disease: yesterday, today, and tomorrow. *Mov. Disord.* **3:** 10–29.

3. Scheinberg, I.H. & D. Gitlin. 1952. Deficiency of ceruloplasmin in patients with hepatolenticular degeneration (Wilson's disease). *Science* **116:** 484–485.

4. Osborn, S.B., C.N. Roberts & J.M. Walshe. 1963. Uptake of radiocopper by the liver. A study of patients with Wilson's disease and various control groups. *Clin. Sci.* **24:** 13–22.

5. Walshe, J.M. & G. Potter. 1977. The pattern of the whole body distribution of radioactive copper (67Cu, 64Cu) in Wilson's Disease and various control groups. *Q. J. Med.* **46:** 445–462.

6. Bearn, A.G. 1960. A genetical analysis of thirty families with Wilson's disease (hepatolenticular degeneration). *Ann. Hum. Genet.* **24:** 33–43.

7. Bull, P.C. *et al.* 1993. The Wilson disease gene is a putative copper transporting P-type ATPase similar to the Menkes gene. *Nat. Genet.* **5:** 327–337.

8. Tanzi, R.E. *et al.* 1993. The Wilson disease gene is a copper transporting ATPase with homology to the Menkes disease gene. *Nat. Genet.* **5:** 344–350.

9. Yamaguchi, Y., M.E. Heiny & J.D. Gitlin. 1993. Isolation and characterization of a human liver cDNA as a candidate gene for Wilson disease. *Biochem. Biophys. Res. Commun.* **197:** 271–277.

10. Cumings, J.N. 1948. The copper and iron content of brain and liver in the normal and in hepato-lenticular degeneration. *Brain* **71:** 410–415.

11. Cumings, J.N. 1951. The effects of B.A.L. in hepatolenticular degeneration. *Brain* **74:** 10–22.

12. Denny-Brown, D. & H. Porter. 1951. The effect of BAL (2,3-dimercaptopropanol) on hepatolenticular degeneration (Wilson's disease). *N. Engl. J. Med.* **245:** 917–925.

13. Walshe, J.M. 1956. Penicillamine, a new oral therapy for Wilson's disease. *Am. J. Med.* **21:** 487–495.

14. Brewer, G.J. *et al.* 1983. Oral zinc therapy for Wilson's disease. *Ann. Intern. Med.* **99:** 314–319.

15. Hoogenraad, T.U., R. Koevoet & E.G. de Ruyter Korver. 1979. Oral zinc sulphate as long-term treatment in Wilson's disease (hepatolenticular degeneration). *Eur. Neurol.* **18:** 205–211.

16. Walshe, J.M. & M. Yealland. 1993. Chelation treatment of neurological Wilson's disease. *Q. J. Med.* **86:** 197–204.

17. Brewer, G.J. *et al.* 1994. Treatment of Wilson's disease with ammonium tetrathiomolybdate. I. Initial therapy in 17 neurologically affected patients. *Arch. Neurol.* **51:** 545–554.

18. Brewer, G.J. *et al.* 1996. Treatment of Wilson disease with ammonium tetrathiomolybdate. II. Initial therapy in 33 neurologically affected patients and follow-up with zinc therapy. *Arch. Neurol.* **53:** 1017–1025.

19. Brewer, G.J. *et al.* 2003. Treatment of Wilson disease with ammonium tetrathiomolybdate: III. Initial therapy in a total of 55 neurologically affected patients and follow-up with zinc therapy. *Arch. Neurol.* **60:** 379–385.

20. Brewer, G.J. *et al.* 2006. Treatment of Wilson disease with ammonium tetrathiomolybdate: IV. Comparison of tetrathiomolybdate and trientine in a double-blind study of treatment of the neurologic presentation of Wilson disease. *Arch. Neurol.* **63:** 521–527.

21. Reilly, M., L. Daly & M. Hutchinson. 1993. An epidemiological study of Wilson's disease in the Republic of Ireland. *J. Neurol. Neurosurg. Psychiatry* **56:** 298–300.

22. Brewer, G.J. 2001. *Wilson's Disease : A Clinician's Guide to Recognition, Diagnosis, and Management*. Kluwer Academic. Boston.

23. Brewer, G.J. & V. Yuzbasiyan-Gurkan. 1992. Wilson disease. *Medicine (Baltimore)* **71:** 139–164.

24. Merle, U. *et al.* 2007. Clinical presentation, diagnosis and long-term outcome of Wilson's disease: a cohort study. *Gut* **56:** 115–120.

25. Ala, A. *et al.* 2005. Wilson disease in septuagenarian siblings: Raising the bar for diagnosis. *Hepatology* **41:** 668–670.

26. Roberts, E.A. & M.L. Schilsky. 2003. A practice guideline on Wilson disease. *Hepatology* **37:** 1475–1492.

27. Walshe, J.M. & M. Yealland. 1992. Wilson's disease: the problem of delayed diagnosis. *J. Neurol. Neurosurg. Psychiatry* **55:** 692–696.

28. Giagheddu, A. *et al.* 1985. Epidemiologic study of hepatolenticular degeneration (Wilson's disease) in Sardinia (1902–1983). *Acta Neurol. Scand.* **72:** 43–55.

29. Machado, A. *et al.* 2006. Neurological manifestations in Wilson's disease: Report of 119 cases. *Mov. Disord.* **21:** 2192–2196.

30. Oder, W. *et al.* 1991. Neurological and neuropsychiatric spectrum of Wilson's disease: a prospective study of 45 cases. *J. Neurol.* **238:** 281–287.

31. Starosta-Rubinstein, S. *et al.* 1987. Clinical assessment of 31 patients with Wilson's disease. Correlations with

structural changes on magnetic resonance imaging. *Arch. Neurol.* **44:** 365–370.

32. Stremmel, W. *et al.* 1991. Wilson disease: clinical presentation, treatment, and survival. *Ann. Intern. Med.* **115:** 720–726.

33. Taly, A.B. *et al.* 2007. Wilson disease: description of 282 patients evaluated over 3 decades. *Medicine (Baltimore)* **86:** 112–121.

34. Soltanzadeh, A. *et al.* 2007. Wilson's disease: a great masquerader. *Eur. Neurol.* **57:** 80–85.

35. Dening, T.R. & G.E. Berrios. 1989. Wilson's disease: clinical groups in 400 cases. *Acta Neurol. Scand.* **80:** 527–534.

36. Denny-Brown, D. 1964. Hepatolenticular degeneration (Wilson's disease). Two different components. *N. Engl. J. Med.* **270:** 1149–1156.

37. Okinaka, S. 1961. Studies on hepatocerebral disease. III. Hepatolenticular degeneration in Japan, with studies on copper metabolism. *Neurology* **11:** 792–799.

38. Svetel, M. *et al.* 2001. Dystonia in Wilson's disease. *Mov. Disord.* **16:** 719–723.

39. Volkmann, J. *et al.* 1992. Impairment of temporal organization of speech in basal ganglia diseases. *Brain Lang.* **43:** 386–399.

40. Lorincz, M.T. 2006. Geriatric chorea. *Clin. Geriatr. Med.* **22:** 879–897, vii.

41. Lang, C. 1989. Is Wilson's disease a dementing condition? *J. Clin. Exp. Neuropsychol.* **11:** 569–570.

42. Lang, C. *et al.* 1990. Neuropsychological findings in treated Wilson's disease. *Acta Neurol. Scand.* **81:** 75–81.

43. Akil, M. & G.J. Brewer. 1995. Psychiatric and behavioral abnormalities in Wilson's disease. *Adv. Neurol.* **65:** 171–178.

44. Dening, T.R. & G.E. Berrios. 1990. Wilson's disease: a longitudinal study of psychiatric symptoms. *Biol. Psychiatry* **28:** 255–265.

45. Dening, T.R., G.E. Berrios & J.M. Walshe. 1988. Wilson's disease and epilepsy. *Brain* **111**(Pt 5): 1139–1155.

46. Wiebers, D.O., R.W. Hollenhorst & N.P. Goldstein. 1977. The ophthalmologic manifestations of Wilson's disease. *Mayo Clin. Proc.* **52:** 409–416.

47. Fleming, C.R. *et al.* 1977. Pigmented corneal rings in non-Wilsonian liver disease. *Ann. Intern. Med.* **86:** 285–288.

48. Prashanth, L.K. *et al.* 2004. Wilson's disease: diagnostic errors and clinical implications. *J. Neurol. Neurosurg. Psychiatry* **75:** 907–909.

49. Goldstein, N.P. *et al.* 1968. Psychiatric aspects of Wilson's disease (hepatolenticular degeneration): results of psychometric tests during long-term therapy. *Am. J. Psychiatry* **124:** 1555–1561.

50. Dening, T.R. & G.E. Berrios. 1989. Wilson's disease. Psychiatric symptoms in 195 cases. *Arch. Gen. Psychiatry* **46:** 1126–1134.

51. Sallie, R. *et al.* 1992. Failure of simple biochemical indexes to reliably differentiate fulminant Wilson's disease from other causes of fulminant liver failure. *Hepatology* **16:** 1206–1211.

52. Ostapowicz, G. *et al.* 2002. Results of a prospective study of acute liver failure at 17 tertiary care centers in the United States. *Ann. Intern. Med.* **137:** 947–954.

53. Ala, A. *et al.* 2007. Wilson's disease. *Lancet* **369:** 397–408.

54. Ross, M.E. *et al.* 1985. Late-onset Wilson's disease with neurological involvement in the absence of Kayser-Fleischer rings. *Ann. Neurol.* **17:** 411–413.

55. Shimoji, A. *et al.* 1987. Wilson's disease with extensive degeneration of cerebral white matter and cortex. *Jpn. J. Psychiatry Neurol.* **41:** 709–717.

56. Ellison, D. & S. Love. 1998. *Neuropathology.* Mosby. Tokyo.

57. Shah, A.B. *et al.* 1997. Identification and analysis of mutations in the Wilson disease gene (ATP7B): population frequencies, genotype-phenotype correlation, and functional analyses. *Am. J. Hum. Genet.* **61:** 317–328.

58. Gu, Y.H. *et al.* 2003. Mutation spectrum and polymorphisms in ATP7B identified on direct sequencing of all exons in Chinese Han and Hui ethnic patients with Wilson's disease. *Clin. Genet.* **64:** 479–484.

59. Kumar, S. *et al.* 2005. Identification and molecular characterization of 18 novel mutations in the ATP7B gene from Indian Wilson disease patients: genotype. *Clin. Genet.* **67:** 443–445.

60. Stapelbroek, J.M. *et al.* 2004. The H1069Q mutation in ATP7B is associated with late and neurologic presentation in Wilson disease: results of a meta-analysis. *J. Hepatol.* **41:** 758–763.

61. Vrabelova, S. *et al.* 2005. Mutation analysis of the ATP7B gene and genotype/phenotype correlation in 227 patients with Wilson disease. *Mol. Genet. Metab.* **86:** 277–285.

62. Magalhaes, A.C. *et al.* 1994. Wilson's disease: MRI with clinical correlation. *Neuroradiology* **36:** 97–100.

63. van Wassenaer-van Hall, H.N. *et al.* 1996. Wilson disease: findings at MR imaging and CT of the brain with clinical correlation. *Radiology* **198:** 531–536.

64. Sinha, S.S. *et al.* 2007. Sequential MRI changes in Wilson's disease with de-coppering therapy: a study of 50 patients. *Br. J. Radiol.* **80:** 7 4–749.

65. Schlaug, G. *et al.* 1994. Dopamine D2 receptor binding and cerebral glucose metabolism recover after

D-penicillamine-therapy in Wilson's disease. *J. Neurol.* **241:** 577–584.

66. Brewer, G.J. *et al.* 1987. Worsening of neurologic syndrome in patients with Wilson's disease with initial penicillamine therapy. *Arch. Neurol.* **44:** 490–493.

67. Prashanth, L.K. *et al.* 2005. Prognostic factors in patients presenting with severe neurological forms of Wilson's disease. *QJM* **98:** 557–563.

68. Czlonkowska, A., J. Gajda & M. Rodo. 1996. Effects of long-term treatment in Wilson's disease with D-penicillamine and zinc sulphate. *J. Neurol.* **243:** 269–273.

69. Hoogenraad, T.U. 2006. Paradigm shift in treatment of Wilson's disease: zinc therapy now treatment of choice. *Brain Dev.* **28:** 141–146.

70. Brewer, G.J., V. Yuzbasiyan-Gurkan & D.Y. Lee. 1990. Use of zinc-copper metabolic interactions in the treatment of Wilson's disease. *J. Am. Coll. Nutr.* **9:** 487–491.

71. Marcellini, M. *et al.* 2005. Treatment of Wilson's disease with zinc from the time of diagnosis in pediatric patients: a single-hospital, 10-year follow-up study. *J. Lab. Clin. Med.* **145:** 139–143.

72. Hockly, E. *et al.* 2002. Environmental enrichment slows disease progression in R6/2 Huntington's disease mice. *Ann. Neurol.* **51:** 235–242.

73. Hoogenraad, T.U. 1998. Zinc treatment of Wilson's disease. *J. Lab. Clin. Med.* **132:** 240–241.

74. Hoogenraad, T.U. & J. Van Hattum. 1988. Zinc therapy as the initial treatment for Wilson's disease. *Arch. Neurol.* **45:** 373–374.

75. Hoogenraad, T.U., J. Van Hattum & C.J. Van Den Hamer. 1987. Management of Wilson's disease with zinc sulphate. Experience in a series of 27 patients. *J. Neurol. Sci.* **77:** 137–146.

76. Anderson, L.A., S.L. Hakojarvi & S.K. Boudreaux. 1998. Zinc acetate treatment in Wilson's disease. *Ann. Pharmacother.* **32:** 78–87.

77. Eghtesad, B. *et al.* 1999. Liver transplantation for Wilson's disease: a single-center experience. *Liver Transpl. Surg.* **5:** 467–474.

78. Schumacher, G. *et al.* 1997. Liver transplantation: treatment of choice for hepatic and neurological manifestation of Wilson's disease. *Clin. Transplant.* **11:** 217–224.

79. Rodriguez, R.T. *et al.* 2007. Manipulation of OCT4 levels in human embryonic stem cells results in induction of differential cell types. *Exp. Biol. Med. (Maywood)* **232:** 1368–1380.

80. Nazer, H. *et al.* 1986. Wilson's disease: clinical presentation and use of prognostic index. *Gut* **27:** 1377–1381.

Ann. N.Y. Acad. Sci. ISSN 0077-8923

ANNALS OF THE NEW YORK ACADEMY OF SCIENCES

The progression of pathology in Parkinson's disease

Glenda Margaret Halliday and Heather McCann

Prince of Wales Medical Research Institute and University of New South Wales, Sydney, Australia

Address for correspondence: Professor Glenda Halliday, Prince of Wales Medical Research Institute, Barker Street, Randwick, NSW 2031, Australia. Voice: +61 2 9399 1104; fax: +61 2 9399 1105. g.halliday@powmri.edu.au

To identify the progression of pathology over the entire course of Parkinson's disease, we longitudinally followed a clinical cohort to autopsy and identified three clinicopathological phenotypes that progress at different rates. Typical Parkinson's disease has an initial rapid loss of midbrain dopamine neurons with a slow progression of Lewy body infiltration into the brain (over decades). Dementia intervenes late when Lewy bodies invade the neocortex. Older onset patients (> 70 years old) dement earlier and have much shorter disease durations. Paradoxically, they have far more α-synuclein-containing Lewy bodies throughout the brain, and many also have additional age-related plaque pathology. In contrast, dementia with Lewy bodies has the shortest disease course, with substantive amounts of Lewy bodies and Alzheimer-type pathologies infiltrating the brain. These data suggest that two age-related factors influence pathological progression in Parkinson's disease—the age at symptom onset and the degree and type of age-related Alzheimer-type pathology.

Keywords: α-synuclein; disease progression; Lewy bodies; Parkinson's disease

Introduction

Idiopathic Parkinson's disease (PD) is a synucleinopathy that damages neurons in particular sites of the brain, causing the cardinal motor signs of bradykinesia, rigidity, resting tremor, and postural instability. As disease duration increases, other signs and symptoms such as cognitive deficits and autonomic failure often occur.[1] Although the etiology of idiopathic PD remains a mystery, the pathological aggregation of the synaptic protein α-synuclein, either in the form of Lewy bodies (LB) or Lewy neurites (LN) is considered diagnostic.[2] In 2003, Braak and colleagues proposed a staging scheme to explain the progression of the α-synuclein pathology in PD and the relationship between the distribution of these pathological inclusions and the onset and severity of clinical signs and symptoms.[3] This was enthusiastically received by the clinical and research community as a much-needed clarification of the stepwise nature of PD, however the retrospective nature of the study has been a cause for concern. This review will examine the concept of such a single pathological phenotype underpinning clinical PD in relationship to both longitudinal and retro-spective clinical and pathological studies in order to further understand the progression of α-synuclein pathology.

The pathological progression of Parkinson's disease as identified by Braak staging

In 2002, Braak and colleagues proposed a staging scheme for the α-synuclein inclusion pathology of PD, publishing several papers in the following years outlining and rationalizing this uniform and systematic progression.[3,4] To summarize, Stages I and II indicate involvement of LB and LN in the olfactory regions and lower brain stem (dorsal motor nucleus of the vagus nerve [DMV] and the intermediate reticular zone, locus ceruleus). Stages III and IV see the α-synuclein aggregations extend to the midbrain, particularly the substantia nigra pars compacta and to the basal forebrain, transentorhinal cortex, and CA2 region of the hippocampus. Stages V and VI involve depositions in the higher order cortical association areas such as the temporal, insular, and anterior cingulate cortices and finally a progression to the entire neocortex.[3,4]

Ann. N.Y. Acad. Sci. 1184 (2010) 188–195 © 2009 New York Academy of Sciences.

The progression of α-synuclein pathology through these anatomical regions has been correlated with the appearance and worsening of motor and other symptoms of PD. Olfactory and autonomic dysfunction and REM sleep disorders are noted as early and often subtle nonmotor features of PD,[5–10] when pathology would be confined to Braak Stages I–III. In Stage IV there is a loss of pigmented neurons in the substantia nigra pars compacta, which heralds the onset of the first recognizable motor symptoms of PD.[3,11] The end stages of the progression have been shown to correlate with cognitive decline,[12,13] although other studies have not found this to be the case within their cohorts.[14–17] A recent assessment of the staging scheme for use in routine neuropathology and brain banking revealed that acceptable intra- and interrater reliabilities were easily achieved, but that severity of stage did not necessarily correspond with the expected presence of the core symptoms of PD (bradykinesia, rigidity, tremor, postural instability),[18] a finding substantiated by others (see below). That the staging scheme can be easily observed pathologically suggests α-synuclein deposits in only certain vulnerable neuronal populations in particular anatomical regions in PD. However, the lack of independent confirmation of the clinical utility of this unifying staging scheme suggests that other paradigms must be considered.

Clinical evidence for a single unifying entity for PD

It has been known for some time that clinical cohorts of patients identified with early PD are heterogeneous, even excluding those who are not responsive to dopamine-replacement therapies. Clinical phenotypes include those with different symptoms (resting tremor vs. akinesia and rigidity and/or postural instability and gait disorder), with differing rates of progression (rapid vs. slow), and with different ages of onset (early vs. late onset), often with overlap between these phenotypes.[19] In particular, significantly greater neurological dysfunction is consistently observed in PD patients of older onset or those with postural instability and gait disorder, compared to those with younger onset or with mainly resting tremor who have a more benign course.[19] In three independent cohort studies using cluster analysis, two to four clinical sub-

types have been consistently identified depending on when in the disease course the patients have been assessed.[20–22] After 10 years only two subtypes are seen, whereas at 5 years there are three subtypes, and a fourth rapidly progressive and underreported motor subtype is found only very early in the disease process.[20–22] Such independent data-driven analyses confirm that clinical PD does not have a uniform starting position or pattern of progression, as expected by the staging scheme defined by Braak and collegues.[3]

The three main clinical phenotypes can be distinguished over time relatively easily. Firstly, there is the early severe akinetic, rigid, dementia-dominant syndrome that fulfils criteria for dementia with Lewy bodies (DLB)[23] but also has the clinical features of PD at onset. Secondly, there is the subset of older onset PD cases (∼70 years and older) in which dementia occurs relatively early in their disease, often within 3–10 years. These cases fulfill current criteria for PD with dementia (PDD).[24] Lastly, there exists a group of younger onset cases (< 70 years old) in which dementia occurs at a very late stage of disease (after 10 and often after 15 years). The overall course in these cases would be considered typical for idiopathic PD.[1] These phenotypes differ substantially in the timing of symptom onset, the age of symptom onset, and the severity of the ensuing cognitive impairment. The obvious cognitive differences alone would suggest that the pattern and progression of cortical neuropathology is likely to also differ substantially between such cases, again calling into question the uniform concept of the Braak staging scheme.[3]

Pathological variability in PD

While pathological studies of cases with levodopa-responsive PD will include cases with the different clinical phenotypes noted above, they all display several similar basic pathological features. In particular, the loss of dopamine-producing neurons in the substantia nigra pars compacta and the presence of abnormal α-synuclein aggregates in the brain are so consistent across cases that they form the diagnostic features of PD.[23] Careful longitudinal studies with autopsy confirmation have identified early cell loss in the ventrolateral nigra as a consistent feature, with the severity of dopamine cell loss correlating with disease duration (Fig. 1A and B).[11,25,26] These

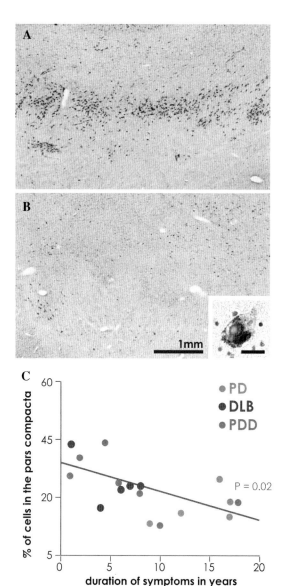

Figure 1. Targeted neuronal loss occurs within the substantia nigra pars compacta in PD. Nissl-stained transverse section of the midbrain from a control shows a normally pigmented cell population in the nigra (A), while in advanced PD there is substantial pigmented cell loss (B) with α-synuclein immunopositive Lewy body inclusions in remaining cells (inset, scale bar represents 25 μm). (C) Graph of the significant relationship between the proportion of neurons remaining in the nigra and the duration of PD showing more cell loss with longer disease durations.[25] Note that more PD patients survive to older age than DLB or PDD patients.

studies show that significant neurodegeneration is already present at clinical diagnosis (Fig. 1C),[25] consistent with a slow, drawn-out process of cell death that must occur preclinically.[3,27–31]

In addition to the loss of midbrain dopamine neurons, all cases have α-synuclein aggregates in the form of LB and LN that are present in brain stem (Fig. 2A and B) and to variable degrees in the entorhinal and cortical regions (consistent with Braak staging of IV–VI). Since the emergence of the Braak staging scheme, several research groups have undertaken retrospective autopsy studies to verify Braak's observations and ascertain any clinical relevance. A large study of cases from the UK Parkinson's Disease Society Tissue Bank reported that 47% of cases did not fit with the caudorostral spread of α-synuclein pathology throughout the brain.[32] Similarly, other studies have substantiated this, finding in autopsy-confirmed PD cases that despite LB pathology in the higher brain stem or cortex there was no involvement of the DMV.[16,33] It has also been found retrospectively that many apparently neurologically normal elderly cases exist where the amount and distribution of α-synuclein pathology should warrant the overt motor symptoms of PD, but for some reason these do not occur.[16,34–40] Whether this is as a result of greater brain reserve or compensatory function in the individual, or whether some are effectively "immune" to the pathology and will never develop PD despite the burden of α-synuclein pathology, or whether they have motor dysfunction that is just thought to be age rather than disease related, remains unclear. Overall these studies suggest substantive clinical variability between cases in the pathological staging scheme.

Despite this variability, the assessment of well-studied clinical cohorts has shown that high densities of LB in the parahippocampus distinguish cases of PDD from those with typical PD,[41] suggesting that more substantial protein deposition occurs with shorter rather than longer disease durations. This is confirmed in a recent autopsy study with prospectively assessed subjects demonstrating more cortical α-synuclein pathology in older PDD patients with shorter disease durations.[42] Cases with Braak Stages IV–VI pathology do have significant cognitive decline[43] that relates to the severity of their parkinsonism.[12,13] However, there is no association between the presence of dementia and survival duration,[13,44]

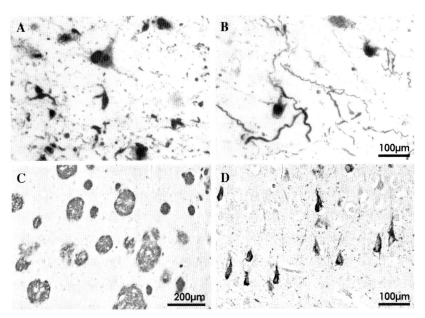

Figure 2. Intracellular α-synuclein immunopositive Lewy bodies (**A**) and Lewy neurites (**B**) are found in the substantia nigra pars compacta in all PD cases, however patients with older onset (**A**) have a higher density than those with younger onset (**B**). Age-related Aβ plaques (**C**) and tau immunopositive neurofibrillary tangles (**D**) also occur more frequently in older-onset cases and may be a significant contributing factor to the clinical heterogeneity observed in PD.

despite the concept that advanced Braak stage of disease equals a higher likelihood of the dementia that occurs at end-stage. Surprisingly, the densities of LB at end stage disease are most related to older age[40] and therefore clinical phenotype[45] rather than to a linear progression of pathology over time.[46] It should be noted that there is an increased amount of cellular α-synuclein in the substantia nigra pars compacta that occurs normally in middle to old age.[47] When the pathological process intervenes it changes this linear increase in cellular α-synuclein into a nonlinear or exponential increase in patients with older onset of PD.[46] This age association is also seen in the demographics of the cohort Braak and colleagues used to pathologically stage PD. Cases with Stage I–II should be on average younger than Stage III–IV cases which should be younger on average than Stage IV–V cases if there is a uniform disease progression over time. This was not observed in the large cohort studied by Braak and colleagues in 2003,[3] where preclinical cases should have been younger on average than PD cases but often were not. As pointed out by Halliday, Del Tredici, and Braak,[29] if these preclinical cases were to progress

to PD it would be an extremely late-onset disease. Overall, there is an age-associated increase in cellular α-synuclein that theoretically predisposes everyone to LB formation over time. In combination with a pathological stimulus, LB formation appears to be significantly enhanced with increasing age of PD onset.

In addition to these consistently observed pathologies, there are a number of other pathologies that occur more variably. The degree of cell loss in a variety of structures is highly variable. For example, loss of hippocampal neurons occurs in DLB but not PDD,[48] whereas loss of basal forebrain cholinergic neurons is marked in all cases of dementia.[49–53] Cell loss in a number of subcortical structures (hypothalamus,[54] pedunculopontine tegmental nucleus,[55,56] locus ceruleus[57]) relates to the degree of nigral cell loss and the extent of motor disability. The amount of age-related Alzheimer-type pathology is also highly variable, but consistent with the age-related changes observed in the general population.[58] In particular, Aβ plaques (Fig. 2C) concentrate in cases with older onset PD,[45] along with neocortical neurofibrillary tangles (Fig. 2D), which occur more frequently in cases with early dementia.[17] In large autopsy samples approximately 10–40% of the population between 70–75 years of age have moderate to frequent Aβ plaques, while smaller numbers have limbic or neocortical neurofibrillary tangles at the same ages.[58] Similarly, the prevalence of cerebrovascular pathology is highly variable but also consistent with an age-related phenomenon.[59] Clinical studies have shown that older age[60] and comorbid illnesses[61] are the major risk factor for the emergence of nonmotor PD symptoms such as somnolence, hallucinations, and dementia. The higher frequency of these more variable pathologies with increasing age is consistent with such additional pathologies significantly contributing to the greater disability and more rapid disease progression observed in cases with older onset of clinical PD.[45]

Longitudinal clinicopathological studies

To date, most studies used to formulate, validate, or refute the staging scheme have been performed either using consecutive autopsy series in the elderly or brain bank/autopsy cases with pathologically confirmed PD, with the clinical information then collected retrospectively. To our knowledge only one study to date follows the longitudinal progression of PD pathology in patients with clinically confirmed, levodopa-responsive PD.[45] In this study, cases were subjects who participated in the Sydney Multicentre Study of PD and who came to autopsy. Standardized clinical and neuropathological assessments over five epochs of time (end-stage clinical diagnosis at 1–5 years, 6–10 years, 11–15 years, 16–20 years, and 20+ years) identified three different clinicopathological groups that were largely consistent with the three clinical groups described earlier.

The first was a group of younger-onset cases (50–60 years of age) with long disease durations (> 15 years) consistent with typical PD. The second was a group with a dominant dementia syndrome (consistent with DLB), and the last was an older onset group (over 70 years of age) with shorter disease duration (< 15 years) and greater disability and dementia (consistent with PDD). Pathologically, the first group followed the Braak staging scheme, with LB load and earlier age of onset correlating with disease duration (Fig. 3). Brain stem LB dominated this group over the first 5 years of disease, by 13 years

50% had a limbic distribution of LB pathology, by 18 years all cases had limbic LB, and by 20 years nearly all were demented (Fig. 3).[45]

The other two groups had an earlier dementia phenotype, with one having severe neocortical α-synuclein and Aβ pathology (consistent with DLB) at the onset of clinical symptoms and the other having similar high densities of LB and less substantial Aβ pathology (consistent with PDD) (Fig. 3).[45] Survival time in these dementia cases negatively correlated with the proportion of cases with significant Aβ plaque load, suggesting that plaque pathology is a contributing factor to this later-onset phenotype.[45] Choosing cases with PD pathology retrospectively from an autopsy series would not have discriminated between these three different clinicopathological groups. However, the assessment of longitudinally followed clinical cohorts reveals good reason for the different clinical phenotypes noted, with older onset complicated by additional age-associated pathologies.

Conclusions

Several conclusions can be drawn from the current literature on the progression of α-synuclein pathology in PD. The foremost is that the time course of pathology can only be understood using a series of epoch pathological evaluation in longitudinally studied patients, rather than the cross-sectional pathological studies dominating the literature, which infer progression without the consideration of time. Unfortunately, the majority of cross-sectional pathological studies are biased toward assessing PD cases that have died at the end stage of disease and are advanced in age, without considering the clinical variability in their sample (particularly age at disease onset). The fact that onset age influences α-synuclein deposition in PD continues to confound the majority of studies, with little research occurring on this important aspect. Data from the longitudinal epoch study suggest two patterns of disease progression that align with clinical phenotype: a cell loss–dominant mechanism typical of younger-onset PD, in which less α-synuclein deposition occurs and a greater period of time expires before the onset of dementia, and a widespread increase in abnormal α-synuclein protein deposition in older onset PD with earlier dementia and other age-related disorders predisposing to nigral

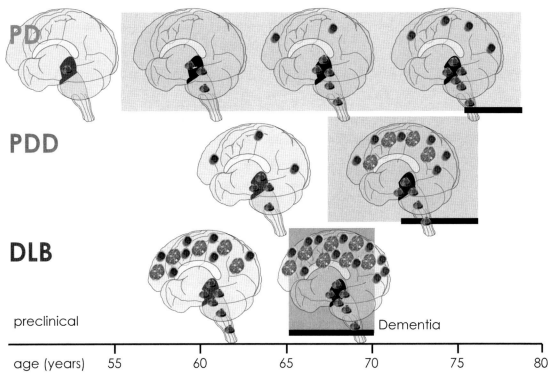

Figure 3. Schematic representation of the progression of pathology in the three main clinical phenotypes of PD from longitudinal epoch data.[45] Dopamine cell loss in the substantia nigra is represented as the solid color over the midbrain region, with darker colors indicating greater cell loss over time. Pink-colored brain stem Lewy bodies and brown-colored cortical Lewy bodies are represented separately. Larger lighter brown cortical plaques are also shown. For each of the three main clinical phenotypes, a preclinical period is indicated as well as the average period of time with dementia. Typical PD phenotype: younger-onset cases have longer disease durations and a slow infiltration of Lewy bodies from the brain stem to the cortex in line with the pathological progression of PD identified by Braak and colleagues.[3] Fifty percent of cases have at least limbic infiltration by 13 years, with 100% progressing at least to this stage by 18 years.[45] Dementia in this phenotype occurs late in association with the cortical infiltration of Lewy bodies. PDD phenotype: an older-onset group with shorter disease durations and dementia by midstage disease have greater amounts of cortical Lewy bodies early in their disease and some coexisting Alzheimer's disease pathology appearing with the onset of dementia. DLB phenotype: a dominant dementia syndrome with severe cortical Lewy body loads often with coexisting Alzheimer's disease pathology, which must occur early in the disease process due to their short disease durations and early onset of dementia.

cell loss and other age-related pathologies. The need for more autopsy studies assessing closely followed cases over defined epochs is vital to elucidating the true progression of pathology in PD and any contributing factors such as age, disease duration, and coexisting illnesses.

Acknowledgments

We wish to thank Heidi Cartwright for the figures.

Conflicts of interest

The authors declare no conflicts of interest.

References

1. Gelb, D.J., E. Oliver & S. Gilman. 1999. Diagnostic criteria for Parkinson disease. *Arch. Neurol.* **56:** 33–39.
2. Pollanen, M.S., D.W. Dickson & C. Bergeron. 1993. Pathology and biology of the Lewy body. *J. Neuropathol. Exp. Neurol.* **52:** 183–191.

3. Braak, H. *et al.* 2003. Staging of brain pathology related to sporadic Parkinson's disease. *Neurobiol. Aging* **24:** 197–211.

4. Braak, H. *et al.* 2006. Stanley Fahn Lecture 2005: The staging procedure for the inclusion body pathology associated with sporadic Parkinson's disease reconsidered. *Mov. Disord.* **21:** 2042–2051.

5. Tissingh, G. *et al.* 2001. Loss of olfaction in de novo and treated Parkinson's disease: possible implications for early diagnosis. *Mov. Disord.* **16:** 41–46.

6. Ponsen, M.M. *et al.* 2004. Idiopathic hyposmia as a preclinical sign of Parkinson's disease. *Ann. Neurol.* **56:** 173–181.

7. Schenck, C.H., S.R. Bundlie & M.W. Mahowald. 1996. Delayed emergence of a parkinsonian disorder in 38% of 29 older men initially diagnosed with idiopathic rapid eye movement sleep behaviour disorder. *Neurology* **46:** 388–393.

8. Stiasny-Kolster, K. *et al.* 2005. Combination of 'idiopathic' REM sleep behaviour disorder and olfactory dysfunction as possible indicator for alpha-synucleinopathy demonstrated by dopamine transporter FP-CIT-SPECT. *Brain* **128:** 126–137.

9. Pfeiffer, R.F. 2003. Gastrointestinal dysfunction in Parkinson's disease. *Lancet Neurol.* **2:** 107–116.

10. Senard, J.M. *et al.* 1997. Prevalence of orthostatic hypotension in Parkinson's disease. *J. Neurol. Neurosurg. Psychiatry* **63:** 584–589.

11. Greffard, S. *et al.* 2006. Motor score of the Unified Parkinson Disease Rating Scale as a good predictor of Lewy body-associated neuronal loss in the substantia nigra. *Arch. Neurol.* **63:** 584–588.

12. Braak, H., U. Rub & K. Del Tredici. 2006. Cognitive decline correlates with neuropathological stage in Parkinson's disease. *J. Neurol. Sci.* **248:** 255–258.

13. Braak, H. *et al.* 2005. Cognitive status correlates with neuropathologic stage in Parkinson disease. *Neurology* **64:** 1404–1410.

14. Colosimo, C. *et al.* 2003. Lewy body cortical involvement may not always predict dementia in Parkinson's disease. *J. Neurol. Neurosurg. Psychiatry* **74:** 852–856.

15. Jellinger, K.A. 2007. Morphological substrates of parkinsonism with and without dementia: a retrospective clinico-pathological study. *J. Neural. Transm. Suppl.* 91–104.

16. Parkkinen, L., T. Pirttila & I. Alafuzoff. 2008. Applicability of current staging/categorization of alpha-synuclein pathology and their clinical relevance. *Acta Neuropathol.* **115:** 399–407.

17. Weisman, D. *et al.* 2007. In dementia with Lewy bodies, Braak stage determines phenotype, not Lewy body distribution. *Neurology* **69:** 356–359.

18. Muller, C.M. *et al.* 2005. Staging of sporadic Parkinson disease-related alpha-synuclein pathology: inter- and intra-rater reliability. *J. Neuropathol. Exp. Neurol.* **64:** 623–628.

19. Jankovic, J. *et al.* 1990. Variable expression of Parkinson's disease: a base-line analysis of the DATATOP cohort. The Parkinson Study Group. *Neurology* **40:** 1529–1534.

20. Post, B., J.D. Speelman & R.J. de Haan. 2008. Clinical heterogeneity in newly diagnosed Parkinson's disease. *J. Neurol.* **255:** 716–722.

21. Lewis, S.J. *et al.* 2005. Heterogeneity of Parkinson's disease in the early clinical stages using a data driven approach. *J. Neurol. Neurosurg. Psychiatry* **76:** 343–348.

22. Graham, J.M. & H.J. Sagar. 1999. A data-driven approach to the study of heterogeneity in idiopathic Parkinson's disease: identification of three distinct subtypes. *Mov. Disord.* **14:** 10–20.

23. McKeith, I.G. *et al.* 2005. Diagnosis and management of dementia with Lewy bodies: third report of the DLB Consortium. *Neurology* **65:** 1863–1872.

24. Emre, M. *et al.* 2007. Clinical diagnostic criteria for dementia associated with Parkinson's disease. *Mov. Disord.* **22:** 1689–1707; quiz 1837.

25. Halliday, G.M. *et al.* 1996. Midbrain neuropathology in idiopathic Parkinson's disease and diffuse Lewy body disease. *J. Clin. Neurosci.* **3:** 52–60.

26. Fearnley, J.M. & A.J. Lees. 1991. Ageing and Parkinson's disease: substantia nigra regional selectivity. *Brain* **114**(Pt 5): 2283–2301.

27. DelleDonne, A. *et al.* 2008. Incidental Lewy body disease and preclinical Parkinson disease. *Arch. Neurol.* **65:** 1074–1080.

28. Dickson, D.W. *et al.* 2008. Evidence that incidental Lewy body disease is pre-symptomatic Parkinson's disease. *Acta Neuropathol.* **115:** 437–444.

29. Halliday, G.M., K. Del Tredici & H. Braak. 2006. Critical appraisal of brain pathology staging related to presymptomatic and symptomatic cases of sporadic Parkinson's disease. *J. Neural. Transm. Suppl.* 99–103.

30. Thal, D.R., K. Del Tredici & H. Braak. 2004. Neurodegeneration in normal brain aging and disease. *Sci. Aging Knowl. Environ.* 2004; pe26.

31. Jellinger, K.A. 2003. Alpha-synuclein pathology in Parkinson's and Alzheimer's disease brain: incidence and topographic distribution–a pilot study. *Acta Neuropathol.* **106:** 191–201.

32. Kalaitzakis, M.E. *et al.* 2008. The dorsal motor nucleus of the vagus is not an obligatory trigger site of

Parkinson's disease: a critical analysis of alpha-synuclein staging. *Neuropathol. Appl. Neurobiol.* **34**: 284–295.

33. Attems, J. & K.A. Jellinger. 2008. The dorsal motor nucleus of the vagus is not an obligatory trigger site of Parkinson's disease. *Neuropathol. Appl. Neurobiol.* **34**: 466–467.

34. Forno, L.S. 1969. Concentric hyalin intraneuronal inclusions of Lewy type in the brains of elderly persons (50 incidental cases): relationship to parkinsonism. *J. Am. Geriatr. Soc.* **17**: 557–575.

35. Parkkinen, L. *et al.* 2001. Alpha-synuclein pathology is highly dependent on the case selection. *Neuropathol. Appl. Neurobiol.* **27**: 314–325.

36. Jellinger, K.A. 2004. Lewy body-related alpha-synucleinopathy in the aged human brain. *J. Neural. Transm.* **111**: 1219–1235.

37. Saito, Y. *et al.* 2004. Lewy body-related alpha-synucleinopathy in aging. *J. Neuropathol. Exp. Neurol.* **63**: 742–749.

38. Zaccai, J. *et al.* 2008. Patterns and stages of alpha-synucleinopathy: Relevance in a population-based cohort. *Neurology* **70**: 1042–1048.

39. Aho, L. *et al.* 2008. Systematic appraisal using immuno-histochemistry of brain pathology in aged and demented subjects. *Dement. Geriatr. Cogn. Disord.* **25**: 423–432.

40. Wakisaka, Y. *et al.* 2003. Age-associated prevalence and risk factors of Lewy body pathology in a general population: the Hisayama study. *Acta Neuropathol.* **106**: 374–382.

41. Harding, A.J. & G.M. Halliday. 2001. Cortical Lewy body pathology in the diagnosis of dementia. *Acta Neuropathol.* **102**: 355–363.

42. Ballard, C. *et al.* 2006. Differences in neuropathologic characteristics across the Lewy body dementia spectrum. *Neurology* **67**: 1931–1934.

43. Hurtig, H.I. *et al.* 2000. Alpha-synuclein cortical Lewy bodies correlate with dementia in Parkinson's disease. *Neurology* **54**: 1916–1921.

44. Papapetropoulos, S. *et al.* 2005. Dementia in Parkinson's disease: a post-mortem study in a population of brain donors. *Int. J. Geriatr. Psychiatry* **20**: 418–422.

45. Halliday, G. *et al.* 2008. The progression of pathology in longitudinally followed patients with Parkinson's disease. *Acta Neuropathol.* **115**: 409–415.

46. Kempster, P.A. *et al.* 2007. Patterns of levodopa response in Parkinson's disease: a clinico-pathological study. *Brain* **130**: 2123–2128.

47. Chu, Y. & J.H. Kordower. 2007. Age-associated increases of alpha-synuclein in monkeys and humans are associ-

ated with nigrostriatal dopamine depletion: Is this the target for Parkinson's disease? *Neurobiol. Dis.* **25**: 134–149.

48. Harding, A.J., B. Lakay & G.M. Halliday. 2002. Selective hippocampal neuron loss in dementia with Lewy bodies. *Ann. Neurol.* **51**: 125–128.

49. Arendt, T. *et al.* 1983. Loss of neurons in the nucleus basalis of Meynert in Alzheimer's disease, paralysis agitans and Korsakoff's Disease. *Acta Neuropathol.* **61**: 101–108.

50. Mattila, P.M. *et al.* 2001. Choline acetytransferase activity and striatal dopamine receptors in Parkinson's disease in relation to cognitive impairment. *Acta Neuropathol.* **102**: 160–166.

51. Rogers, J.D., D. Brogan & S.S. Mirra. 1985. The nucleus basalis of Meynert in neurological disease: a quantitative morphological study. *Ann. Neurol.* **17**: 163–170.

52. Ruberg, M. *et al.* 1986. Acetylcholinesterase and butyryl-cholinesterase in frontal cortex and cerebrospinal fluid of demented and non-demented patients with Parkinson's disease. *Brain Res.* **362**: 83–91.

53. Tagliavini, F. *et al.* 1984. The basal nucleus of Meynert in idiopathic Parkinson's disease. *Acta Neurol. Scand.* **70**: 20–28.

54. Thannickal, T.C., Y.Y. Lai & J.M. Siegel. 2008. Hypocretin (orexin) and melanin concentrating hormone loss and the symptoms of Parkinson's disease. *Brain* **131**: e87.

55. Rinne, J.O. *et al.* 2008. Loss of cholinergic neurons in the pedunculopontine nucleus in Parkinson's disease is related to disability of the patients. *Parkinsonism Relat. Disord.* **14**: 553–557.

56. Perry, E.K. *et al.* 1995. Alteration in nicotine binding sites in Parkinson's disease, Lewy body dementia and Alzheimer's disease: possible index of early neuropathology. *Neuroscience* **64**: 385–395.

57. Zweig, R.M. *et al.* 1993. The locus ceruleus and dementia in Parkinson's disease. *Neurology* **43**: 986–991.

58. Braak, H. & E. Braak. 1997. Frequency of stages of Alzheimer-related lesions in different age categories. *Neurobiol. Aging* **18**: 351–357.

59. Jellinger, K.A. & J. Attems. 2008. Prevalence and impact of vascular and Alzheimer pathologies in Lewy body disease. *Acta Neuropathol.* **115**: 427–436.

60. Aarsland, D. *et al.* 2007. The effect of age of onset of PD on risk of dementia. *J. Neurol.* **254**: 38–45.

61. Biglan, K.M. *et al.* 2007. Risk factors for somnolence, edema, and hallucinations in early Parkinson disease. *Neurology* **69**: 187–195.

Ann. N.Y. Acad. Sci. ISSN 0077-8923

ANNALS OF THE NEW YORK ACADEMY OF SCIENCES

Familial pain syndromes from mutations of the Na$_v$1.7 sodium channel

Tanya Z. Fischer[1,2,3] and Stephen G. Waxman[1,2,3]

[1]Department of Neurology and [2]Center for Neuroscience & Regeneration Research, Yale University School of Medicine, New Haven, Connecticut, USA. [3]Rehabilitation Research Center, Veterans Administration Connecticut Healthcare System, West Haven, Connecticut, USA

Address for correspondence: Stephen G. Waxman, M.D., Ph.D., Department of Neurology, LCI 707, Yale School of Medicine, 333 Cedar Street, New Haven, CT 06510. Voice: 203-785-6351; fax: 203-785-2238. stephen.waxman@yale.edu

The literature currently suggests that voltage-gated sodium channels play a major role in the pathogenesis of neuropathic pain. Alterations in the expression and targeting of specific sodium channels within injured dorsal root ganglia neurons appear to predispose the neurons to abnormal firing properties, allowing for the development of neuropathic pain. Mutations of one particular sodium channel (Na$_v$1.7) have been shown to cause inherited neuropathic pain in humans, specifically in erythromelalgia and paroxysmal extreme pain disorder. Inherited erythromelalgia is the first human pain syndrome to be understood at a molecular level, having been linked to gain-of-function mutations of Na$_v$1.7. Conversely, a loss-of-function of the Na$_v$1.7 channel can produce channelopathy-associated insensitivity to pain. Therefore, the Na$_v$1.7 channel may provide a unique target for the pharmacotherapy of pain in humans. In this review article we summarize current knowledge regarding several different disease manifestations arising from changes within the Na$_v$1.7 channel.

Keywords: neuropathic pain; sodium channels; erythromelalgia; paroxysmal extreme pain disorder; channelopathy-associated insensitivity to pain; dorsal root ganglion; voltage clamp

Introduction

Primary nociceptive or pain-signaling sensory neurons, specifically within dorsal root ganglia (DRG) and trigeminal ganglia, constitute the peripheral entry point of the pain pathway. Usually, these neurons are relatively quiescent. When stimulated, these neurons produce a series of action potentials, allowing information about the external sensory world to be transmitted to the brain. Injury to these neurons causes them to become hyperexcitable, thus giving rise to abnormal, unprovoked spontaneous action potentials or pathological bursting, which results in chronic pain.[1–4]

In mammalian neurons, voltage-gated sodium channels produce action potentials in response to membrane depolarization. Sodium channels are composed of a single α-subunit and several auxiliary β-subunits.[5] The α-subunit endows the channel with voltage sensitivity and forms the ion-selective pore, while the β-subunits appear to influence channel gating and targeting.[6–10] Here we focus on sodium channel α-subunits which,

for brevity, we will refer to as sodium channels (Na$_v$). Although the literature indicates that there are multiple sodium channels, only seven (Na$_v$1.1, Na$_v$1.2, Na$_v$1.3, Na$_v$1.6, Na$_v$1.7, Na$_v$1.8, and Na$_v$1.9) have been found in the nervous system.[11] These different sodium channels share a common structure but are encoded by different genes and manifest distinct voltage-dependent and kinetic properties. Sodium channels are expressed in a regionally and temporally specific pattern in the nervous system. Interestingly, the majority of neurons express multiple sodium channel isoforms, with different ensembles of sodium channel isoforms endowing different types of neurons with unique functional properties.[12]

Multiple sodium channels in dorsal root ganglia neurons

It has been well established through early electrophysiologic studies that DRG neurons produce multiple, distinct sodium currents, which can be distinguished from one another by their differences in voltage dependence, kinetics, and sensitivity to the neurotoxin tetrodotoxin (TTX).[13–16] Importantly, multiple distinct sodium currents have been recorded from individual neurons, suggesting that multiple types of sodium channels are present within them.[17,18]

Of the known neuronally expressed sodium channels, Na$_v$1.7, Na$_v$1.8, and Na$_v$1.9 are preferentially expressed in DRG and trigeminal ganglia neurons,[19–22] most of which are nociceptive. The Na$_v$1.7 channel is expressed in almost all DRG neurons at various levels,[20] while the Na$_v$1.8 and Na$_v$1.9 channels are primarily expressed in small DRG neurons that include nociceptors.[18,19,21] The Na$_v$1.8 and Na$_v$1.9 channels are also distinguished from the Na$_v$1.7 channel by their resistance to TTX.[18,19] Expression of the Na$_v$1.8 and Na$_v$1.9 channels are both downregulate in DRG neurons after sciatic nerve transection but are elevated under inflammatory conditions.[21,23] Although Na$_v$1.3 channels are not expressed above background levels in adult DRG neurons, the Na$_v$1.3 channel has been shown to be upregulated in DRG neurons following injury.[24,25] Therefore, along with the Na$_v$1.8 and Na$_v$1.9 channels, Na$_v$1.3 has been suggested to play a role in neuropathic pain.

Multiple studies have shown the importance of voltage-gated ion channels in the perception and transmission of pain.[26,27] For example, a mouse knockout model of the voltage-gated Na$_v$1.8 channel results in animals with deficits of thermal pain perception[28] and visceral pain perception[29] but not neuropathic pain.[30] When Na$_v$1.7 is selectively knocked out of nociceptive neurons, the mice display markedly reduced inflammatory pain responses and a deficit in heat-induced pain threshold, while the mechanical pain and cold-evoked thresholds appear to be intact.[31] On the other hand, in mice, global knockout of Na$_v$1.7 has been found to be lethal,[31] possibly due to a failure to feed. Interestingly, when both Na$_v$1.7 and Na$_v$1.8 channels were knocked out of mice, alterations only in inflammatory pain were seen.[30]

In humans, point mutations within the *SCN9A* gene, which codes for the Na$_v$1.7 channel, have been associated with two different pain syndromes caused by a "gain-in-function" of the channel: inherited erythromelalgia (IEM) and paroxysmal extreme pain disorder (PEPD). Conversely, several cases have been described in the literature of otherwise healthy patients with a congenital inability to experience pain, arising from nonsense mutations of Na$_v$1.7, which produce truncated, nonfunctional proteins.[32–34] These various studies, both in animals and in humans, have helped to establish ion channels, especially Na$_v$1.7, as a major factor of peripheral nociception.

Inherited erythromelalgia

IEM, originally described by S. Weir Mitchell in 1878,[35] is characterized by intense episodic burning pain associated with redness and warmth of the affected extremities. In the absence of an underlying cause (such as in myeloproliferative diseases or as a side effect of medication), it is termed primary erythromelalgia and in many instances occurs as an autosomal dominant trait (Mendelian Inheritance in Man 133020).[36] Clinical onset of the inherited form of this disease has been reported as early as 1 year of age, often manifesting itself before the end of the first decade of life. Attacks are described by patients as a burning pain (which patients describe as excruciating, "like hot lava poured into my body") with accompanying redness in the distal extremities (feet, sometimes hands) in response to warm stimuli or moderate exercise.[36] A characteristic feature is relief obtained by immersing the extremities in ice, which can lead to ulceration and gangrene. In the absence of a clear etiology, treatment has been empirical and is partially effective at best. IEM shares a number of clinical features with, and is sometimes confused with, reflex sympathetic dystrophy (RSD) since both are characterized by severe pain and vasomotor disturbances, but in contrast to RSD, erythromelalgia is bilateral and symmetric.[35–38] Since attacks are episodic and can be counted, IEM appears to provide a human model that is especially tractable for therapeutic trials.

Mutations of Na$_v$1.7: genetic analysis and expression studies

Importantly, IEM is the first known inherited painful neuropathy to be examined at a molecular level. Until recently the pathogenesis of this disease was unknown. Hypotheses encompassing vascular shunting, neuropathic etiologies, microvascular etiologies, and inflammatory etiologies have all been suggested.

In 2004, Yang and coworkers,[39] using linkage analysis, identified two independent point mutations in the gene encoding Na$_v$1.7 in two separate families in China with IEM. A single amino-acid substitution (F1449V) was subsequently identified in the Na$_v$1.7 channel in another large American family.[40] In each of these kindreds, all affected family members carried this mutation, while it was absent in unaffected family members and in the alleles from an ethnically matched control group. A number of other mutations, all in Na$_v$1.7, have subsequently been found in other families with IEM.[41–47] Thus far, penetrance appears to be close to 100% for IEM mutations.[39,40]

Consistent with a role in painful neuropathy, Na$_v$1.7 channels are preferentially expressed in nociceptive DRG neurons and their nerve endings.[22,48,49] In these neurons, Na$_v$1.7 produces "threshold currents" close to resting potential, amplifying small depolarizations such as generator potentials,[50,51] while other sodium channel isoforms contribute most of the current underlying all-or-none action potentials.[52] IEM mutations of Na$_v$1.7 have been shown to cause a hyperpolarizing shift in activation and slow deactivation[43] (Fig. 1A and B). The hyperpolarizing shift in the voltage dependence of activation of the Na$_v$1.7 channel (which makes it easier to open the channel) and the slowed deactivation (which keeps the channel open longer once it is activated), in turn, are expected to decrease the threshold for action potential generation in sensory neurons, thus increasing neuronal excitability. The response of Na$_v$1.7 channels to slow ramp depolarizations (e.g., 0.2 mV/ms depolarizations from -100 to -20 mV) (Fig. 1D) are also significantly enhanced compared with wild-type (WT) channels.[43] Because the ramp currents are evoked close to the resting potential of DRG neurons,[13,53] the larger ramp currents in DRG neurons expressing IEM mutations of Na$_v$1.7 are poised to amplify the response to small depolarizing inputs. This, in turn, would increase excitability. Na$_v$1.7 channels are present in small, mostly nociceptive, sensory neurons,[48] suggesting that changes in activation, deactivation, and ramp current amplitude contribute to the pain experienced by IEM patients.

Subsequent studies[40,46,54] used current-clamp recording to directly show that this mutation renders sensory neurons hyperexcitable. When DRG neurons, a cell type known to express Na$_v$1.7 channels,[22,48,49] are transfected with WT Na$_v$1.7 channels, they produce all-or-none action potentials in response to injections of 135 pA or greater (Fig. 2A). However, in DRG neurons expressing the L858H IEM mutant channel, a much lower current input is required for the generation of an action potential (Fig. 2B). The current threshold is significantly decreased, by more than 40%, in cells expressing IEM mutant channels, such as the L858H Na$_v$1.7 mutation, compared with WT Na$_v$1.7 channels (Fig. 2C). IEM mutations also enhance repetitive firing in DRG neurons (Fig. 3B) compared with WT cells (Fig. 3A). These experiments show that an IEM mutation of Na$_v$1.7 can produce hyperexcitability (decreased threshold and enhanced repetitive firing) within DRG neurons, providing a molecular explanation for the pain experienced in patients with IEM.

Our group has found *de novo* "founder" mutations that increase DRG neuron excitability in several sporadic cases of erythromelalgia, and thus has indicted Na$_v$1.7 mutations in some individuals who do not have a family history of the disorder.[45,46] In addition, several mutations in the gene for Na$_v$1.7 have been found, which appear to modulate the channel's sensitivity to local anaesthetics.[44,55,56] Choi and colleagues[55] identified a new Na$_v$1.7 mutation, V872G, in a patient who reported pain relief with mexiletine and observed that the mutation resulted in stronger use-dependent current fall-off when the channels were exposed to mexiletine. Fischer and colleagues[44] reported a family with carbamazepine (CBZ)-responsive IEM and demonstrated that the mutation confers CBZ-sensitivity in the mutant channel.

While missense mutations in Na$_v$1.7 channel have been found in many families with IEM, this disease may be genetically heterogeneous because some cases of familial early-onset[57] or adult-onset[58] IEM do not have mutations in the coding exons of *SCN9A*. To date, mutations within the coding regions of the Na$_v$1.8 channel and the Na$_v$1.9 channel have not been observed in these cases of IEM, suggesting that other target genes or mutations in the noncoding regions of *SCN9A*, the gene encoding Na$_v$1.7, may result in the IEM phenotype.

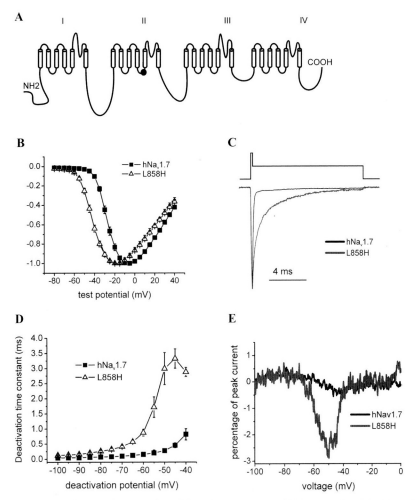

Figure 1. The L858H mutation produces a gain-of-function in Na$_v$1.7. (**A**) Schematic of the Na$_v$1.7 channel. The L858H mutation substitutes a single amino acid within the domain II/S4-S5 linker. (**B**) Cells expressing the mutant L858H channel display a hyperpolarizing shift in activation. (**C**) Representative tail currents of WT and L858H channels, showing that the mutant channel causes slow deactivation. (**D**) Time constants for tail current deactivation are increased for L858H Na$_v$1.7 channels. (**E**) Representative ramp currents in HEK293 cells expressing WT or L858H channels, showing that cells expressing the mutant channel generate larger currents in response to small, slow depolarizations. This may, in turn, allow for an earlier initiation of the action potential by the mutant channel. (Adapted with permission from Cummins and colleagues.[43] Panels B–D are from Fig. 1, and Panel E is from Fig. 3 of that article.)

Paroxysmal extreme pain disorder

A second autosomal dominant pain disorder, resulting from a different set of gain-of-function mutations that impair inactivation of Na$_v$1.7, is PEPD.[59–61] Severe pain in PEPD patients, accompanied by autonomic manifestations such as skin flushing, can start as early as infancy.[62] The pain attacks are most severe in the lower part of the body and can be triggered by a bowel movement or probing of the perianal area; they may also be accompanied by tonic nonepileptic seizures, bradycardia, and/or apnea, which appears to be more common in infancy and young children.[62] The cause for the seizure-like activity and cardiac symptoms is not well understood at this time. As the person ages, the

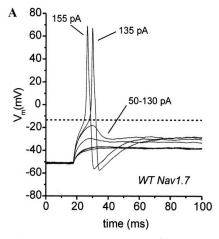

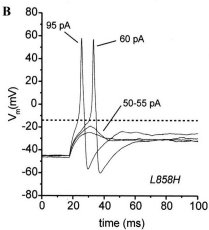

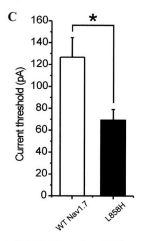

Figure 2. L858H renders DRG neurons hyperexcitable. Representative traces from cells expressing WT Na$_v$1.7 (A) and the L858H IEM mutant channel (B) show that action potentials were evoked with smaller depolarizing stimuli in cells housing the mutant channel. (C) The average current threshold for action potential firing of DRG neurons expressing WT Na$_v$1.7 channels is significantly greater than that of neurons expressing L858H mutant channels, indicating that the L858H mutation renders sensory neurons hyperexcitable. (Adapted with permission from Rush and colleagues.[54] Panels A–C are from Fig. 1 of that article.)

pain symptoms often change, with pain primarily affecting the ocular and maxillary and/or mandibular areas rather than the rectal area. These attacks are often triggered by temperature changes (such as cold winds), eating, and/or emotional upsets (such as crying).[62] Pain episodes usually last seconds to minutes but may last for hours in extreme cases. Between episodes, patients with PEPD complain of constipation, which can be seen as early as infancy. It has been speculated that this may be due to the patient's fear of inducing a pain attack by the passage of stool.[62] Interestingly, most patients with PEPD have a favorable response to treatment with CBZ.[60] As with IEM, not all patients with the diagnosis of PEPD carry mutations in Na$_v$1.7.[60]

Mutations of Na$_v$1.7: genetic analysis and expression studies

The first described PEPD mutations, located in domain III and IV of Na$_v$1.7, were reported in 2006 to impair fast-inactivation without altering channel activation, leading to a persistent current that is attenuated by CBZ.[60] Dib-Hajj and collaborators[59] extended the initial analysis to examine other gating properties of the M1627K mutant Na$_v$1.7 channel from a family with PEPD, showing that the mutant channel recovers from fast-inactivation faster than the WT channel and produces larger currents in response to ramp stimuli. Figure 4 shows whole cell currents from representative human embryonic kidney (HEK) cells expressing WT Na$_v$1.7 (Fig. 4B) and the M1627K mutant channel (Fig. 4C), elicited with a series of depolarizing test pulses. The peak current-voltage relationship between the WT channels and the mutant channels were about the same (Fig. 5A), and the time constants for deactivation were not altered for the M1627K channel (Fig. 5B), indicating that the M1627K mutation does not alter Na$_v$1.7 activation properties. However, the voltage-dependence of steady-state fast-inactivation

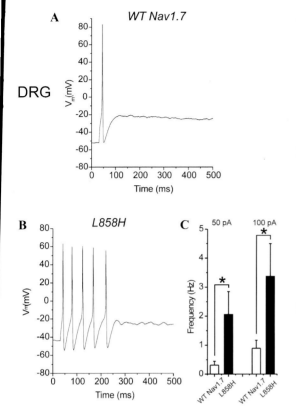

Figure 3. The L858H mutation increases firing frequency in DRG neurons. (**A**) Representative DRG neuron expressing WT Na_v1.7 fires a single action potential in response to a current injection. (**B**) Representative DRG neuron expressing L858H fires five action potentials in response to the same current injection. (**C**) For the entire population of DRG neurons studied, the firing frequency evoked by 50-pA current stimuli was 0.32 ± 0.13 Hz after transfection with WT channels and 2.06 ± 0.79 Hz after transfection with L858H, and the firing frequency evoked by 100-pA stimuli was 0.89 ± 0.28 Hz after transfection with WT and 3.37 ± 1.13 Hz after transfection with L858H (*, $P < 0.05$). (Adapted with permission from Rush and colleagues.[54] Panels A–C are from Fig. 3 of that article.)

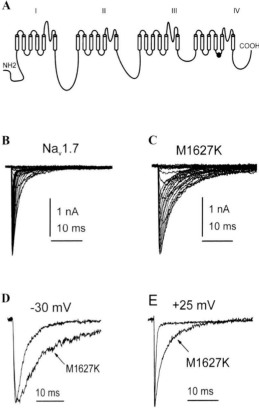

Figure 4. Currents produced by PEPD mutant M1672K decay slower than WT Nav1.7 currents. (**A**) Schematic of the Na_v1.7 channel. The M1627K substitution is located in the domain IV/S4-S5 linker. Representative WT (**B**) and M1627K (**C**) Nav1.7 currents are shown. Cells were held at −100 mV and currents were elicited with 50-ms test pulses to potentials ranging from −80 to 40 mV. For better comparison, WT and M1627K currents elicited with −30 mV (**D**) and +25 mV (**E**) depolarizations are shown superimposed. Although the rate of activation is not apparently altered, the decay phase is slowed for mutant channels, indicating an abnormality of channel inactivation. (Adapted with permission from Dib-Hajj and colleagues.[59] Panels B–E are from Fig. 2 of this article.)

was dramatically shifted in the depolarizing direction by the M1627K mutation (Fig. 5C). Similar changes in fast-inactivation have been seen with some[40,45,46] but not all IEM mutations.[42,43,47,56] The ramp currents elicited with slow ramp depolarizations in the M1627K PEPD mutation were significantly larger for the mutant channels than for the WT channels (Fig. 5D). Using current clamp,

Dib-Hajj and collaborators demonstrated that the M1627K mutation reduces the threshold for generation of single action potentials and increases the number of action potentials in DRG neurons in response to graded stimuli,[59] thus showing that the mutant channel renders DRG neurons hyperexcitable (Fig. 6). These data provide a link between altered channel properties and the pain symptoms

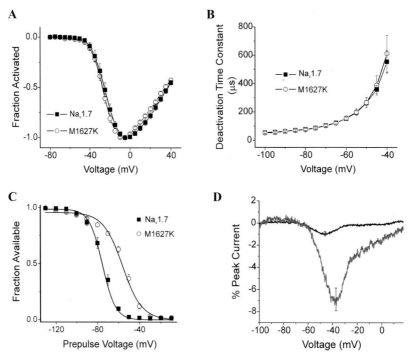

Figure 5. The M1627K mutation alters inactivation properties of Nav1.7. (**A**) Normalized peak current-voltage relationship for WT and M1627K channels, showing that channel activation is not substantially altered by the M1627K mutation. (**B**) The time constants for deactivation, which reflect the channel's transition from an open to a closed state, were also not significantly altered between cells expressing WT Nav1.7 or M1627K channels. (**C**) Steady-state fast-inactivation of the M1627K Nav1.7 channels is shifted in a depolarizing direction. (**D**) The average relative ramp current (ramp current divided by peak transient current amplitude) is larger for M1627K than for WT. (Adapted with permission from Dib-Hajj and colleagues.[59] Panels A–C are from Fig. 3 and Panel D is from Fig. 6 of that article.)

experienced by PEPD patients. Why IEM patients experience pain in the feet and hands, triggered by warmth, while PEPD patients experience pain in the perirectal area, triggered by rectal stimuli and then perimandibular and/or periocular pain, is not currently known.

The A1632E mutation—part of a continuum between IEM and PEPD

In 2008 a new mutation in Na$_v$1.7, A1632E, was described[63] in a patient with a unique mixture of symptoms, which included clinical characteristics of both IEM and PEPD. This mutation alters a conserved amino acid within the linker between transmembrane segments S4 and S5 of domain IV, which is close to the PEPD mutation M1627K.[59,60] The amino acid sequence within this loop is highly

conserved among most sodium channels, excluding Na$_v$1.9. The patient described with this particular mutation had had apnea, bradycardia, and poor feeding since birth. The bradycardia episodes were often precipitated by touching, feeding, urination, or defecation. As the patient grew older, the patient also complained of episodes of pain described as "hot needles" in the feet, hands, and head, often precipitated by warmth and attenuated by cooling.

The A1632E mutation from this patient was shown to have biophysical characteristics common to both IEM and PEPD mutations, altering activation and inactivation (Fig. 7A), deactivation (Fig. 7B), and slow ramp currents (Fig. 7C) of the channel.[63] Figure 8 shows diagrammatically how this particular mutation exhibits electrophysiological properties commonly seen in patients with either PEPD or IEM characteristics.[63] The A1632E

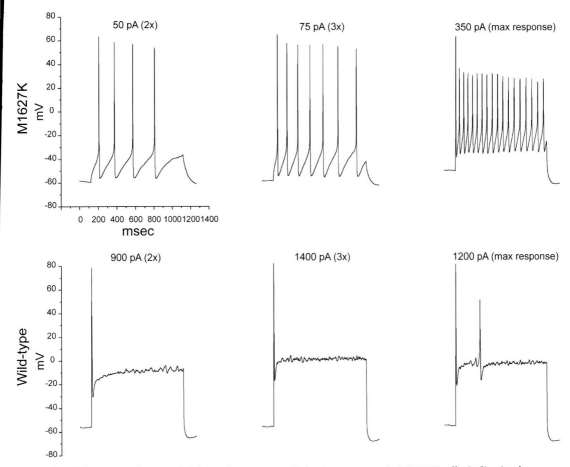

Figure 6. Higher rates of neuronal firing at lower current injections are seen in M1627K cells, indicating hyperexcitability of the mutant channel. The *upper panels* are the responses of a DRG neuron expressing M1627K channels, which can be compared to responses of cells housing WT Nav1.7 channels. Cells expressing the mutant channel live at a higher firing frequency in response to stimuli at 2× and 3× threshold and show increased maximal firing rates. (Adapted with permission from Dib-Hajj and colleagues.[59] This is Fig. 9 from that article.)

mutation and its associated phenotype suggest that IEM and PEPD mutations may be part of a physiological continuum that can produce a continuum of clinical pictures.

Channelopathy-associated insensitivity to pain

Subsequent to the identification of the role of the Na$_v$1.7 sodium channel in IEM, Cox and coworkers[33] reported several families in which loss-of-function mutations of Na$_v$1.7 were associated with profound insensitivity to pain; other sensory modalities were preserved and the remainder of the patients' central and peripheral nervous systems were

intact by report. Affected individuals displayed painless burns, fractures, and injuries of the lips and tongue, and were reported never to have felt pain in any part of the body, in response to any injury or noxious stimulus. The patients did not appear to exhibit autonomic or motor abnormalities, and reportedly had normal tear formation, sweating ability, reflexes, and intelligence. Cox and coworkers[33] found that in all three of the studied families, distinct, homozygous nonsense mutations of Na$_v$1.7 produced truncated, nonfunctional proteins. Patch-clamping experiments, done in HEK 293 cells co-expressing either WT or mutant channels together with β_1 and β_2 subunits, showed a loss-of-function in cells containing the mutant

A

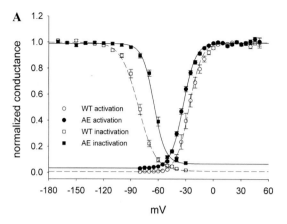

B

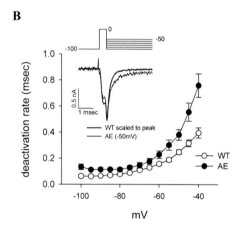

C

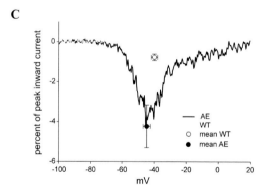

Figure 7. A1632E shifts both activation and fast inactivation of the mutant channel, as previously observed in IEM and PEPD mutations, respectively. (**A**) Activation and fast inactivation curves for WT and mutant cells are shown. The mutant cells exhibit hyperpolarized activation and impaired fast inactivation when compared with cells expressing the WT channel. (**B**) The A1632E mutation also slows deactivation, thus causing the channel to close more slowly than the WT channel. This feature has been observed in Na$_v$1.7 mutations that produce IEM.

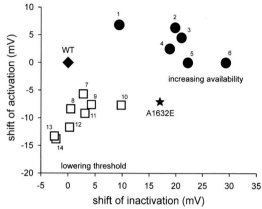

Figure 8. A comparison of IEM and PEPD mutations. This diagram plots the shifts seen in known IEM mutations (*open squares*) and PEPD mutations (*gray circles*). The WT control is plotted as a black diamond at (0,0). The *dotted lines* through (0,0) demarcate between positive and negative shifts and indicate the outcome for the shifts. The A1632E mutation from a patient with clinical characteristics of both IEM and PEPD is plotted with the star symbol and shows shifts in activation and inactivation common to both IEM and PEPD mutants. The identity of each numbered symbol is as follows: 1, T1464I (Fertleman *et al.*, 2006); 2, V1298F (Jarecki *et al.*, 2008); 3, V1299F (Jarecki *et al.*, 2008); 4, I1461T (Jarecki *et al.*, 2008); 5, M1627K (Fertleman, 2006); 6, I1461T (Fertleman, 2006); 7, I136V (Cheng *et al.*, 2008); 8, S241T (Lampert *et al.*, 2006); 9, F1449V (Dib-Hajj, 2005); 10, A863P (Harty *et al.*, 2006); 11, L858F (Han *et al.*, 2006); 12, F216S (Choi *et al.*, 2006); 13, L858H (Cummins *et al.*, 2004); and 14, I848T (Cummins *et al.*, 2004). (Adapted with permission from Estacion and colleagues.[63] This is Fig. 8 in that article.)

channels.[33] Additional families with similar loss-of-function mutations of Na$_v$1.7 and a similar clinical picture were subsequently reported by Ahmad and colleagues[32] and Goldberg and colleagues.[34] The

Example data traces comparing the deactivation during repolarization to −50 mV are shown in the inset. (**C**) The ramp response is enhanced by the A1632E mutant channels. (Adapted with permission from Estacion and colleagues.[63] Panels A and B are from Fig. 2 and Panel C is from Fig. 3 of that article.)

remarkably dense loss of pain sensibility in these patients provides strong evidence for a central function of Na$_v$1.7 in human pain.

Conclusion

It is becoming clear that gain-of-function mutations of Na$_v$1.7 cause syndromes characterized by severe pain[39–47,55,59,60,63–65] while loss-of-function mutations in Na$_v$1.7 produce insensitivity to pain.[32–34] Upregulated expression of Na$_v$1.7, together with Na$_v$1.8, another sodium channel isoform that works together with Na$_v$1.7 to produce high-frequency firing of DRG neurons, occurs within injured axons in human painful neurons.[66] These observations in humans, together with observations in rodent models that show upregulation of Na$_v$1.7 within nociceptive DRG neurons in response to inflammation within their peripheral projection fields,[67] and in which knockout of Na$_v$1.7 in nociceptors is associated with attenuated inflammatory pain responses,[31] establish Na$_v$1.7 as a critically important molecule along the pain pathway, where it appears to set the gain on pain responses.[27] The recent observations in humans have accelerated the search for Na$_v$1.7-specific blockers as potential pain therapeutics. Whether these agents, once identified, will alleviate pain in a clinically useful manner remains to be established.

Conflicts of interest

The authors declare no conflicts of interest.

References

1. Devor, M. 1994. The pathophysiology of damaged peripheral nerves. In *Textbook of Pain*, 2nd edn. P.D. Wall, R. Melzack, Eds.: 79–101. Churchill Livingstone. Edinburgh.

2. Nordin, M., B. Nystrom, U. Wallin & K.E. Hagbarth. 1984. Ectopic sensory discharges and paresthesiae in patients with disorders of peripheral nerves, dorsal roots and dorsal columns. *Pain* **20:** 231–245.

3. Ochoa, J.L. & H.E. Torebjork. 1980. Paraesthesiae from ectopic impulse generation in human sensory nerves. *Brain* **103:** 835–853.

4. Zhang, J.M., D.F. Donnelly, X.J. Song & R.H. Lamotte. 1997. Axotomy increases the excitability of dorsal root ganglion cells with unmyelinated axons. *J. Neurophysiol.* **78:** 2790–2794.

5. Catterall, W.A., A.L. Goldin & S.G. Waxman. 2005. International Union of Pharmacology. XLVII. Nomenclature and structure-function relationships of voltage-gated sodium channels. *Pharmacol. Rev.* **57:** 397–409.

6. Chen, C., V. Bharucha, Y. Chen, *et al.* 2002. Reduced sodium channel density, altered voltage dependence of inactivation, and increased susceptibility to seizures in mice lacking sodium channel beta 2-subunits. *Proc. Natl. Acad. Sci. USA* **99:** 17072–17077.

7. Qu, Y., R. Curtis, D. Lawson, *et al.* 2001. Differential modulation of sodium channel gating and persistent sodium currents by the beta1, beta2, and beta3 subunits. *Mol. Cell. Neurosci.* **18:** 570–580.

8. Yu, F.H., R.E. Westenbroek, I. Silos-Santiago, *et al.* 2003. Sodium channel beta4, a new disulfide-linked auxiliary subunit with similarity to beta2. *J. Neurosci.* **23:** 7577–7585.

9. Isom, L.L. 2000. I. Cellular and molecular biology of sodium channel beta-subunits: therapeutic implications for pain? I. Cellular and molecular biology of sodium channel beta-subunits: therapeutic implications for pain? *Am. J. Physiol. Gastrointest. Liver Physiol.* **278:** G349–G353.

10. Isom, L.L., K.S. De Jongh, D.E. Patton, *et al.* 1992. Primary structure and functional expression of the beta 1 subunit of the rat brain sodium channel. *Science* **256:** 839–842.

11. Felts, P.A., S. Yokoyama, S. Dib-Hajj, *et al.* 1997. Sodium channel alpha-subunit mRNAs I, II, III, NaG, Na6 and hNE (PN1): different expression patterns in developing rat nervous system. *Brain Res. Mol. Brain Res.* **45:** 71–82.

12. Waxman, S.G. 2000. The neuron as a dynamic electrogenic machine: modulation of sodium-channel expression as a basis for functional plasticity in neurons. *Philos. Trans. R. Soc. Lond. B Biol. Sci.* **355:** 199–213.

13. Caffrey, J.M., D.L. Eng, J.A. Black, *et al.* 1992. Three types of sodium channels in adult rat dorsal root ganglion neurons. *Brain Res.* **592:** 283–297.

14. Elliott, A.A. & J.R. Elliott. 1993. Characterization of TTX-sensitive and TTX-resistant sodium currents in small cells from adult rat dorsal root ganglia. *J. Physiol.* **463:** 39–56.

15. Kostyuk, P.G., N.S. Veselovsky & A.Y. Tsyndrenko. 1981. Ionic currents in the somatic membrane of rat dorsal root ganglion neurons-I. Sodium currents. *Neuroscience* **6:** 2423–2430.

16. Roy, M.L. & T. Narahashi. 1992. Differential properties of tetrodotoxin-sensitive and tetrodotoxin-resistant

sodium channels in rat dorsal root ganglion neurons. *J. Neurosci.* **12:** 2104–2111.

17. Cummins, T.R. & S.G. Waxman. 1997. Downregulation of tetrodotoxin-resistant sodium currents and up-regulation of a rapidly repriming tetrodotoxin-sensitive sodium current in small spinal sensory neurons after nerve injury. *J. Neurosci.* **17:** 3503–3514.

18. Dib-Hajj, S.D., L. Tyrrell, T.R. Cummins, *et al.* 1999. Two tetrodotoxin-resistant sodium channels in human dorsal root ganglion neurons. *FEBS Lett.* **462:** 117–120.

19. Akopian, A.N., L. Sivilotti & J.N. Wood. 1996. A tetrodotoxin-resistant voltage-gated sodium channel expressed by sensory neurons. *Nature* **379:** 257–262.

20. Black, J.A., S. Dib-Hajj, K. McNabola, *et al.* 1996. Spinal sensory neurons express multiple sodium channel alpha-subunit mRNAs. *Brain Res. Mol. Brain Res.* **43:** 117–131.

21. Dib-Hajj, S.D., J.A. Black, T.R. Cummins, *et al.* 1998. Rescue of alpha-SNS sodium channel expression in small dorsal root ganglion neurons after axotomy by nerve growth factor in vivo. *J. Neurophysiol.* **79:** 2668–2676.

22. Toledo-Aral, J.J., B.L. Moss, Z.J. He, *et al.* 1997. Identification of PN1, a predominant voltage-dependent sodium channel expressed principally in peripheral neurons. *Proc. Natl. Acad. Sci. USA* **94:** 1527–1532.

23. Dib-Hajj, S., J.A. Black, P. Felts & S.G. Waxman. 1996. Down-regulation of transcripts for Na channel alpha-SNS in spinal sensory neurons following axotomy. *Proc. Natl. Acad. Sci. USA* **93:** 14950–14954.

24. Black, J.A., T.R. Cummins, C. Plumpton, *et al.* 1999. Upregulation of a silent sodium channel after peripheral, but not central, nerve injury in DRG neurons. *J. Neurophysiol.* **82:** 2776–2785.

25. Waxman, S.G., J.D. Kocsis & J.A. Black. 1994. Type III sodium channel mRNA is expressed in embryonic but not adult spinal sensory neurons, and is reexpressed following axotomy. *J. Neurophysiol.* **72:** 466–470.

26. Baker, M.D. & J.N. Wood. 2001. Involvement of Na+ channels in pain pathways. *Trends Pharmacol. Sci.* **22:** 27–31.

27. Waxman, S.G. 2006. Neurobiology: a channel sets the gain on pain. *Nature* **444:** 831–832.

28. Akopian, A.N., V. Souslova, S. England, *et al.* 1999. The tetrodotoxin-resistant sodium channel SNS has a specialized function in pain pathways. *Nat. Neurosci.* **2:** 541–548.

29. Laird, J.M., V. Souslova, J.N. Wood & F. Cervero. 2002. Deficits in visceral pain and referred hyperalgesia in Nav1.8 (SNS/PN3)-null mice. *J. Neurosci.* **22:** 8352–8356.

30. Nassar, M.A., A. Levato, L.C. Stirling & J.N. Wood. 2005. Neuropathic pain develops normally in mice lacking both Nav1.7 and Nav1.8. *Mol. Pain.* **1:** 24.

31. Nassar, M.A., L.C. Stirling, G. Forlani, *et al.* 2004. Nociceptor-specific gene deletion reveals a major role for Nav1.7 (PN1) in acute and inflammatory pain. *Proc. Natl. Acad. Sci. USA* **101:** 12706–12711.

32. Ahmad, S., L. Dahllund, A.B. Eriksson, *et al.* 2007. A stop codon mutation in SCN9A causes lack of pain sensation. *Hum. Mol. Genet.* **16:** 2114–2121.

33. Cox, J.J., F. Reimann, A.K. Nicholas, *et al.* 2006. An SCN9A channelopathy causes congenital inability to experience pain. *Nature* **444:** 894–898.

34. Goldberg, Y.P., J. MacFarlane, M.L. MacDonald, *et al.* 2007. Loss-of-function mutations in the Nav1.7 gene underlie congenital indifference to pain in multiple human populations. *Clin. Genet.* **71:** 311–319.

35. Mitchell, S.W. 1878. On a rare vaso-motor neurosis of the extremities, and on the maladies with which it may be confounded. *Am. J. Med. Sci.* **76:** 17–36.

36. van Genderen, P.J., J.J. Michiels, J. & P. Drenth. 1993. Hereditary erythermalgia and acquired erythromelalgia. *Am. J. Med. Genet.* **45:** 530–532.

37. Drenth, J.P. & S.G. Waxman. 2007. Mutations in sodium-channel gene SCN9A cause a spectrum of human genetic pain disorders. *J. Clin. Invest.* **117:** 3603–3609.

38. Novella, S.P., F.M. Hisama, S.D. Dib-Hajj & S.G. Waxman. 2007. A case of inherited erythromelalgia. *Nat. Clin. Pract. Neurol.* **3:** 229–234.

39. Yang, Y., Y. Wang, S. Li, *et al.* 2004. Mutations in SCN9A, encoding a sodium channel alpha subunit, in patients with primary erythermalgia. *J. Med. Genet.* **41:** 171–174.

40. Dib-Hajj, S.D., A.M. Rush, T.R. Cummins, *et al.* 2005. Gain-of-function mutation in Nav1.7 in familial erythromelalgia induces bursting of sensory neurons. *Brain* **128:** 1847–1854.

41. Cheng, X., S.D. Dib-Hajj, L. Tyrrell & S.G. Waxman. 2008. Mutation I136V alters electrophysiological properties of the Na(v)1.7 channel in a family with onset of erythromelalgia in the second decade. *Mol. Pain* **4:** 1.

42. Choi, J.S., S.D. Dib-Hajj & S.G. Waxman. 2006. Inherited erythermalgia: limb pain from an S4 charge-neutral Na channelopathy. *Neurology* **67:** 1563–1567.

43. Cummins, T.R., S.D. Dib-Hajj & S.G. Waxman. 2004. Electrophysiological properties of mutant Nav1.7 sodium channels in a painful inherited neuropathy. *J. Neurosci.* **24:** 8232–8236.

44. Fischer, T.Z., E.S. Gilmore, M. Estacion, *et al.* 2009. A novel Nav1.7 mutation producing carbamazepine-responsive erythromelalgia. *Ann. Neurol.* **65:** 773–741.

45. Han, C., A.M. Rush, S.D. Dib-Hajj, *et al.* 2006. Sporadic onset of erythermalgia: a gain-of-function mutation in Nav1.7. *Ann. Neurol.* **59:** 553–558.

46. Harty, T.P., S.D. Dib-Hajj, L. Tyrrell, *et al.* 2006. Na(V)1.7 mutant A863P in erythromelalgia: effects of altered activation and steady-state inactivation on excitability of nociceptive dorsal root ganglion neurons. *J. Neurosci.* **26:** 12566–12575.

47. Lampert, A., S.D. Dib-Hajj, L. Tyrrell & S.G. Waxman. 2006. Size matters: Erythromelalgia mutation S241T in Nav1.7 alters channel gating. *J. Biol. Chem.* **281:** 36029–36035.

48. Djouhri, L., R. Newton, S.R. Levinson, *et al.* 2003. Sensory and electrophysiological properties of guinea-pig sensory neurones expressing Nav 1.7 (PN1) Na+ channel alpha subunit protein. *J. Physiol.* **546:** 565–576.

49. Sangameswaran, L., L.M. Fish, B.D. Koch, *et al.* 1997. A novel tetrodotoxin-sensitive, voltage-gated sodium channel expressed in rat and human dorsal root ganglia. *J. Biol. Chem.* **272:** 14805–14809.

50. Cummins, T.R., J.R. Howe & S.G. Waxman. 1998. Slow closed-state inactivation: a novel mechanism underlying ramp currents in cells expressing the hNE/PN1 sodium channel. *J. Neurosci.* **18:** 9607–9619.

51. Herzog, R.I., T.R. Cummins, F. Ghassemi, *et al.* 2003. Distinct repriming and closed-state inactivation kinetics of Nav1.6 and Nav1.7 sodium channels in mouse spinal sensory neurons. *J. Physiol.* **551:** 741–750.

52. Renganathan, M., T.R. Cummins & S.G. Waxman. 2001. Contribution of Na(v)1.8 sodium channels to action potential electrogenesis in DRG neurons. *J. Neurophysiol.* **86:** 629–640.

53. Harper, A.A. & S.N. Lawson. 1985. Electrical properties of rat dorsal root ganglion neurones with different peripheral nerve conduction velocities. *J. Physiol.* **359:** 47–63.

54. Rush, A.M., S.D. Dib-Hajj, S. Liu, *et al.* 2006. A single sodium channel mutation produces hyper- or hypoexcitability in different types of neurons. *Proc. Natl. Acad. Sci. USA* **103:** 8245–8250.

55. Choi, J.S., L. Zhang, S.D. Dib-Hajj, *et al.* 2009. Mexiletine-responsive erythromelalgia due to a new Na(v)1.7 mutation showing use-dependent current falloff. *Exp. Neurol.* **216:** 383–389.

56. Sheets, P.L., J.O. Jackson, 2nd, S.G. Waxman, *et al.* 2007. A Nav1.7 channel mutation associated with hereditary erythromelalgia contributes to neuronal hyperexcitability and displays reduced lidocaine sensitivity. *J. Physiol.* **581:** 1019–1031.

57. Drenth, J.P., R.H. Te Morsche, S. Mansour & P.S. Mortimer. 2008. Primary erythermalgia as a sodium channelopathy: screening for SCN9A mutations: exclusion of a causal role of SCN10A and SCN11A. *Arch. Dermatol.* **144:** 320–324.

58. Burns, T.M., R.H. Te Morsche, J.B. Jansen & J.P. Drenth. 2005. Genetic heterogeneity and exclusion of a modifying locus at 2q in a family with autosomal dominant primary erythermalgia. *Br. J. Dermatol.* **153:** 174–177.

59. Dib-Hajj, S.D., M. Estacion, B.W. Jarecki, *et al.* 2008. Paroxysmal extreme pain disorder M1627K mutation in human Nav1.7 renders DRG neurons hyperexcitable. *Mol. Pain* **4:** 37.

60. Fertleman, C.R., M.D. Baker, K.A. Parker, *et al.* 2006. SCN9A mutations in paroxysmal extreme pain disorder: allelic variants underlie distinct channel defects and phenotypes. *Neuron* **52:** 767–774.

61. Jarecki, B.W., P.L. Sheets, J.O. Jackson, 2nd & T.R. Cummins. 2008. Paroxysmal extreme pain disorder mutations within the D3/S4-S5 linker of Nav1.7 cause moderate destabilization of fast inactivation. *J. Physiol.* **586:** 4137–4153.

62. Fertleman, C.R., C.D. Ferrie, J. Aicardi, *et al.* 2007. Paroxysmal extreme pain disorder (previously familial rectal pain syndrome). *Neurology* **69:** 586–595.

63. Estacion, M., S.D. Dib-Hajj, P.J. Benke, *et al.* 2008. NaV1.7 gain-of-function mutations as a continuum: A1632E displays physiological changes associated with erythromelalgia and paroxysmal extreme pain disorder mutations and produces symptoms of both disorders. *J. Neurosci.* **28:** 11079–11088.

64. Drenth, J.P., R.H. te Morsche, G. Guillet, *et al.* 2005. SCN9A mutations define primary erythermalgia as a neuropathic disorder of voltage gated sodium channels. *J. Invest. Dermatol.* **124:** 1333–1338.

65. Waxman, S.G. & S. Dib-Hajj. 2005. Erythermalgia: molecular basis for an inherited pain syndrome. *Trends Mol. Med.* **11:** 555–562.

66. Black, J.A., L. Nikolajsen, K. Kroner, *et al.* 2008. Multiple sodium channel isoforms and mitogen-activated protein kinases are present in painful human neuromas. *Ann. Neurol.* **64:** 644–653.

67. Black, J.A., S. Liu, M. Tanaka, *et al.* 2004. Changes in the expression of tetrodotoxin-sensitive sodium channels within dorsal root ganglia neurons in inflammatory pain. *Pain* **108:** 237–247.

Ann. N.Y. Acad. Sci. ISSN 0077-8923

ANNALS OF THE NEW YORK ACADEMY OF SCIENCES

Epilepsy in the elderly

Ilo E. Leppik[1] and Angela K. Birnbaum[2]

[1]Department of Neurology, University of Minnesota, and MINCEP Epilepsy Care, Minneapolis, Minnesota, USA. [2]Department of Experimental and Clinical Pharmacology, University of Minnesota, Minneapolis, Minnesota, USA

Address for correspondence: Ilo E. Leppik, M.D., 7500 Western Ave, Golden Valley, MN, 55427. Voice: 763-546-3328; fax: 763-546-1013. leppi001@umn.edu

The elderly, often defined as those 65 years or older, are the most rapidly growing segment of the population, and onset of epilepsy is higher in this age group than in any other. This paper reviews recent developments, including a new proposed definition of epilepsy, a transgenic mouse model of Alzheimer's disease that exhibits complex partial seizures, evidence that the highest incidence of epilepsy may occur after admission to a nursing home, a challenge to the vitamin D hypothesis of osteoporosis associated with antiepileptic drugs (AEDs), evidence that the genetic complement of hepatic isoenzymes is more predictive of metabolic rate than age, and data showing that there is considerable variability in serum levels of AEDs in many nursing home residents during constant dosing conditions.

Keywords: epilepsy; elderly; nursing homes; treatment

Introduction

The elderly, often defined as those 65 years or older, are the most rapidly growing segment of the U.S. population. Demographic predictions indicate that their numbers will increase from an estimated 40 million in 2010 to 71.5 million in 2030.[1] Epidemiologic studies have shown that the incidence of epilepsy is significantly higher in the elderly than in any other age cohort.[2,3] During 1995, for example, approximately 181,000 persons in the United States developed epilepsy, 68,000 of whom were over the age of 65.[4] The incidence of epilepsy is high in the pediatric cohort and declines in younger adults but begins to increase after age 55. The prevalence rate in community-dwelling elderly in the United States is approximately 1.5%, considerably higher than the approximately 0.5% in younger adults. High rates of epilepsy in the elderly have also been reported from other developed countries.[5,6] In Finland, the number of elderly persons with epilepsy is now greater than those in the pediatric cohort, a reversal from just a few decades ago. Thus, due the projected increase in the number of elderly persons, as well as their propensity to develop epilepsy, these individuals will represent an increasingly large group of patients needing expert care pertaining to this disorder.

Definition of epilepsy and seizures

At the present time, there is a debate within the epilepsy community regarding the precise definition of epilepsy.[7] Until recently, it has been accepted that an individual should not be diagnosed with epilepsy until he or she experienced two or more seizures. The definition of two unprovoked seizures is used in epidemiologic studies, texts, and often in practice. However, with the diagnostic tools now available, specific central nervous disease processes can be readily identified. Epidemiologic studies have shown that persons with certain conditions, such as stroke or brain tumor, have a high probability of experiencing additional seizures after an initial ictal event. Often, there is also a desire to treat to prevent morbidity or mortality from further seizures. A committee of the International League Against Epilepsy (ILAE) has proposed that epilepsy be defined as a condition of the central nervous system (CNS) predisposed to seizure activity.[8] The counterargument is that many persons with a CNS lesion may never have another seizure, and diagnosing and treating everyone using the proposed definition may lead to overtreatment and unnecessarily labeling many people as having epilepsy. However, it is now necessary to use an ICD-9 code with every prescription. The code for epilepsy is 345.xx, but

Ann. N.Y. Acad. Sci. 1184 (2010) 208–224 © 2009 New York Academy of Sciences.

there is another code, 780.3, which is for seizure not otherwise specified. Thus, if one wishes to treat after a single seizure but does not wish to diagnose a person as having epilepsy, 780.3 may be used. This is of particular importance to the physician who wishes to decrease the risk of falls resulting in fractures or severe cardiac stress, but not use the epilepsy code. But treating after a single seizure will likely reduce the number of patients having a second seizure. Epidemiologic studies that use the two unprovoked seizure criteria may thus be compromised.

Causes of epilepsy

The most common identifiable comorbidity of epileptic seizures in the elderly is a previous stroke. Overall, from 30% to 40% of all epileptic seizure cases in the elderly are in persons who have had a stoke.[2] In a prospective study of 1897 patients suffering from stroke, seizures occurred in 168 (8.9%) during a 9-month follow-up period.[9] Of the 265 patients within the study who suffered a hemorrhagic stroke, 28 (10.6%) suffered a seizure; of 1632 patients who suffered an ischemic stoke, 140 (8.6%) suffered a seizure.[9] Thus, those who suffered a hemorrhagic stroke had a twofold increased risk for a seizure as compared to those who suffered an ischemic stroke. During the 9 months of follow-up in this study, epilepsy, as defined by the onset of a second seizure, occurred in 47 out of 1897 (2.5%) persons. A longer observation period might have detected a higher rate. Some retrospective studies have indicated that the eventual risk of experiencing seizures after suffering a stroke may be as high as 20%.[10] It has been estimated that each year more than 730,000 persons in the United States have a stroke. Projecting these data, the incidence of new seizures after stroke may exceed 36,000 cases per year.[10]

One confusing factor is that a transient ischemic attack (TIA) will sometimes lead to simple partial seizures whose pattern is similar to the deficit of the TIA. This may create a diagnostic dilemma and concern that another TIA is occurring. The major clinical differential feature between a TIA and a simple partial seizure is the length of the event. Simple partial seizures rarely last more than a few minutes, whereas TIAs last much longer, usually hours.

Brain tumor, head injury, and Alzheimer's disease are other major causes of epilepsy in the elderly. It is suspected that people with Alzheimer's disease who experience brief periods of increased confusion may be having unrecognized partial complex seizures.[11] Although the probable comorbid condition and presumed cause can be identified in many cases, in approximately half of the cases the precise cause cannot be determined and the etiology is termed cryptogenic (*crypt* = hidden, *genic* = cause).

Neurobiology of aging and epilepsy

Although rodent models have a long history of contributing to the understanding of epilepsy, they have not been utilized to study issues of the aging brain and epilepsy. There are many reasons for this, but perhaps the most salient are the issues of obtaining appropriate-aged animals.[12] The National Institute on Aging has an aged rodent colony of a limited number of strains. They also maintain a tissue bank from aged rodent colonies and have a number of human cell lines that include samples from patients with convulsive disorders. However, the genetic background of animals is crucial because there are major species differences in susceptibility to seizures.[12] For example, C57BL/6 mice are completely resistant to audiogenic seizures, whereas DBA/2 mice have a very low threshold to this type of stimulus.[13] There are also major strain differences in susceptibility to maximal electroshock seizures (MES). To study the effects of aging on epilepsy, one would need to select an appropriate genetic strain and raise them through the life cycle to old age. The cost of this would be considerable, and one would need a long grant cycle to accomplish this.

One difficulty in studying the effect of aging on epilepsy is the heterogeneity of this disorder. The mechanism of developing epilepsy after a stroke may differ significantly from the process by which persons with Alzheimer's disease become susceptible to seizures. Even within the stroke category, hemorrhagic strokes may have a different mechanism than ischemic stroke. Then there are the large number of persons who have cryptogenic epilepsy. Nevertheless, there are a number of changes in the aging brain that may alter the seizure threshold.

In aging rodents, significant synaptic loss in the middle and inner molecular layers of the dentate gyrus has been demonstrated.[14] Changes in the volume of human hippocampi can also be seen in humans using magnetic resonance imaging (MRI) scans.[15] However, the effect of these processes on epileptogenisis is not easily understood. Long-term potentiation (LTP) is the long-lasting augmentation of synaptic responses after brief trains of high-frequency stimulation of monosynaptic pathways. There appears to be no significant difference in the extent of LTP between young and old animals in the Shaffer collateral-CA1 synapse and the perforant path–granular cell synapse.[16] This may be due to the fact that NMDA receptor–dependent LTP is markedly reduced in aged animals while voltage-dependent, calcium channel–dependent LTP is significantly increased.[17] Thus, the overall result of these two components of LTP may not show a change as a function of "normal" aging. However, in old memory-impaired rats LTP declines much faster than in younger rats. Kindling was initially used as a model to study learning. Thus it is interesting to note that the process of kindling to spontaneous epilepsy is retarded in aged animals.[18] This set of studies found a striking relationship between rate of kindling and memory: old rodents with poor memory kindled slowly, whereas old rodents with good memory kindled rapidly.[18] A human study of secondary epileptogenisis reported that older persons were much less likely to develop an independent secondary focus than younger ones.[19] These studies suggest that the increased incidence of seizures in elderly patients may be due more to the frequency of various insults to the brain rather than an increase in susceptibility to epileptogenisis.

Because stroke (hemorrhagic and ischemic) is the major cause of symptomatic epilepsy in the elderly, study of animal models in this field may lead to important insights into developing strategies for the prevention of epilepsy after a stroke. Middle cerebral artery occlusion (MCAO) and photothrombosis with concomitant electroencephalography (EEG) recoding have been the most widely used models of ischemic infarction. In one study MCAO resulted in multiple generalized or focal ictal discharges within 2 h of the insult, but clinical seizures were not observed.[20] Another study of MCAO, however, found no evidence for clinical or EEG seizures in animals followed for 1 year.[21] On the other hand, large photothrombotic infarctions are associated with electroencephalographic seizures. Another model uses glutamate excitotoxicity injury–induced epileptogenisis in hippocampal neuronal cultures. This has led to the Ca^{2+}

hypothesis of epileptoginisis.[22] It is hoped that a better understanding of the mechanisms of epilptogenisis may eventually lead to new therapeutic interventions. Recently a transgenic mouse model of Alzheimer's disease was found to have spontaneous nonconvulsive seizures accompanied by electroencephalographic changes reminiscent of human temporal lobe epilepsy.[23]

Diagnosis

The diagnosis of epilepsy is difficult in the elderly for many reasons. A good history may be difficult to obtain, many seizures may be subtle complex partial events, and seizures may be provoked. In the VA study #428 of new onset epilepsy in a community-dwelling cohort, many subjects eventually diagnosed as having epilepsy had been initially misdiagnosed.[24] Because most seizures in the elderly are caused by a focal area of damage to the brain, the most common seizure types are localization related. Complex partial seizures are the most common seizure type, accounting for nearly 40% of all seizures in the elderly population.[25] Both simple and complex seizures may spread and develop into generalized tonic–clonic seizures.

When considering the diagnosis of epilepsy, a clear distinction must be made between epileptic seizures—those arising from brain pathology—and nonepileptic seizures (provoked seizures)—those arising within a normal brain due to an alteration in physiology, such as hypoxia. It is imperative that provoked seizures be ruled out before concluding that the seizure was epileptic. Other causes of seizure activity, such as cardiac insufficiency, metabolic conditions, convulsive syncope (micturation syncope, cough syncope), must be eliminated as etiological factors because a misdiagnosis can have serious consequences. Evaluation after a single seizure must therefore be comprehensive. A thorough history must be obtained, focusing on events of the previous day or days, in order to identify any precipitating or predisposing factors that may have led to the onset. An electrocardiogram (EKG) should be utilized in order to rule out possible cardiac conditions. Laboratory tests for metabolic disorders should be done, as well as a review of prescription drugs, over-the-counter agents, and natural products being used by the patient. Unfortunately, many natural products designed to stimulate weight loss or improve memory may have proconvulsant properties. Further, withdrawal from CNS depressants such as benzodiazepines or alcohol may provoke seizures. Stimulants such as methamphetamine and cocaine may cause convulsions. Unfortunately, abuse of drugs is not absent in the elderly, and a drug screen should be considered.

Computed tomography and magnetic resonance imaging

The use of cortical imaging studies is highly predictive of seizures.[26] Structural studies, such as computed tomography (CT) that screen for intracerebral hemorrhage, brain tumor, and encephalomalacia, should be performed following a convulsion. CT scans serve as an appropriate imaging tool for the initial emergency study. Because of its X-ray modality, it is capable of detecting tissue contrasts; therefore, it is effective in locating blood, areas of encephalomalacia, and calcified lesions. The CT scan is unable to appropriately visualize subtle changes in tissue density. Glial tumors, subtle changes within the hippocampus, and other significant lesions may not be well visualized by a CT scan. Detection of these lesions requires MRI, which is more appropriate for identifying subtle changes in brain tissue. An MRI should be requested if an obvious pathology is not detected by the initial CT scan.

Electroencephalogram

EEG serves many useful roles in the diagnosis of epilepsy. Detection of interictal patterns can confirm the presence of physiologically abnormal brain, solidifying the diagnosis of an epileptic as opposed to a nonepileptic seizure. Additionally, interictal patterns can provide information on the severity of the epilepsy. Frequent interictal activity would suggest a more aggressive epileptogenic process and reinforce the impetus for treatment. The presence of interictal activity on EEGs can also identify the epileptogenic region, providing additional clues to the etiology of the patient's disorder. Patients who experience periodic lateralized epileptiform discharges (PLEDs) after a stroke are also prone to develop epileptic seizures.[27] Those with focal spikes have a 78% risk for developing epileptic seizures.[28] It is recommended that an EKG rhythm strip be obtained during an EEG in order to help identify artifacts and to provide additional evidence to exclude a cardiac cause for the seizure.

Complex issues

Problems faced by the elderly suffering from epilepsy are different and more complex than those faced by younger adults also suffering from the same disorder. These problems involve medical complexities, such as correct diagnoses, selection of the most appropriate medication(s), and presence of comorbid illnesses, as well other societal factors like emotional stability and economic responsibilities.

Falls, fractures, and bone health

The presence of epilepsy increases the risk for falls and fractures by two- to sixfold. Osteoporosis and bone fractures are commonly seen in the elderly population, and thus an elderly person with epilepsy is at increased risk. Lack of exercise, inadequate nutrition, impairment of mobility, and neurological conditions leading to poor balance and protective reflexes may all play a role. Large prospective studies in women and men have associated use of both PHT and gabapentin with decreased bone mineral density.[29,30] The fact that nonenzyme-inducing AEDs such as gabapentin and valproate both affect bone mineral density, while carbamazepine, a strong inducer, does not brings into question the commonly held belief that the influence of AEDs on bone health is only through vitamin D metabolism. However, vitamin D supplementation is recommended for all elderly, with or without epilepsy. Not well studied is the possible influence of AED toxicity (ataxia, neuropathy, nystagmus, sedation) on falls. Because the elderly are more sensitive to AED side effects, care should be taken to avoid AED concentrations in the higher range effective for younger adults, and levels below the usually effective range may be appropriate.

Elderly are not a homogenous population

The elderly are not a single cohort. Thus, broad statements about these persons may not be relevant to each individual patient. Just as medical issues involving persons up to 18 years of age cannot be properly interpreted without using newborn, infant, child, and adolescent subcategories, elderly people should also be subdivided into appropriate cohorts. One system divides this group into the young-old

Table 1. Categorization of elderly with epilepsy according to health status. Each cohort may require a different approach.

Young-Old Healthy	Middle-Old Healthy	Old-Old Healthy
Young-Old Multiple with Medical Problems	Middle-Old Multiple Medical Problems	Old-Old Multiple Medical Problems
Young-Old Frail	Middle-Old Frail	Old-Old Frail
FE	FE	FE

Modified from Ref. 31.

(65–74 years of age); the middle-old (75–84 years of age); and the old-old (≥85 years of age). However, because the elderly develop health issues at different ages, further subdivisions, such as the elderly healthy who have epilepsy (EH), the elderly with multiple medical problems (EMMP), and the frail elderly, those usually found residing in nursing homes (NHs) (FE), have also been proposed (Table 1).[31]

Adding to the complexity are the major differences between the community-dwelling elderly, those living independently, and the elderly residing in NHs. Drug side effects, efficacy, absorption, and other factors may be markedly different between a 93-year-old healthy person living independently and a 68-year-old frail person residing in an NH. In addition, issues regarding healthcare delivery will differ between the community-dwelling elderly and those residing in an NH. Thus, studies should be designed to address specific populations, and reports should specify the populations studied.[32]

Also seen as significantly problematic is the selection of an appropriate AED, which requires the consideration of many factors. Such factors include changes in organ function, increased susceptibility to adverse effects, use of other medications known to interact with AEDs, and economic limitations associated with the patient. Further, pharmaceutical treatment for the elderly carries greater risks than in younger persons. In addition to their use in epilepsy, AEDs are prescribed for a variety of other disorders affecting the elderly, including pain and psychiatric disorders. AEDs rank fifth among all drug categories in their capacity to illicit adverse reactions.[33] Yet very little research has been done within this vulnerable population and only general recommendations can be made at this time.

Pharmacoepidemiology of antiepileptic drug use in community-dwelling elderly

The largest study of AED use in U.S. community-dwelling elderly people was coordinated by Berlowitz.[34,35] This study's cohort identified 1,130,155 veterans ≥65 years of age from the Veteran Administrations (VA) national database between 1997 and 1999. Of these, 20,558 (1.8%) were identified as having epilepsy by exhibiting an ICD-9-CM diagnostic code representative of this condition. Approximately 80% of those with epilepsy were receiving one AED, whereas 20% were being treated with two or more. PHT was used as monotherapy by almost 70% of the cohort, whereas phenobarbital was used as monotherapy by approximately 10%. Another 5% were using phenobarbital in combination with PHT. Carbamazepine was used by just more than 10%, and newer AEDs (gabapentin and lamotrigine) were used by less than 10%.[35] Levetiracetam was not available at the time of this survey. Smaller studies of AED use in community-dwelling non-VA elderly patients have shown similar distributions of AED use, with PHT by far the most widely used AED in the United States by this population. These studies, done almost a decade ago, from this writing and may not reflect current practice.

Pharmacoepidemiology of AED use in nursing homes

As people age, their need for NH care increases due to greater frailty and the likely onset of age-related diseases. For patients ≥65 years of age, there is a lifetime risk of 43% to 46% of becoming an NH resident.[36] Accordingly, at any one time 4.5% of the U.S. elderly population resides within an NH.[37] In epidemiological research concerning NHs, it is necessary to make distinctions between residents and admissions. A resident cohort includes all residents in the facility at a specified time and usually represents a cross-sectional sample that consists of a mixture of newly admitted residents and those who have been in the NH for different periods of time. In contrast, an admissions cohort includes all people admitted to a facility during a specified time period.[38]

In a study of U.S. NH residents residing within various facilities during the spring of 1995, the mean age of the 21,551 persons studied was 83.78 years (SD = 8.13 years).[38] The sample had the following age group distribution: young-old 15%, middle-old 36%, and old-old 49%. This distribution is similar to the data provided by the U.S. Census Bureau which, in 2000 described the admittance of 1,555,800 persons to NH facilities.[37] Of the residents in the NH sample studied by Garrard and colleagues, 10.5% had one or more AED orders on the day of study and 9.2% had a seizure indication (epilepsy or seizure disorder) documented in their computerized medical record. PHT was used by 6.2% of the residents, followed by carbamazepine (1.8%), phenobarbital (1.7%), clonazepam (1.2%), valproic acid (VPA) (0.9%), and all other AEDs combined (1.2%). These percentages exceed 10.5% due to AED polytherapy. If these results are extrapolated to all 1,557,800 U.S. elderly NH residents in 2000, as many as 163,569 elderly NH residents were likely to have been receiving at least one AED.[37] In the Garrard and colleagues study, age was inversely related to AED use. Of the young-old cohort, 23.7% were prescribed an AED (16.4% for seizure indication and 7.3% for other). Of the middle-old, 12.2% were prescribed an AED (8.3% for seizure indication and 3.9% for nonseizure indication). However, of the old-old cohort only 5.8% were prescribed an AED (3.7% for seizure indication and 2.1% for other). Notably, this finding was unexpected because studies of community-dwelling elderly show that the incidence of epilepsy/seizure disorder rises with advancing age. Thus, one of the major findings concerning AED use in U.S. NHs is that the young-old are three to four times more likely to be prescribed an AED than the old-old, either prior to, or after admission. A similar pattern was reported from a study in Italy.[39] The reason for this inverse relationship between community-dwelling elderly and NH residents is unknown and needs to be further investigated. One hypothesis is that younger

NH residents have a higher prevalence of the disorders predisposing to them epilepsy than older residents.

In a study of NH admissions using a longitudinal design to explore AED use at the time of admission, two groups were used: the first including all persons aged $\geq$ 65 years of age admitted between January 1 and March 31, 1999 to one of the 510 Beverly Enterprises NH facilities in 31 states ($n = 10,318$); while the second was a follow-up cohort ($n = 9516$) of those in the admissions group who were not using an AED at the time of NH admission.[38] The cohort not receiving AEDs at the time of admission was followed for 3 months or until NH discharge, whichever occurred first, after their initial admission date. Approximately 8% ($n = 802$) of the admissions group used one or more AEDs at entry, and among these, more than half (58%) had an epilepsy/seizure disorder indication. The AEDs used by newly admitted individuals with an epilepsy/seizure disorder ($n = 585$) included PHT ($n = 315$; 54%), VPA ($n = 57$; 10%), carbamazepine ($n = 52$; 9%), and gabapentin ($n = 27$; 5%).

Among the 9516 residents within the follow-up cohort of the Garrard study who were not using an AED at admission, 260 (3%) were started on an AED within 3 months of admission. Factors associated with the initiation of AEDs during this period included epilepsy/seizure, manic depression (bipolar disease), age group, cognitive performance (Minimum Data Set-Cognition [MDS-COGS]), and peripheral vascular disease (PVD). Thus, many patients admitted without a diagnosis of epilepsy were given this diagnosis after entry to the NH. Based on this study, it seems that the incidence of newly diagnosed epilepsy after admission to the NH far exceeds numbers relevant to other age-group populations. A crude estimate would be 600/100,000 per 3 months, or four to six times that reported for community-dwelling elderly. AEDs used by those in the cohort that had AEDs started after admission and who had an epilepsy/seizure indication were PHT 48%, gabapentin 13%, carbamazepine 12%, VPA 8%, phenobarbital 7%, and other 12%. There was also an inverse relationship between age group and initiation of an AED. Compared to the young-old, those in the middle-old age group were 33% less likely to have been prescribed an AED ($P < 0.05$), whereas the old-old were 50% less likely to have been prescribed an AED.[38]

Table 2. Frequency of use of comedications with potential pharmacokinetic or pharmacodynamic interactions with antiepileptic drugs in 4,291 residents of nursing homes

Drug Category	% use with AEDs
Antidepressants	18.9
Antipsychotics	12.7
Benzodiazepams	22.4
Thyroid supplements	14.0
Antacids	8.0
Calcium Channel Blockers	6.9
Warfarin	5.9
Cimetidine	2.5

From Lackner *et al.*, 1998.

Another issue is that many elderly persons are taking other drugs (Table 2). In addition to AEDs, the average elderly NH patient takes six medications concomitantly, greatly increasing the risk for side effects and drug–drug interactions.[40]

Clinical pharmacology of AEDs in the elderly

The theoretical basis for expecting age-related changes in drug pharmacokinetics was described many years ago but has not been widely applied to AEDs. Drug concentration at the site of action determines the magnitude of both desired and toxic responses. The unbound drug concentration in serum is in direct equilibrium with the concentration at the site of action and provides the best correlation to drug response.[41] Total serum drug concentration is useful for monitoring therapy when the drug is not highly protein bound (less than 75%) or when the ratio of unbound to total drug concentration remains relatively stable. Three of the major AEDs (VPA, PHT, and carbamazepine) are highly bound, and their protein binding may be altered in the elderly. Age-related physiologic changes that appear to have the greatest effect on AED pharmacokinetics involve protein binding and a reduction in liver volume and blood flow.[42–44] Reduced serum albumin and increased α1-acid glycoprotein (AAG) concentrations in the elderly alter protein binding of some drugs.[41–43] By age 65, many individuals have low normal albumin concentrations or are considered hypoalbuminemic. Albumin concentration may be further reduced by conditions such as malnutrition, renal insufficiency, and rheumatoid arthritis. The concentration of AAG, a reactant serum protein, increases with age, and further elevations occur during pathophysiologic stress, such as stroke, heart failure, trauma, infection, myocardial infarction, surgery, and chronic obstructive pulmonary disease.[43]

Administration of enzyme-inducing AEDs also increases AAG.[45] When the concentration of AAG rises, the binding of weakly alkaline and neutral drugs such as carbamazepine to AAG can increase, causing higher total serum drug concentrations and decreased unbound drug concentrations. Because of the complexity of confounding variables and the lack of correlation between simple measures of liver function and drug metabolism, the effect of age on hepatic drug metabolism remains largely unknown.[46,47] Interestingly, genetic determinants of hepatic isoenzymes may be more important than age in determining a person's clearance rate.[48]

Renal clearance is the major route of elimination for a number of newer AEDs. It is well known that among elderly people renal capacity decreases by approximately 10% per decade.[49] However, there is a substantial amount of individual variability because clearance is also highly dependent upon the patient's general state of health.[50] Thus, purely age-based dose recommendations may not be appropriate and measurements of serum creatinine and estimations of creatinine clearance may lead to more accurate dosing.

Despite the theoretical effects of age-related physiologic changes on drug disposition and the widespread use of AEDs in the elderly, few studies on AED pharmacokinetics in the elderly have been published. The available reports generally involve single-dose evaluations in small samples of the young-old. Also, there is a lack of data regarding AED pharmacokinetics in the old-old, those individuals who may be at greatest risk for therapeutic failure and adverse reactions. A recent series of studies used stable-labeled isotopes of PHT to determine the precise pharmacokinetics of this AED in elderly.[51]

Variability of plasma AED levels in nursing homes

In compliant patients, the variability of plasma AED concentrations over time is relatively small. One study showed that in institutionalized younger adults, the variability between serial PHT measurements over time was on the order of 10%.

Within the same study, compliant clinic patients experienced variability of approximately 20%.[52] Approximately 5–10% of this variability may be due to interlaboratory variability in measurement of drug concentrations, although laboratories not following rigid quality control standards may experience even larger amounts of variability. The remainder of noted variability could arise from day-to-day alterations in absorption and metabolism or differences in AED dose content. The variability for carbamazepine and valproate is on the order of 25%, possibly due to their shorter half-lives, which may increase sample time variability.[53]

A small study found that PHT levels might fluctuate in the NH elderly.[54] This was confirmed in an analysis of serial serum PHT levels in NH patients across the United States who had experienced no change in dose, formulation, or medication.[55] Some patients experienced a difference in concentration of two- to threefold from the lowest to the highest level. Interestingly, some had very little fluctuation similar to the younger adults previously mentioned.[55] Similar but less severe fluctuations were also observed for carbamazepine and VPA. These findings suggest that elderly frail of any age group NH residents may experience a greater variability than seen in elderly outpatients in absorption of drugs. Factors that contribute to this variability in concentration must be identified and strategies should be developed in order to minimize this phenomenon. This phenomenon also exists for valproate and carbamazepine, but to a lesser degree.[55] Attempting to adjust doses based on serum drug levels, unfortunately, only serves to increase the amplitude of the oscillations (personal observation, IEL). Thus, the best strategy at this time may be to obtain serial levels to identify persons who fluctuate and those who do not and consider using AEDs that may not fluctuate. At this time, however, it is not known if the newer AEDs are less prone to variability. Prospective studies are also needed to determine if these changes in concentrations relate to clinically significant outcomes (Fig. 1).

Clinical trials of AEDs in the elderly

All major AEDs have an FDA indication for use for the seizure types most likely to be encountered in the elderly. However, there are little data relating specifically to these drugs in the elderly, and those that

are available have been limited to the community-dwelling elderly. One post-hoc VA cooperative study of carbamazepine and valproate found that elderly patients often had seizure control associated with lower AED levels than those seen in younger subjects. Notably, these elderly patients also experienced side effects at lower levels compared with those seen in younger subjects.[56]

A multicenter, double-blind, randomized comparison between lamotrigine and carbamazepine in newly diagnosed epileptic elderly patients (mean age 77 years) in the United Kingdom showed that the main difference between the two groups was the rate of dropout due to adverse events, with lamotrigine incurring an 18% dropout rate and carbamazepine a 42% dropout rate.[57] The VA Cooperative Study #428, an 18-center, parallel, double-blind trial on the use of gabapentin, lamotrigine, and carbamazepine in patients ≥60 years of age found that drug efficacy did not differ, but that the two newer AEDs had better tolerability than carbamazepine.[24]

Choosing AEDs for the elderly

At the present time, there are few data regarding the clinical use of AEDs in the elderly. The paucity of information makes it very difficult to recommend specific AEDs with any confidence that outcomes will be optimal. A drug that is optimal for the EH group may not be appropriate for the EMMP or FE groups due to the differences in pharmacokinetic or pharmacodynamic properties in these populations.

To date, PHT is still the most commonly used AED in both the community-dwelling and NH elderly within the United States, although expert opinion may disagree with this practice.[35] In the following sections, discussion is based first on the most commonly used AEDs for which there are more data, and is then followed by an alphabetical review of other AEDs. Table 3 provides a summary of the properties of most AEDs.

Phenytoin

PHT is effective for localization-related epilepsies and thus has an efficacy profile appropriate for the elderly. Evidence for this can be gathered from a VA cooperative study that included elderly patients and found PHT to be as effective as carbamazepine,

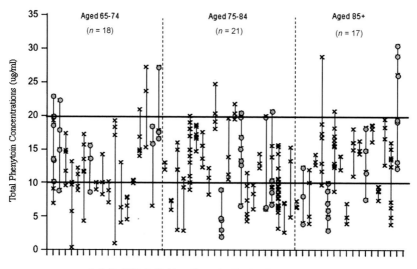

Figure 1. Variability of serum phenytoin (PHT) concentrations in elderly nursing home residents. The subjects were included in the figure if: they had no change in PHT dose over all of the measurements, they were on no medications which could alter PHT clearance, and had standing orders for routine serial PHT measurements. Each vertical column incorporates the concentrations from a single subject. Subjects are arranged in order of ascending age. Levels in each subject varied randomly over time. Note that although many subjects had large variations over time, some had little fluctuation. Data regarding medical condition of subjects was not available. This problem is now being investigated by a prospective study to determine the causes and consequences of fluctuating levels. Used by permission from authors and publisher.[100] Circles represent use of Dilantin suspension, the crosses represent Diantin Capseals. Generic phenytoin was not available at the time of the study.

phenobarbital, and primidone, but that PHT and carbamazepine were better tolerated.[58] PHT has a narrow therapeutic range, is approximately 90% bound to serum albumin, and undergoes saturable metabolism, which has the effect of producing non-linear changes in serum concentrations when the dose is changed or absorption is altered. Clinical studies in elderly patients have shown decreases in PHT binding to albumin and increases in free fraction. The binding of PHT to serum proteins correlates with the albumin concentration, which is typically low normal to subnormal in the elderly. One study compared the pharmacokinetics of PHT at steady state after oral administration in 34 elderly (60–79 years of age) persons, 32 middle-aged (40–59 years of age) persons, and 26 younger adult (20–39 years of age) persons with epilepsy.[59] All subjects had normal albumin concentrations and liver function and received no other medications known to alter hepatic metabolism, including other AEDs. The maximum rate of metabolism (V_{max}) declined with age, and significantly lower values

were seen in the elderly group compared with the younger adults.[59] Other earlier and smaller studies have also shown that PHT metabolism is reduced in the elderly. Therefore, smaller maintenance doses of PHT may be needed to attain desired unbound serum concentrations. Relatively small changes in dose (<10%) are recommended when making dosing adjustments. Several studies have shown that elderly persons in NHs receive lower daily doses of PHT than younger adults. However, total daily dose (mg/day) does not consider the weights of the patients and would suggest that elderly are slower metabolizers than the younger patients. But since PHT clearance is related to body weight, recalculating these values by weight (mg/kg/day) gives similar values for the young and elderly.[60] This might suggest that metabolism does not decrease greatly with age. A study using stable labeled (non-radioactive) PHT to very precisely measure PHT clearance found that advancing age was not as much a factor as had been previously reported.[51] In addition, a gender effect was found in this

Table 3. AED pharmacokinetics in the elderly

Drug	Protein binding	Elimination	Comments
Carbamazepine	75–85%	hepatic CYP 3A4/5	Protein binding decreased with age Levels increased by erythromycin, prophoxyphene, and grapefruit juice Decreases levels of calcium channel blockers (dilitiazem, verapamil) Decreases effect of warfarin, Decreases tricyclic antidepressant levels
Felbamate	<10%	hepatic	
Gabapentin	<10%	renal	Elimination correlates with creatinine clearance No drug interactions
Lamotrigine	55%	hepatic-glucuronide conjugation	Levels decreased by inducing agents—carbamazepine, phenytoin, some hormones, and others yet to be determined. Levels increased by vaproate
Levetiracetam	<10%	renal	Very water soluble, IV formulation available No drug interactions
Oxcarbazepine	40%	hepatic	Causes hyponatremia
Phenobarbital	50%	Hepatic renal	Induces metabolism of many drugs
Phenytoin	80–93%	hepatic CYP 2C9 CYP 2C19	Protein binding decreased with reduced serum albumin and renal failure Decreases levels of calcium channel blockers (dilitiazem, verapamil) Complicated interaction with warfarin Decreases tricyclic antidepressant levels Interacts with diabetes and arthritis medications Decreases effectiveness of cancer chemotherapy
Topiramate	9–17%	hepatic and renal	Inhibits CYP 2C19 and increase serum Phenytoin and other drug levels Induces CYP-3A4 isoenzymes
Valproic acid	87–95%	hepatic multiple pathways	Protein binding decreased in elderly Inhibits glucuronidation and may increse levels of lamotirigine and other drugs Decreases platelet function
Zonisamide	40%	Hepatic CYP 3A4	Weight loss and nephrolithiasis are issues

population, as women required higher doses than men of PHT to achieve similar serum concentrations.[60] Thus, in the elderly a starting daily dose of 3 mg/kg appears to be appropriate, rather than the 5 mg/kg per day used in younger adults.[61] This 3-mg/kg dose is only 160 mg/day for a 52 kg woman, or 200 mg/day for a 66 kg man. Use of lower doses in the elderly may reflect age-related changes in the therapeutic or toxic effects more than a significant decline in hepatic functioning.

Due to the high protein binding of PHT, unbound PHT concentrations may be a better indicator of efficacy and toxicity than total concentrations. Measurement of unbound PHT concentrations is essential for elderly patients who have (1) decreased serum albumin concentration; (2) total PHT concentrations that are near the upper boundary of the therapeutic range; (3) total concentrations that decline over time; (4) a low total concentration relative to the daily dose; or (5) total concentrations that do not correlate with clinical response. A range of 5 mg/L to 15 mg/L total may be more appropriate than the 10 to 20 mg/L used for younger adults as a therapeutic range for the elderly.[61]

PHT has many drug–drug interactions and should be used cautiously in EMMP patients receiving other medications. VPA, which is also highly protein bound, competes with PHT for albumin binding sites and inhibits PHT's metabolism. Carbamazepine induces PHT metabolism and necessitates higher PHT doses. There is also some indication that SSRI antidepressants may inhibit the cytochrome 2C family of P450 enzymes responsible for metabolizing PHT.[62] Fluoxetine and norfluoxetine are more potent inhibitors of this enzyme, followed by sertraline and paroxetine. The latter two SSRI antidepressants may prove to be a safer choice in the elderly. Coumadin also has a very complicated interaction with PHT, and often doses of both need to be manipulated.[61]

PHT has some effects on cognitive functioning, especially at higher serum concentrations.[63] However, it is not known if the elderly will be more sensitive to this problem. In addition, PHT may cause imbalance and ataxia. It is likely that EMMP patients, especially those with CNS disorders, may be more sensitive to this medication.[64] In a study involving elderly persons, among the various lifestyles, demographic, and health factors that contributed to an increased risk, PHT was the only drug that was associated with a significant increase in fractures.[65] However, this study could not determine if this was due to falls from ataxia or seizures, or was an effect due to bone changes.

PHT is also known to be a mild blocker of cardiac conduction and should be used cautiously in persons with conduction defects, especially heart blocks. In spite of its limitations, PHT is the least expensive major AED. This, as well as its long record of use, may account for it presently being the most widely used AED.

Carbamazepine

Carbamazepine is effective for localization-related epilepsies, and thus has an efficacy profile appropriate for the elderly. Evidence from two large VA co-operative studies showed it to be as effective as PHT, phenobarbital, primidone, and valproate, but better tolerated than the latter three.[58,66] Two studies of new-onset epilepsy in the community-dwelling elderly found it to be as effective as lamotrigine but noted that it had a higher incidence of side effects.[24,57]

The apparent clearance of carbamazepine has been reported to be 20% to 40% lower in the elderly as compared with younger adults.[67,68] A population analysis of patients from ambulatory neurology clinics at three medical centers also showed that the apparent oral clearance of carbamazepine was 25% lower in patients who were more than 70 years old.[68] Decreases in clearance result in prolonged elimination half-life. These changes in carbamazepine pharmacokinetics indicate that lower and less frequent dosing in elderly patients may be appropriate. Lower doses of carbamazepine have been observed in older (>85 years) elderly NH residents as compared with elderly in the younger age group (65–74 years); however, doses were similar after adjusting for a patient's weight.[69] Observed carbamazepine concentrations in the Birnbaum study were lower or below the suggested therapeutic range used in treating younger adults.

Carbamazepine has some significant drug–drug interactions with medications that inhibit the cytochrome P450 enzyme, CYP3A4, responsible for carbamazepine metabolism. Among the inhibitors are erythromycin, fluoxetine, ketoconazole, propoxyphene (Darvon), and cimetidine (Tagamet). Grapefruit interacts with carbamazepine by inhibiting the intestinal enzyme that metabolizes some of the carbamazepine before it is absorbed. Thus, with grapefruit, more carbamazepine will be absorbed, resulting in higher concentrations and possible toxicity. Elderly healthy patients will need to be cautioned about these interactions and should be instructed to inform the physician whenever they are beginning a new medication, including any over-the-counter medications. Many other drug interactions do occur, so carbamazepine is one AED that will need to be used cautiously in EMMP patients receiving other medications.

Carbamazepine also induces the CYP3A4 system, reducing the effectiveness of other drugs. St. John's Wort, an herbal remedy used for depression, is a powerful inducer of CYP3A4 and may significantly lower the concentration of carbamazepine.

Carbamazepine has some effects on cognitive functioning, especially at higher levels. However, it is not known if the elderly are especially sensitive to this problem. In addition, carbamazepine may cause imbalance and ataxia. It is possible that EMMP patients, especially those with CNS disorders, may be more sensitive to these effects. One of the major concerns with carbamazepine is its effect on sodium levels.[70] Hyponatremia is a well-known phenomenon seen with carbamazepine use and may cause significant problems in younger adults, especially if there is polydypsia. The hyponatremia associated with carbamazepine is more pronounced as a person becomes older.[71] This may become more problematic if a person is on a salt restriction diet or a diuretic. Because of the mild neutropenia associated with carbamazepine use in younger adults, the effects of this AED on hematopoetic parameters in the elderly will need to be studied. Carbamazepine is also known to affect cardiac rhythms and should be used cautiously, if at all, in persons with rhythm disturbances.

One of the pharmacokinetic problems of carbamazepine is its short half-life and its possible need to be taken multiple times a day. In the elderly, however, the half-life may be longer, and slow-release formulations may overcome the need to dose multiple times each day as well as some of the side effects associated with a rapid time to a high peak (short T_{max} and high C_{max}).

Phenobarbital

Phenobarbital is effective for localization-related epilepsies and has an efficacy profile appropriate for the elderly. However, a VA cooperative study demonstrated that phenobarbital and primidone are not as well tolerated as carbamazepine or PHT.[58] Thus, although phenobarbital is the least expensive of all AEDs, its side effects profile, which may worsen cognition and depression, make it an undesirable drug for the elderly, especially in the NH setting, where declines in cognition are already present.

Valproic acid

Only a few studies have compared the pharmacokinetics of VPA in young and old patients.[72,73] Total VPA clearance is similar in young and elderly individuals; however, unbound clearance is higher in the elderly.

Much like PHT, VPA is associated with reduced protein binding and unbound clearance in the elderly. As a result, the desired clinical response may be achieved with a lower dose. A nationwide elderly NH study showed that VPA dose and total VPA concentrations decrease within elderly age groups.[74] The apparent clearance of VPA in elderly NH residents has also been shown to be 27% lower in women, 41% greater with the co-administration of an inducer such as carbamazepine or PHT, and 25% greater when the syrup formulation was used.[69] Because the serum elimination half-life may be prolonged, the dosing interval can be extended. If the albumin concentration has fallen or the patient's clinical response does not correlate with total drug concentration, measurement of the unbound drug should be considered. Because of its effects on mood stabilization, it may be especially appropriate for elderly patients with a dual diagnosis.

Felbamate

Felbamate is effective for localization-related epilepsies and appears to have a broader spectrum of effectiveness than some of the other AEDs. Elderly subjects had a lower mean clearance (31.2 vs. 25.1 mL/min; 90% CI: –11.4 to –0.9; $P = 0.02$) than adults in a study involving 24 elderly healthy volunteers.[75] Felbamate is primarily metabolized by the liver and is known to have a number of drug–drug interactions, both inhibitory and inductive, and therefore may not be a good choice for EMMP patients.

Gabapentin

Gabapentin is effective for localization-related epilepsies and has an efficacy profile appropriate for the elderly. Gabapentin is not metabolized by the liver, but rather renally excreted; therefore, there are no drug–drug interactions.[76] Thus it may be especially useful in EMMP patients. There is, however, a reduction of renal function that correlates with advancing age, so doses may need to be adjusted in both EH and EMMP patients. Levels must be monitored after initiation and doses adjusted accordingly. However, gabapentin does appear to have some sedative side effects, especially at higher levels, and the elderly may be especially sensitive to this problem.

Gabapentin has a short half-life that requires it to be given multiple times a day. In the elderly, however, the half-life may be longer due to a reduction in renal elimination. Because gabapentin is effective in treating neuralgic pain, it may be additionally beneficial for someone suffering from both epilepsy and pain.

VA Cooperative Study #428 compared carbamazepine with gabapentin and lamotrigine. Efficacies were similar but withdrawal related to side effects was highest for carbamazepine.[24] This suggests that the newer AEDs may be better tolerated.

Lamotrigine

Lamotrigine is effective for localization-related epilepsies and has an efficacy profile appropriate for the elderly. However, very few studies regarding lamotrigine and its effects on the elderly have been published. Lamotrigine is primarily metabolized by the liver using the glucuronidation pathway, which is thought to be less affected by age than the P450 system.[77] Data from a population pharmacokinetic study of 163 epilepsy patients, which included only 30 subjects more than 65 years of age, 10 subjects between 70 and 76 years of age, and no subjects from the old-old age group, showed that age did not affect lamotrigine apparent clearance.[78] Based on a study of 150 elderly subjects, the dropout rate due to adverse events was lower with lamotrigine (18%) than with carbamazepine (42%). The difference was attributable to the finding that lamotrigine subjects had fewer rashes (lamotrigine 3%, carbamazepine 19%) and fewer complaints of somnolence (lamotrigine 12%, carbamazepine 29%).[57] Clinicians may want to consider other factors when dosing lamotrigine for elderly patients. Results of the VA Cooperative #428 Study in elderly community-dwelling epilepsy patients aged 59–92 years showed that lamotrigine apparent clearance can be effected by blood urea nitrogen and serum creatinine ratio, weight, and PHT use.[79]

Lamotrigine clearance is increased by approximately 2–3 times with co-administration of PHT and carbamazepine; whereas lamotrigine clearance decreases twofold with co-administration of VPA.[80] However, these drug interaction studies included very few elderly subjects. Therefore, the extent of the changes in clearance with administration of co-medications in the elderly is not known, and caution may need to be observed in EMMP patients who are on other drugs.

Levetiracetam

Levetiracetam has been approved as adjunctive therapy for partial-onset seizures in adults. Levetiracetam is extremely water soluble, which allows for rapid and complete absorption after oral administration. Levetiracetam is not metabolized by the liver and thus is free of nonlinear elimination kinetics, auto induction kinetics, and drug–drug interactions. Lack of protein binding (<10%) also avoids the problems of displacing highly protein-bound drugs and the monitoring of unbound concentrations. Also, lack of drug interactions would make it useful for treating elderly epilepsy patients, particularly those patients who have other illnesses and are taking other medications.[81] Notably, the manufacturer reports a decrease of 38% in total body clearance and an increased half-life up to 2.5 h longer in elderly subjects (age 61–88 years) who exhibited creatinine clearances ranging from 30–74 mL/min. However, doses do need to be adjusted depending on the renal function of the patient as measured by serum creatinine and levetiracetam concentrations.[82]

One prospective phase IV study indicates a favorable efficacy profile in the elderly.[83] Levetiracetam also appears to have a favorable safety profile. It was initially studied as a potential agent for treating cognitive disorders in the elderly, and thus a considerable amount of data regarding its tolerability in this age group are available. Analysis of 3252 elderly persons involved in studies of levetiracetam for epilepsy and other conditions demonstrated that levetiracetam was well tolerated by the elderly.[84]

Oxcarbazepine

Oxcarbazepine is rapidly metabolized by first-pass metabolism to 10-hydroxcarbazepine (10-OH-carbazepine or MHD); MHD is considered the active compound. MHD is further metabolized by glucuronidation and excreted by the kidneys.[85] The most extensive elderly oxcarbazepine study involved low doses of oxcarbazepine given to 12 young and 12 elderly healthy male volunteers and 12 young and 12 elderly healthy female volunteers. At low doses of oxcarbazepine (300–600 mg/day) a significantly higher maximum concentration, higher area under the curve parameters, and a lower elimination rate constant were observed in the elderly volunteers.[86]

Oxcarbazepine can affect the cytochrome P450 system by inducing the CYP3A4 enzyme, which is responsible for the metabolism of dihydropyridine calcium antagonists and many other substances.[87,88] However, oxcarbazepine appears to have a more powerful effect on sodium balance than carbamazepine, and this effect has been shown to increase with age resulting in more pronounced hyponatremia in this age group.[71]

Pregabalin

Pregabalin is related to gabapentin but is more potent, with doses of only one-fifth those of gabapentin needed for therapeutic effect. Its absorption also appears to be more predictable because of the lower amounts transported across the intestinal system. Although it may prove to be a favorable AED for the elderly, its cost and lack of experimental and clinical data may limit its use.

Tiagabine

Tiagabine is effective for localization-related epilepsies, has an efficacy profile appropriate for the elderly, and is primarily metabolized by the liver (CYP3A4). Comedications that affect CYP3A4 substrates will also affect the metabolism of tiagabine, giving it a drug interaction profile similar to carbamazepine. A major feature of tiagabine is its potency; usually, effective doses are 20 to 60 mg per day, and effective concentrations are 100 to 300 nanograms per milliliter, or as much as 100-fold lower than other AEDs.

Topiramate

Topiramate is effective for localization-related epilepsies and thus has an efficacy profile appropriate for the elderly. Topiramate is approximately 20% bound to serum proteins and is both metabolized by the liver and excreted unchanged in the urine. The enzymes involved in topiramate's metabolism have not been identified; however, the cytochrome P450 system may be involved. Topiramate clearance may decrease with age, causing higher than expected serum concentrations when doses used in younger

adults are given to elderly patients. In addition, topiramate metabolism can be induced in the presence of inducing comedications such as carbamazepine and PHT.[89] There is also some indication that topiramate can inhibit CYP2C19 activity.[90] Thus, levels will need to be monitored to ensure that the topiramate dose given does not result in higher than expected serum concentrations. Topiramate does have effects on cognitive functioning, especially at higher levels. However, it is not known if the elderly will be unusually sensitive to this problem.

Zonisamide

Zonisamide is effective for localization-related epilepsies.[91] Protein binding is approximately 40%, and its major elimination pathway is hepatic as a substrate of CYP 3A4. It may thus have interactions with other drugs using this pathway. In addition to the usual AED side effects of of somnolence and dizziness, zonisamide may be associated with weight loss. It has an association with the development of renal calculi in approximately 1–2% of patients during chronic use.[92]

Drug interactions with non-AEDs

Co-medications are frequently used by patients in NHs receiving AEDs (Table 2). Thus, it is imperative to note that concomitant medications taken by elderly patients can alter the absorption, distribution, and metabolism of AEDs, thereby increasing the risk of toxicity or therapeutic failure.

Calcium-containing antacids and sucralfate reduce the absorption of PHT.[93,94] The absorption of PHT, carbamazepine, and valproate may be reduced significantly by oral antineoplastic drugs that damage gastrointestinal cells.[95,96] In addition, PHT concentrations may be lowered by intravenously administered antineoplastic agents.[96] The use of folic acid for treatment of megaloblastic anemia may decrease serum concentrations of PHT, and enteral feedings can also lower serum concentrations in patients receiving orally administered PHT.[97]

Many drugs displace AEDs from plasma proteins, an effect that is especially serious when the interacting drug also inhibits the metabolism of the displaced drug; this occurs when valproate interacts with PHT. Several drugs used on a short-term basis (including propoxyphene and erythromycin) or as a maintenance therapy (such as cimetidine, diltiazem, fluoxetine, and verapamil) significantly inhibit the metabolism of one or more AEDs that are metabolized by the P450 system. Certain agents can induce the P450 system or other enzymes, causing an increase in drug metabolism. The most commonly prescribed inducers of drug metabolism are PHT, phenobarbital, carbamazepine, and primidone. Ethanol, when used chronically, also induces drug metabolism.[98]

The interaction between antipsychotic drugs and AEDs is complex. Hepatic metabolism of certain antipsychotics such as haloperidol can be increased by carbamazepine, resulting in diminished psychotropic response. Antipsychotic medications, especially chlorpromazine, promazine, trifluoperazine, and perphenazine can reduce the threshold for seizures; and, the risk of seizure is directly proportional to the total number of psychotropic medications being taken, their doses, any abrupt increases in doses, and the presence of organized brain pathology.[99] The epileptic patient taking antipsychotic drugs may need a higher dose of antiepileptic medication to control seizures. In contrast, central nervous system depressants are likely to lower the maximum dose of AEDs that can be administered before toxic symptoms occur.

Dosing

Drug adherence (compliance) is a potential challenge in the elderly due to multiple medications, memory problems, and visual issues. In general, twice daily dosing is preferable to once daily. In long-term care facilities, drug adherence may be less of an issue than with community-dwelling elderly patients; however, reductions in staff and time spent on the multiple administration of medicines may help to reduce errors and cost.

Conclusions

In the elderly population, the problem of epilepsy is a growing one. Unfortunately little research has been done to determine the basic mechanisms underlying this disorder. Research has been hampered by a lack of appropriate models. Adding to the confusion is that there are many associated conditions that may predispose the brain to seizures. Are the mechanisms leading to poststroke epilepsy different from those predisposing to seizures in persons with Alzheimer's disease? Should different drugs be used

for the various presentations? Elderly epileptic patients face issues that may alter the approach of AED treatments. Information obtained from studies of younger adults may at times be applicable to the elderly, but not in all instances. Community-dwelling elderly, relatively healthy except for epilepsy, may have similar patterns of response to AEDs similar to younger patients. But AED levels may fluctuate significantly in the elderly NH population, and dose changes based on a single level may exacerbate these already unstable levels. This has been shown for the older AEDs, but whether the newer or water-soluble AEDs are better still needs to be demonstrated. Although age may influence hepatic clearance, earlier studies may have overestimated the degree of this effect; accordingly, the genetic make up of a patient's isoenzymes may play a much greater role than previously suspected. Of the newer AEDs, gabapentin, lamotrigine, and levetiracetam are the most widely researched and utilized. As drug patents expire, costs may lessen and lead to increasing use. However, much more research to develop evidence is needed to determine the best treatments for EH, EMMP, and FE cohorts.

Conflicts of interest

The authors declare no conflicts of interest.

References

1. *Administration on Aging*. 2005. Washington, DC.
2. Hauser, W. & D. Hesdorffer. 1990. *Epilepsy, Frequency, Causes and Consequences*. Demos Publications. New York, NY.
3. Hauser, W.A., J.F. Annegers & W.A. Rocca. 1996. *Mayo. Clin. Proc.* **71:** 576–586.
4. *Epilepsy Foundation of America*. 1999. *Epilepsy, a Report to the Nation*. Epilepsy Foundation of America. Landover, MD.
5. de la Court, A., M.M. Breteler, H. Meinardi, *et al.* 1996. *Epilepsia* **37:** 141–147.
6. Sillanpaa, M., R. Kalviainen, T. Klaukka, *et al.* 2006. *Epilepsy Res.* **71:** 206–215.
7. Fisher, R.S. & I. Leppik. 2008. *Epilepsia* **49**(Suppl 9): 7–12.
8. Fisher, R.S., W. van Emde Boas, W. Blume, *et al.* 2005. *Epilepsia* **46:** 470–472.
9. Bladin, C.F., A.V. Alexandrov, A. Bellavance, *et al.* 2000. *Arch. Neurol.* **57:** 1617–1622.

10. Silverman, I.E., L. Restrepo & G.C. Mathews. 2002. *Arch. Neurol.* **59:** 195–201.

11. Leonard, A.S. & J.O. McNamara. 2007. *Neuron* **55:** 677–678.

12. Kelly, K.M., N.L. Nadon, J.H. Morrison, *et al.* 2006. *Epilepsy Res.* **68S:** S5–S20.

13. Seyfried, T.N., G.H. Glaser, R.K. Yu & S.T. Palayoor. 1986. *Adv. Neurol.* **44:** 115–133.

14. Geinisman, Y., L. de Toledo-Morrell, F. Morrell & R.E. Heller. 1995. *Prog. Neurobiol.* **45:** 223–252.

15. Du, A.T., N. Schuff, D. Amend, *et al.* 2001. *J. Neurol. Neurosurg. Psych.* **71:** 441–447.

16. Barnes, C.A. 2001. *Int. Rev. Neurobilo.* **45:** 339–354.

17. Shankar, S., & T.J. Teyler. 1998. Robbins. *Neurophysiol.* **79:** 334–341.

18. de Toledo-Morrell, L. & F.S. Morrell. 1984. *Behav. Neurosci.* **98:** 902–907.

19. Leppik, I.E., K.M. Kelly, L. de Toledo-Morrell, *et al.* 2006. *Epilepsy Res.* 68S: S21–S37.

20. Hartings J.A., A.J. Williams & F.C. Tortella. 2003. *Exp. Neurol.* **179:** 139–149.

21. Karhunen H., A. Pitkanae, T. Virtanen, *et al.* 2003. *Epilepsy Res.* 54.

22. DeLorenzo, R.J., D.A. Sun, & D. LS. 1998. *Proc. Natl. Acad. Sci. USA* **95:** 14482–14487.

23. Palop, J.J., J. Chin, E.D. Roberson, *et al.* 2007. *Neuron* **55:** 697–711.

24. Rowan, A.J., R.E. Ramsay, J.F. Collins, *et al.* 2005. *Neurology* **64:** 1868–1873.

25. Hauser, W.A. 1992. *Epilepsia* **33**(Suppl 4): S6–S14.

26. Gupta, S.R., M.H. Naheedy, D. Elias & F.A. Rubino. 1988. *Stroke* **19:** 1477–1481.

27. Holmes, G. 1980. *Clin. Electroencephalogrl.* **11:** 83–86.

28. Holmes, G.L. 1980. *Clin. Electroencephalogr.* **11:** 83–86.

29. Ensrud, K.E., T.S. Walczak, T.L. Blackwell, *et al.* 2008. *Neurology* **71:** 723–730.

30. Ensrud, K.E., T.S. Walczak, T. Blackwell, *et al.* 2004. *Neurology* **62:** 2051–1057.

31. Leppik, I.E. 2006. *Epilepsy Res.* **68**(Suppl 1): S1–S4.

32. Leppik, I.E., M.J. Brodie, E.R. Saetre, *et al.* 2006. *Epilepsy Res.* **68**(Suppl 1): S71–S76.

33. Moore, S.A. & T.W. Teal. 1985. Adverse drug reaction surveillance in the geriatric population: a preliminary review. In *Proceedings of the Drug Information Association Workshop Geriatric Drug Use: Clinical and Social Perspectives.* Pergamon Press. Washington, DC.

34. Perucca, E., D. Berlowitz, A. Birnbaum, *et al.* 2006. *Epilepsy Res.* **68**(Suppl 1): S49–S63.

35. Pugh, M., J. Cramer, J. Knoefel, *et al.* 2003. *J. Am. Geriatr. Soc.* **52:** 417–422.

36. Kemper, P. & C.M. Murtaugh. 1991. *N. Engl. J. Med.* **324:** 595–600.

37. Hetzel, L. & A. Smith. 2001. The 65 years and over population: 2000, Census 2000 Brief; Census Bureau, C2KBR/01-10. Washington, DC.

38. Garrard, J., S. Harms, N. Hardie, *et al.* 2003. *Ann. Neurol.* **54:** 75–85.

39. Galimberti, C.A., F. Magri, B. Magnani, *et al.* 2006. *Epilepsy Res.* **68:** 1–8.

40. Lackner, T.E., J.C. Cloyd, L.W. Thomas & I.E. Leppik. 1998. *Epilepsia* **39:** 1083–1087.

41. Wallace, S. & R. Verbeeck. 1987. *Clin. Pharmacokinet.* **12:** 91–97.

42. Greenblatt, D.J. 1979. *J. Am. Geriatr. Soc.* **27:** 20–22.

43. Verbeeck, R.K., J.A. Cardinal & S.M. Wallace. 1984. *Eur. J. Clin. Pharmacol* **27:** 91–97.

44. Wynne, H.A., L.H. Cope, E. Mutch, *et al.* 1989. *Hepatology* **9:** 297–301.

45. Tiula, E. & P.J. Neuvonen. 1982. *N. Engl. J. Med.* **307:** 1148.

46. Cusack, B.J. 1988. *J. Clin. Pharmacol.* **28:** 571–576.

47. Dawling, S. & P. Crome. 1989. *Clin. Pharmacokinet.* **17:** 236–263.

48. Ahn, J.E., J.C. Cloyd, R.C. Brundage, *et al.* 2008. *Neurology* **71:** 38–43.

49. Rowe, J.W., R. Andres, J.D. Tobin, *et al.* 1976. *J. Gerontol.* **31:** 155–163.

50. Fehrman-Ekholm, I. & L. Skeppholm. 2004. *Scand. J. Urol. Nephrol.* **38:** 73–77.

51. Ahn, J., J. Cloyd, R. Brundage, *et al.* 2008. *Neurology* **71:** 38–43.

52. Leppik, I.E., J.D. Cloyd, R.J. Sawchuk & S.M. Pepin. 1979. *Ther. Drug. Mon.* **1:** 475–483.

53. Graves, N.M., G.B. Holmes & I.E. Leppik. 1988. *Epilepsy Res. Suppl.* **1:** 91–99.

54. Mooradian, A.D., L. Hernandez, I.C. Tamai & C. Marshall. 1989. *Arch. Intern. Med.* **149:** 890–892.

55. Birnbaum, A., N.A. Hardie, I.E. Leppik, *et al.* 2003. *Neurology* **60:** 555–559.

56. Ramsay, R., A. Rowan, J. Slater, *et al.* 1994. *Epilepsia* **35:** 91.

57. Brodie, M.J., P.W. Overstall & L. Giorgi. 1999. *Epilepsy Res.* **37:** 81–87.

58. Mattson, R.H., J.A. Cramer, J.F. Collins, *et al.* 1985. *N. Engl. J. Med.* **313:** 145–151.

59. Bauer, L.A. & R.A. Blouin. 1982. *Clin. Pharmacol. Ther.* **31:** 301–304.

60. Birnbaum, A.K., N.A. Hardie, J.M. Conway, *et al.* 2003. *Am. J. Geriatr. Pharmacother.* **1:** 90–95.

61. Leppik, I.E. 2006. *Contemporary Diagnosis and Management of the Patient with Epilepsy*, 6th edn. Handbooks in Healthcare. Newton, PA.

62. Nelson, M.H., A.K. Birnbaum & R.P. Remmel. 2001. *Epilepsy Res.* **44:** 71–82.

63. Thompson, P., F.A. Huppert & M. Trimble. 1981. *Br. J. Clin. Psychol.* **20:** 155–162.

64. Bourdet, S.V., B.E. Gidal & B.K. Alldredge. 2001. *J. Am. Pharm. Assoc. (Wash.)* **41:** 421–436.

65. Bohannon, A.D., J.T. Hanlon, R. Landerman & D.T. Gold. 1999. *Am. J. Epidemiol.* **149:** 1002–1009.

66. Mattson, R.H., J.A. Cramer & J.F. Collins. 1992. *N. Engl. J. Med.* **327:** 765–771.

67. Cloyd, J.C., T.E. Lackner & I.E. Leppik. 1994. *Arch. Fam. Med.* **3:** 589–598.

68. Graves, N.M., R.C. Brundage, Y. Wen, *et al.* 1998. *Pharmacotherapy* **18:** 273–281.

69. Birnbaum, A.K., J.M. Conway, N.A. Hardie, *et al.* 2007. *Epilepsy Res.* **77:** 31–35.

70. Henry, D.A., D.H. Lawson, P. Reavey & S. Renfrew. 1977. *Br. Med. J.* **1:** 83–84.

71. Dong, X., I.E. Leppik, J. White & J. Rarick. 2005. *Neurology* **65:** 1976–1978.

72. Bryson, S.M., N. Verma, P.J. Scott & P.C. Rubin. 1983. *Br. J. Clin. Pharmacol.* **16:** 104–105.

73. Perucca, E., R. Grimaldi, G. Gatti, *et al.* 1984. *Br. J. Clin. Pharmacol.* **17:** 665–669.

74. Birnbaum, A.K., N.A. Hardie, J.M. Conway, *et al.* 2004. *Epilepsy Res.* **62:** 157–162.

75. Richens, A., C.R. Banfield, M. Salfi, *et al.* 1997. *Br. J. Clin. Pharmacol.* **44:** 129–134.

76. Richens, A. 1993. *Clinical Pharmacokinetics of Gabapentin.* Royal Society of Medicine Services. London.

77. Peck, A.W. 1991. *Epilepsia* **32**(Suppl 2): S9–S12.

78. Hussein, Z. & J. Posner. 1997. *Br. J. Clin. Pharmacol.* **43:** 457–465.

79. Rowan, A., R. Ramsay, J. Collins, *et al.* 2005. *Neurology* **64:** 1868–1873.

80. Yuen, A.W., G. Land, B.C. Weatherley & A.W. Peck. 1992. *Br. J. Clin. Pharmacol.* **33:** 511–513.

81. Patsalos, P.N. & J.W. Sander. 1994. *Drug. Saf.* **11:** 37–67.

82. French, J. 2001. *Epilepsia* **42**(Suppl 4): 40–43.

83. Morrell, M.J., I. Leppik, J. French, *et al.* 2003. *Epilepsy Res.* **54:** 153–161.

84. Cramer, J.A., I.E. Leppik, K.D. Rue, *et al.* 2003. *Epilepsy Res.* **56:** 135–145.

85. Faigle, J.W. & M.G. 1990. *Behav. Neurol.* **3:** 21–30.

86. van Heiningen, P.N., M.D. Eve, B. Oosterhuis, *et al.* 1991. *Clin. Pharmacol. Ther.* **50:** 410–419.

87. Klosterskov Jensen, P., V. Saano, P. Haring, *et al.* 1992. *Epilepsia* **33:** 1149–1152.

88. Zaccara, G., P.F. Gangemi, L. Bendoni, *et al.* 1993. *Ther. Drug. Monit.* **15:** 39–42.

89. Sachdeo, R.C., S.K. Sachdeo, S.A. Walker, *et al.* 1996. *Epilepsia* **37:** 774–780.

90. Levy, R., F. Bishop, A. Streeter, *et al.* 1995. *Epilepsia* **36**.

91. Leppik, I.E., L.J. Willmore, R.W. Homan, *et al.* 1993. *Epilepsy Res.* **14:** 165–173.

92. Wroe, O. 2007. *Curr. Med. Res. Opin.* **23:** 1765–1773.

93. Nation, R.L., A.M. Evans & R.W. Milne. 1990. *Clin. Pharmacokinet* **18:** 131–150.

94. Nation, R.L., A.M. Evans & R.W. Milne. 1990. *Clin. Pharmacokinet.* **18:** 37–60.

95. Bollini, P., R. Riva, F. Albani, *et al.* 1983. *Epilepsia* **24:** 75–78.

96. Neef, C. & I. de Voogd-van der Straaten. 1988. *Clin. Pharmacol. Ther.* **43:** 372–375.

97. Haley, C.J. & J. Nelson. 1989. *Dicp – Ann Pharmacother* **23:** 796–798.

98. Sandor, P., E.M. Sellers, M. Dumbrell & V. Khouw. 1981. *Clin. Pharmacol. Ther.* **30:** 390–397.

99. Cold, J.A., B.G. Wells & J.H. Froemming. 1990. *Dicp – Ann. Pharmacother.* **24:** 601–606.

100. Birnbaum, A., N. Hardie, I. Leppik, *et al.* 2003. *Neurology* **60:** 555–559.